A PRESCRIPTION FOR ALCOHOLICS
Medications for Alcoholism

The first book about Medication Assisted Treatment for alcoholism with baclofen, topiramate, naltrexone, acamprosate, nalmefene, gabapentin and more.

LINDA BURLISON

ADDICTION PUBLISHING

ISBN 978-0-9971076-1-6 Electronic Book Text
ISBN 978-0-9971076-0-9 Paperback

A prescription for alcoholics : medications for the treatment of alcoholism / by Linda Burlison. – 1st Edition 1.5

Library of Congress Control Number: 2016902230
Addiction Publishing,New York, N.Y.

Ordering
Special discounts are available on quantity purchases. For details, contact the publisher. Orders by trade bookstores and wholesalers welcome.

Publisher
Addiction Publishing
http://www.AddictionPublishing.com
linda@aprescriptionforalcoholism.com

Book Website
http://www.APrescriptionForAlcoholics.com

WHAT THE EXPERTS SAID

"It is highly disturbing that this drug is not made available to the patients that need it."[1]

–Report in Pharmacology & Therapeutics, 2006

•••

"There is an enormous gap between the number of alcohol use disorder patients [alcoholics] who would potentially benefit from medications and the number of patients who actually receive medications ... a recent study ... showed that nationally, only 3% of Veterans Health Administration patients with alcohol use disorder received treatment medications."[2]

–Report in American Journal of Psychiatry, 2014

•••

"There is no other comparable example in medicine where you *have* evidence-based treatments that are *not available.*"[3]

–Dr. Shelly Greenfield, MD, Chief Academic Officer, McLean Hospital; Professor of Psychiatry, Harvard Medical School, 2012

•••

"People with addictive disorders continue to be offered, with great certitude and frequently at great cost, 'treatments' that are unsubstantiated by data or already known to be without beneficial effects…Meanwhile, advances that may be modest but have solid scientific support are arrogantly rejected by treatment providers in ways that would cause an uproar in other areas of medicine."[4]

–Dr. Markus Heilig, M.D., Ph.D., Former Chief of the Laboratory of Clinical Studies, and a Clinical Director at the US Institute of Alcohol Abuse, 2015

···

"No experimental studies unequivocally demonstrated the effectiveness of AA or [12-step] approaches for reducing alcohol dependence… People considering attending AA or TSF [Twelve Step] programs should be made aware that there is a lack of experimental evidence on the effectiveness of such programs."[5]

–2006 Cochrane Review (Cochrane is one of the most credible and trusted scientific/medical review organizations in the world)

···

"I'm not trying to eliminate AA…I'm just saying it should be prescribed to that tiny group who can make use of it… It's terribly harmful when you send 90 percent of the people for the wrong treatment advice."[6]

–Toronto Star article quoting Dr. Lance Dodes, Retired Professor of Psychiatry, Harvard Medical School, 2014

···

"Medication-assisted treatment has shown much promise in reducing alcohol use and promoting abstinence in patients diagnosed with alcohol use disorder. Considerable research evidence and consensus among experts support the use of pharmacologic treatments…

A number of FDA-approved medications have been shown to be important elements of such treatment.

Although some patients do not benefit from medication-assisted treatment, most do. For each patient deemed an appropriate candidate for medication-assisted treatment, multiple pharmacologic agents offer a variety of options so that treatment can be tailored to each patient's needs and circumstances."[7]

–Free Guide from the Center for Substance Abuse Treatment, Substance Abuse and Mental Health Services Administration, US Department of Health and Human Services, 2013

IMPORTANT LEGAL NOTICES

Affiliations & Endorsements

The publisher and author are not affiliated with, do not endorse, nor recommend any products, brands, brand names, medications, substances, trademarks, companies, individuals, institutions, journals, doctors, writers, scientists, authors, personnel, or any industry (collectively, 'Third Parties') mentioned herein.

Third Parties mentioned herein belong to their respective owners, and are used without permission. Their use and any reference to, comment on, or mention of a Third Party is not intended to imply any endorsement of or direct (or indirect) affiliation with the Third Party.

Views expressed are solely the author's own. No Third Party has authorized, sponsored, or endorsed the content herein.

Risk

The reader ('you') expressly acknowledge and agree that neither the author nor the publisher nor its corporation ('we') are responsible for the results of your decisions resulting from the use of the Book, *'A Prescription for Alcoholics–Medications for Alcoholism'* ('the Book') or associated materials including forums or associated websites ('Related Materials'). Collectively, the Book and Related Materials shall be referred to as 'the content'.

Your use of the content acknowledges acceptance of these restrictions, disclaimers, and limitations. Use of the content is at your own risk.

We make no claim as to the accuracy of this information. You acknowledge that we have no control of or responsibility for your use of the content; have no knowledge of the specific or unique circumstances under which the content may be used by you; undertake no obligation to supplement or update the content of the book or related materials.

You assume all risk for selection and use of the content provided and for ensuring the appropriateness of using and relying upon the information in view of attendant circumstances, indications, and contraindications.

No Representation or Warranty

Except for warranties which may not be disclaimed as a matter of law, we make no representation or warranties whatsoever, express or implied, including but not limited to: representations or warranties regarding the accuracy or nature of the content; warranties of title; noninfringement; merchantability or fitness for a particular purpose; completeness; accuracy; reliability; completeness, suitability or availability with respect to the content of this book. We do not warrant that the information is true, current or non-misleading.

Every effort has been made to ensure that all information is accurate and complete, but no guarantee is made to that effect. We shall not be responsible for any errors, misstatements, inaccuracies or omissions regarding content. The content does not endorse any drug, pharmacy, diagnose patients, or recommend treatment.

References are provided for informational purposes only and do not constitute an endorsement of any websites or other sources. The websites listed may change. We are not medical or healthcare professionals.

ACKNOWLEDGMENTS

Thank-you Naomi for being such a beautiful, amazing, loving person. I love you and am so proud of you, today and forever.

•••

Thank-you so much for your help, love and encouragement: Glenn, Mike, Andrew, Paul M., Colin, Carm, Kira, Abha, Jenn, Alicia, Paul B., Rich, Ed, Brock, Ted and Emma.

DEDICATION

In loving memory of Randy.

TABLE OF CONTENTS

PREFACE

WHERE TO START

I struggled with how to organize this book.

On one hand, I felt the extensive data and research I've gathered on medications (which appear in Part 4) should be first, because if you or someone you love–who needs medical treatment for alcoholism–puts this book down before getting that far, then this book has failed.

On the other hand, I felt it was crucial to tell the story of *why* people who could have been helped by these medications have been struggling and dying for years without ever knowing of them.

And for anyone who is early in the treatment process (either for themselves, or for a loved one), I feel it's critical for you to be aware of some of the perspectives I write about here so that you can make an informed decision about treatment choices.

You probably will not hear these perspectives in most programs or treatment centres.

I also wanted to share with you how I came to write this book.

Finally I decided to leave it up to you.

This book has five parts, and you can start with any one of them depending upon what you are most interested in. I encourage you to jump to what you feel will be most helpful to you.

Here is what you'll find in each part:

Part 1: Background & The Bottom Line

Start here if you'd like to know why you may never have heard of these medications before and what needs to change so alcoholics start receiving proper medical care.

Here we also look at the roles of the 'players' in the system—doctors, pharmaceutical companies, 12-step groups (AA) and more.

If you feel hearing what might be considered 'anti-AA' perspectives will deter you from reading the rest of the book, then you may wish to start elsewhere.

This section takes us through a journey of where we've been, where we are, and what we need to do next. It also explains a little about why I chose to write this book for you.

Part 2: How Alcoholism Works

Start here if you'd like a better understanding of the brain disease called alcoholism.

This section includes an in-depth explanation of how alcoholism works inside the brain; the stages of alcoholism identified by researchers; and a list of clues to your genetic vulnerability.

If you have never thought about alcoholism from a true medical perspective before, this chapter may be of help to you.

Part 3: Your Medication Journey

If you are considering taking medication to treat alcoholism, but are wondering where to begin, start here.

You'll learn everything you need to know to obtain treatment with medication including finding a doctor and obtaining medication.

This section includes information on determining goals, tracking results, developing a medication strategy, combining medications, determining what type of alcoholism you may have, how to obtain medication, and many other considerations.

Part 4: Medications For Alcoholism

Start here if you would like in-depth information about specific medications and the research that backs them up.

Here you'll find over 200 pages of detailed, meticulously researched information on drugs that can treat alcoholism.

This section is divided into four lists:

1) The A-List–Most Important Medications Today

2) The B-List–Medications Worth Consideration Today

3) The D-List–Eleven Drugs that May Increase Drinking

4) The Futures List–Sixty+ Drugs to Watch

This section has been specifically written with doctors and skeptics in mind.

I recommend that you photocopy sections of Part 4 to bring to your doctor, and also visit the book's website (APrescriptionForAlcoholics.com) to access and print the most important research highlighted for each medication.

After reading part 1, if you find you are still skeptical, I suggest jumping to section 4 and scanning through the 'Significant Research Findings' listed for most of the medications in this section–and then perhaps even reading some of the research referenced there yourself.

Part 5: Randy's Story & Resources

This book and all of the insights and advice it contains was written based on my own personal experiences with my dear friend Randy.

If you would like to know more about Randy's story then I invite you to read Part 5 of the book.

SPREAD THE WORD

If this book or the medications in it have made a difference to you, please consider helping to spread the word.

You can do this by:

- Sharing the free chapter found on the website with a friend (www.APrescriptionforAlcoholics.com)

- Passing the book on to someone you know.

- Donating a few copies to a library, school, doctor's office or recovery program.

- Posting about the book on social media.

PART

I

PART 1: BACKGROUND & THE BOTTOM LINE

01 | INTRODUCTION

"When a well-packaged web of lies has been sold gradually to the masses over generations, the truth will seem utterly preposterous and its speaker a raving lunatic."

–Donald James Wheal

PUZZLE PIECES

My friend Randy was an alcoholic. And like many people who care about someone with this devastating disease, I looked high and low for solutions for his alcoholism.

It's just what we do.

Alcoholism was a cage Randy lived his life in, and I wanted to help him escape so he could live the life he was meant to live.

As I was searching for a solution, I came across research about medications that were showing promise in helping alcoholics.

And I came across many stories—very credible-sounding stories—of people for whom medication was working.

Over months, I put together a picture of this world. It was like a jigsaw puzzle—one research article here talking about one medication, another article there on a different medication. A disappointing dead end here, a hopeful new pathway there.

I learned a new language so that I could understand what I was reading—'neuroplasticity', 'allele,' 'homeostasis,' 'neuroadaptation'...no wonder we don't understand alcoholism very well—it comes with its own vocabulary.

I also learned alcoholism is responsible for more deaths worldwide each year than any other illness.[89]

And I learned the little-known fact that there are numerous FDA-approved medications available that are as effective and safe in alcoholism as common anti-depressants are in fighting depression.

But the medical profession hasn't paid attention to this research.

So the tiny percentage of people who actually receive treatment (around eight percent[10]), are shepherded into 12-step program-based treatments which reinforce dangerous misperceptions about the disease and have a dismal 90-95% failure rate[6] and no scientific evidence of effectiveness.[5]

'Write the book you want to read,' is a phrase I recently came across. So I did.

It's true that you can only help an alcoholic who wishes to be helped. But if you know one, or you are one, at least you can find all of this information in one place now.

I've pulled together all of the research on all of the medications that have been shown to help alcoholics, so that you don't have to.

Along the Way

Along the way in my own journey with the alcoholic in my life I saw tragic gaps in our system.

I realized that my own beliefs about alcoholism were outdated and misinformed. I came to see that outdated beliefs reinforce the system we have in place right now—which doesn't work.

I hope you'll question your own beliefs as you read this book because some commonly-held beliefs about alcohol addiction are helping to kill a lot of people.

I also hope that the book will contribute to an informed conversation about how we can stop treating alcoholism like a shameful personality disorder and start treating it like the neurobiological disease that it is.

There is too much needless suffering for alcoholics and their loved ones. It's time to put an end to that.

This Book is Based on Research

Please put aside any assumptions you may have that just because you may not have heard about the medications this book is based on that they do not work.

Thousands of lives (but just a tiny number in comparison to those they could have helped) have been saved because of the drugs in this book.

It is tragic, though, how many alcoholics still die without ever learning that medication was even an option.

There is *solid medical research* supporting the safety and effectiveness of many of the drugs reviewed in this book.

And when I write the phrase 'solid medical research,' I'm not referring to the kind of thing you hear on a late night infomercial or one random study done in 1975 pulled out of a third rate archive somewhere.

I'm referring to hundreds of studies completed by the top research and medical bodies in the world, conducted and written about by the top addiction researchers in the world and published in the top medical journals.

I wrote this book using the life work of over 2000 scientists. I have collected and read over 700 of the studies written by these individuals and have provided summaries of key findings for many of them later in the book.

A sampling of sources of these studies include:

- The three bodies responsible for regulating and determining which medications can be prescribed in North America and Europe: American FDA, Health Canada, Europe's EMA (European Medicines Agency);

- The US National Library of Medicine (www.nlm.nih.gov and livertox.nih.gov);

- Work published in journals such as the European Pharmaceutical Review, the British Journal of Medicine and Medical Research, the Journal of Clinical Psychopharmacology, the American Journal of Psychiatry, the New England Journal of Medicine, The Journal of Addiction Medicine, JAMA, the Cochrane Database of Systematic Reviews, The American Journal of Drug and Alcohol Abuse, The International Journal of Neuropsychopharmacology, Pharmacology Biochemistry and Behavior, and many others.

- Research conducted by the top addiction scientists and doctors in the world. People like Giovanni Addolorato, Bankole A. Johnson, George F. Koob, Markus Heilig, Barbara J. Mason, David Nutt, Rainer Spanagel, Robert M. Swift, Wim van den Brink, Raymond F. Anton, Lara A. Ray, Albert J. Arias, Renaud De Beaurepaire, Jonathan Chick, Ciraulo A. Domenic, James C Garbutt, Antoni Gual, George A. Kenna, Henry R. Kranzler, Lorenzo Leggio, Karl Mann, Helen M. Pettinati, David Sinclair and hundreds of others.

- Research endorsed by the top addiction medicine institutions and organizations in the world such as the National Institute on Alcohol Abuse and Alcoholism (NIAAA), National Institute on Drug Abuse (NIDA), The Scripps Research Institute (TSRI), the Canadian Association for Addiction and Mental Health (CAMH), American Psychiatric Association (APA), the American College of Neuropsychopharmacology (ACNP) and many others.

THIS BOOK IS FOR YOU

WHO CAN THIS BOOK HELP?

It has been pointed out to me that there are many people who do not define themselves as alcoholic, but instead see themselves as a 'heavy drinker' or a 'binge drinker', or define their drinking using another term altogether.

Some people notice that they are beginning to think about alcohol a great deal, or are starting to notice a disturbing pattern in their consumption, but would not call themselves alcoholic.

While I researched and wrote this book with the severe alcoholic in mind, whether you are one, or are just someone who feels they may be heading in the wrong direction, the medications in this book may be able to help you.

I use the terms 'alcoholic,' 'alcoholism,' 'alcohol dependence,' and 'addiction' throughout the book.

Some people now prefer the term 'Alcohol Use Disorder', which is often just shortened to 'AUD'.

While 'AUD' may be the term adopted in the years ahead, I felt it was important to use terms that most people are familiar with.

Definitions are important. But ultimately, I'm most concerned about letting people who can benefit from medication know about them. If alcohol dependence is becoming a problem, or is already a problem, this book is for you.

As one addiction expert says, "If you can't live with it, and can't live without it, you're in trouble. That is the only definition of addiction that matters."[11]

DEAR ALCOHOLIC

If you are suffering from alcoholism, the last thing I want to do is give you false hope. There is no magic bullet for most people, and these medications don't work for everyone.

Many of them have side effects, but they are usually tolerable and have been shown to disappear after safe discontinuation.

The vast majority of them are completely non-addictive and are safely prescribed by doctors for other medical purposes.

If you are one of the few who have tried a medication before, this book may shed light on why it did or did not work for you and can offer ideas about next steps or combinations to try.

The good news is that these medications can save lives. Maybe one of them will be yours.

So, if you are an alcoholic, I hope that you will ask yourself one question as you read this book:

What do I have to lose?

WHAT WE KNOW FOR SURE

It ain't what you don't know that gets you into trouble.

It's what you know for sure that just ain't so.

—Mark Twain/The Big Short

I know many people who believe strongly in AA (Alcoholics Anonymous). And I know many people who believe in people that believe strongly in AA. If you are one of those people, this section is for you.

Many of these individuals are the salt of the earth. They'd give the shirt off their backs if you needed it.

Is it possible, as this book proposes, that all these good people could be so wrong?

Unfortunately, yes.

It reminds me of the bird washers.

Have you ever heard the stories about people that go to oil spills, put their lives aside and spend day and night cleaning and caring for birds who are covered by oil from the spill?

The people who do this work are good-hearted people who just want to help. I thank goodness that there are people like that in the world because they make it a better place.

It was surprising to me to hear about studies the other day that show that more than 99% of the cleaned birds die anyway.[12]

After the traumatic capture and cleaning process, many of the birds die slowly and painfully, out of sight, a week or two later, from liver and kidney damage.

Now, imagine being one of those well-intended, caring people who spend many hope-filled hours cleaning distressed birds, and then hearing the news that instead of helping them to live, you were actually just torturing one bird at a time on its way to an inevitable demise.

I probably would *not* want to accept what I was told.

I would probably try to cast doubt on those studies and defend my own actions.

I would cite examples of birds I knew I had helped, who had lived out long, wonderfully spiritual lives after the cleaning.

Initially, I'd probably do anything to feel like what I had been doing was the right thing.

It's human nature: we don't want to realize we have done something wrong—especially when life and death are at stake, and when we have done that thing with all our heart and soul and best intentions.

That is an uncomfortable, even painful feeling.

Eventually, if I were a former bird-scrubber, with enough evidence, I would probably come to accept the truth.

If my ego could handle it, I might start to advocate for a different way to help the birds. I would know that my heart was always in the right place, but that my actions were simply guided by my best intentions and the information I had at the time.

•••

Alcoholism is polarizing.

When we are polarized, we close our minds.

Are you a health care professional, an AA member or someone who can't believe that medication could help an alcoholic? This book will certainly challenge your beliefs.

This book may tell you some things you don't want to hear, and which might make you feel uncomfortable. You may even feel angry at me right now.

But I'm just the bearer of information. I challenge you to put aside your skepticism for a few days. Stop listening to other bird scrubbers for a week; read the book, read the research, and then make your own conclusions.

As you read this book, if you are a skeptic, you may from time to time, need to think of yourself as that well-intentioned bird-scrubber, helping yourself or the alcoholics(s) in your life in the best way you could.

As you read, you might feel uncomfortable because you may begin to think that something you believed to be true–something you participated in–isn't so true, and while you had nothing but the best intentions, you might realize that there is a better way.

Instead of running from that uncomfortable feeling, I hope you can use it as rocket fuel for the good that you do next.

The goodness of our hearts can stay the same while what we do next can be very different.

WHAT THIS BOOK DOESN'T COVER

This book focuses on pharmaceutical medications for alcoholism.

This book doesn't bring a magic cure for alcoholism for everyone. The word 'Cure' isn't on the cover. These drugs aren't a cure any more than antidepressants are considered a 'cure' for depression.

Anyone involved with alcoholism knows that it is a complex disease and one that seems to breed false hope.

We see our alcoholic abstaining and becoming healthier and voicing their commitment to sobriety and then all of a sudden, they relapse and our hopes disappear again. That can be a sad and bitter pill to swallow.

I want to give you hope–because there is hope. But I want to provide you with accurate data and facts that also temper that hope with reality. This is not a sales pitch for medication or yet another form of treatment.

But I hope you read the information that is available, and make up your own mind.

WITHDRAWAL MEDICATION

There are three categories of medication for alcoholics–those for withdrawal, those to deter drinking; and those that fight characteristics of the disease itself (extending abstinence, reducing cravings, reducing drink consumption).

Withdrawn medications need to be used more often. Alcohol Withdrawal Syndrome (AWS) can be fatal and should be treated medically. However, this book does not focus on them.

Drinking deterrents (like disulfiram) are useful for some, but dangerous for many others. A few are mentioned in the book.

This book focusses primarily on the third category: medication that fights the disease at its root–in the brain. These are medications that can slow or halt the progression of the disease itself.

TREATMENT OF CONCURRENT DISORDERS

Many individuals suffer from multiple concurrent disorders–for example, many alcoholics experience depression and anxiety, and a high percentage of people with schizophrenia are also addicted to alcohol.

Some researchers hypothesize that the cause of alcoholism for many individuals is a related mental illness that they have tried to medicate with alcohol.

There is significant research now that looks at concurrent disorders, and while this research has not been excluded from the book, and in fact, some of the research highlighted touches on concurrent disorders, the primary focus of research and information in this book is for the treatment for alcoholism alone.

02 | SAD STORIES

*"I'm sick of seeing people suffer needlessly and die
needlessly.
The assumptions upon which the North American approach
to addiction has been based since the early 20th century are
mistaken, nasty, and stupid—when it comes right down to it,
they amount to genocide."*[13]
—Dr. Peter Ferentzy, Addiction Scientist

NOT A COMEDY ROUTINE

There is a popular talk-show on TV that sometimes features a character named Sue, who often appears on the show drinking from a bottle of wine.

She seems to be drinking large quantities of alcohol and making poor, sometimes dangerous decisions. Sue falls off of things, wobbles around on too-high heels and acts promiscuously and inappropriately. In one show, with a glass of wine in one hand she topples off a roof to her death.

It's all a lighthearted act, just to make us laugh, and part of me says that it's harmless. I wouldn't have thought twice about it a few years ago.

But another part of me looks at Sue and isn't laughing. I've heard too many sad stories about the real Sues out there.

We don't laugh at cancer or other painful diseases, so why do we laugh at alcoholism? Perhaps we don't connect the often clown-like behavior of the alcoholic to the realities of the disease.

Maybe we need to connect the dots.

CONNECTING THE DOTS

Alcohol dependence is chronic, severe mental disorder characterized by bouts of compulsive and uncontrolled drinking, and an inability to cut down drinking despite the knowledge of its harmful, sometimes fatal consequences.

Worldwide, the World Health Organization says 3.3 million deaths can be attributed to alcohol abuse or dependence each year.[9] They estimate that alcohol is the international number one killer, ahead of AIDS.[8]

Nearly 18 million Americans suffer from alcoholism[14] and the United States spends nearly $35 billion a year[15] on alcohol- and substance-abuse treatment.

And every year, 88,000[14] people in the United States die from this disease anyway.

That's more people than can fit into the Houston Astrodome.

And those are just the ones that die.

Alcoholism is a family disease–it devastates families–so imagine for every person in that Astrodome that has died, there are children, parents, siblings, spouses–people, whose families have been torn apart because one member of it just can't seem to stop lifting that bottle to their mouth.

And alcoholism isn't just a disease–it's a disease maker.

Two hundred different potentially fatal health conditions are brought on by alcoholism.

Alcohol is the root cause of 50% of deaths from liver cirrhosis, 30% of deaths from all oral and pharynx cancers, 25% of deaths from all pancreatitis, 23% of deaths from all laryngeal cancers, 22% of deaths from all oesophageal cancers, 22% of deaths from interpersonal violence, 22% of all deaths from self-harm, 14% of all deaths from poisoning, and on and on and on.[9]

In the UK, 80% of deaths from liver diseases are due to alcohol and while deaths from all other major diseases have seen a gradual decrease, there has been a relentless increase in liver disease related deaths in the last twenty years with mortality rates increasing a staggering five-fold.

Alcohol is the most common reason for death in men under 50 and 20% of all deaths in men aged 16-44 are due to alcohol.[16]

It's an epidemic that respected professor and former chief drug adviser to the government, Dr. David Nutt, called a "public health emergency."[17][18]

Nutt's 2010 research in the respected Lancet looked at 100 drugs and compared the harm they cause to the individual who uses them as well as that caused to those beyond the misuser.

Overall, alcohol was found to be significantly more harmful to the drinker and to others around them than even heroin and crack cocaine.

Its impact on others beyond the alcoholic is born out in statistics in areas such as child abuse and drunk driving fatalities.

In the United States, it's estimated that drunk driving costs $199 billion per year. In 2013, over 10,000 people died and 290,000 were injured in drunk driving crashes.

Alcoholism is a major factor in these accidents since despite the significant repercussions if convicted of drunk driving, one-third of all drivers arrested or convicted are repeat offenders, and the average drunk driver has driven drunk 80 times before their first arrest.[19]

Alcoholism rips families apart and results in isolation, loss of self-esteem, and physical, mental, financial suffering that is beyond measure.

The American Academy of Child & Adolescent Psychiatry estimates that one in five adult Americans have lived with an alcoholic relative while growing up and that most children of alcoholics have experienced neglect or abuse.[20]

And alcoholics have an extremely high risk of suicide—5,080 times that of the general population.[21]

Addiction isn't a comedy routine.

As French-American cardiologist and former alcoholic, the late Dr. Olivier Ameisen wrote:

"Addiction is a living nightmare in which you wake up *to* the horror, not *from* it."[22]

MY LIFE IN BEER MARKETING

Hi, I'm Linda and I'm a former beer marketer. But don't discount me yet.

It's not the tragic epidemic of alcoholism described in the last chapter that motivated me to write this book.

As with many people, I ignore most problems until they hit me in the face and become personal.

I'll tell you what made this personal soon, but first I can perhaps best explain my qualifications for writing this book by telling you what I am not.

I am not a doctor, who has bought into my community's dogma;

I'm not a scientist who has sought research funding from a pharmaceutical company or committed my life to a particular research direction, or a pharma executive trying to pitch the next profitable drug;

I'm not an AA member committed to the AA way; I don't make a living selling a counselling program, a herbal supplement or a meditative retreat. I'm not a part of the alcoholism research or medical or rehab community in any way.

I'm also not an alcoholic who needs to rely on the system for help or is afraid to 'out' myself at work or in my community.

I don't have to be careful about who I offend for fear that I won't be funded again, that an important organization will boycott my clinic; or the only friends I have in the world won't call me again.

My lack of qualification and sponsorship means that in some ways I am the ideal person to write this book, because as a friend pointed out to me, sometimes it takes someone who is completely and utterly outside the system to hold up a mirror to it.

I'm simple: I see a devastating problem with enormous magnitude. And I see solutions that aren't being used to fix this problem. And I think enough is enough.

•••

Ten years ago, before I knew anything about alcoholism, I worked for a great guy I'll call Mark, and we did alcohol marketing together.

For a time, we worked in the head office of one of the two major Canadian breweries, and under Mark's leadership built and managed all of their beer brand websites for them.

A few years later I worked (at an advertising agency this time) for the other major Canadian brewery, doing similar work. During these years, I was the first person in Canada (maybe North America) to create and run search engine marketing campaigns to promote beer brands, and the agency I worked at was the first to run social media campaigns for beer companies.

One of the things I learned back then was that our target group for much of that marketing was men who consumed 13+ drinks per day. (The only exception was the social media marketing, which aimed at a much younger demographic).

We spent half our time trying to figure out how to reach more of them. I sometimes wondered if that was ethical–weren't we targeting alcoholics?

More recently I came across the statistic that 15% of drinkers consume 75%[23] of all alcohol and the top 10% of drinkers average nearly 9 drinks a day[23]–so now I know we *were* targeting alcoholics. It was an inconvenient truth in the business of alcohol marketing then, as it is now.

Ten years later, as I started writing this book, I was once again working for Mark and found myself asking him for time off from work (we long ago stopped working on any alcohol marketing), so that I could write a book about alcoholism and its treatments.

By that time, I had a very close friend who was dying of alcoholism, and Mark's dad had already died from it.

SAD STORIES

In an attempt to understand alcoholism and how to deal with it, I used to go to support groups for the families and friends of people with alcoholism. I attended quite a lot of AA meetings too with my friend Randy.

They were hopeful meetings full of kind people. But they offered no solutions.

One day, I began to research and learn about alcoholism. I read the medical and scientific research about it. And the more I learned, the harder it became for me to attend these meetings. It became more difficult to look at the faces of the people there.

There was a sweet elderly couple that could be your grandparents that cried about their daughter's addiction.

There was an angry suburban mother with two little boys whose sister was killed by a drunk driver when she was four and whose father and husband are both alcoholics. Alcoholism has a funny way of 'clustering'.

There was a lady–the wife of a wealthy doctor–whose daughter was in the hospital just after I started writing this book. The daughter was a beautiful girl. She was my age. Later I learned she had gone to the high school where some of my friends had gone, where she had starred in the school's musicals. Her mother–stressed and overwhelmed–could have been my mother–anyone's mother.

I remember the mom coming to a meeting in the winter in such distress one day that she wore mismatched boots on her feet. It was hard not to notice as we sat in a circle.

I put the daughter's obituary with her pretty face on the wall next to my desk many months ago as a reminder to keep on writing.

There were usually 20 people sitting in the room, all of whom had such sad stories. But they weren't at the meetings for solutions. They were there to learn to follow the serenity prayer and 'accept the things they could not change.'

I found it very hard to keep attending because the most frustrating and tragic thing was that the more I learned, the more I knew it didn't have to be that way.

I'm not a 'bleeding heart' kind of a person.

But I cannot stand seeing the stupid, needless waste of human life, and the pain it leaves behind when it is sitting right next to me in the same circle.

These people and thousands of people like them were why I wrote this book.

It's Personal

"If I can turn her death, and that of many others, into a victory of some kind, then maybe it'll all make sense.
Or, maybe it'll just seem a little less stupid."[11]

Randy was a severe alcoholic. And of course he was the reason I started attending those meetings and researching medications for alcoholism in the first place.

I wish, with all my heart that I could say that the medications in this book saved Randy and that he now lives the amazing life he was always meant to live.

Maybe in a parallel universe he has a beautiful wife, a house with a picket fence, a fast boat, and a dog named Kali.

But in this universe we don't see him anymore.

I sat down and began to write the book in February 2015. About 300 pages into its writing, my dear friend took his life.

He couldn't do it anymore. He didn't want to hurt his friends and family any longer. He couldn't live with it, and he couldn't stop drinking, so he stopped the only way he could.

Randy died, as his alcoholic father had and as too many alcoholics do, by his own hand, leaving a trail of pain, trouble, debt, legal and financial problems, heartache and loss behind him.

And in the strange repeating pattern which is alcoholism, Randy left a son behind too.

The sadness inside me at his loss is not something that words can describe. Guilt made me feel I should have done more.

I took a month off from the book, told his friends, organized his funeral, looked after his belongings, cried a lot of tears and started writing again.

His funeral, held in August 2015, was standing-room only. He called himself a monster, but he was, in fact, a special and rare individual and he was indeed loved as a fellow human being, not a monster. He was a man who, even in the weeks before he died, lit up a room with his good looks and smile, musical talents, and ability to charm those around him.

When Randy died, it occurred to me that it would not be very inspiring to read a book about medications for alcoholism where the 'main character' was not saved by the solution the book proffered.

But this book isn't about proof of efficacy from one person. Nor should it be–the whole point of drawing conclusions from scientific research is that it is repeatable and statistically significant.

So had he survived alcoholism, Randy's single successful data point would have been just as immaterial to this book as is his death.

There is too much medical research backing these medications–the data exists, and I don't mean it exists in the form of a few stray outliers. It is solid. Read it, and I challenge you to tell me it is not.

Randy was tormented by alcoholism and desperate for help. He was a committed AA member and tried to get real help for his alcoholism for 20+ years.

He ashamedly tucked his tail between his legs after numerous destructive binges and walked back through the doors of those rooms over and over again.

He also tried to get help from many non-AA organizations, attending programs at hospitals and treatment centers.

During this time, he was never once offered one of the medications in this book, unprompted, by any medical professional he ever saw.

And he saw dozens–doctors, psychiatrists, social works, occupational therapists, health care workers and all manner of addiction specialists–if not over a hundred of them as his illness progressed.

After facing many difficult and frankly ridiculous roadblocks in even obtaining them, Randy responded well to one of the medications discussed later. I believe strongly that had he received long-term

Medication Assisted Treatment (MAT) many years ago before the disease progressed so far, he would have had a fighting chance.

By the time he died, however, he was a severe, long-term alcoholic.

And unfortunately, even after jumping through hoops to get treatment from the leading addiction treatment organization in our country, bringing with him pages of research, he could not find a doctor there willing to support him in prescribing the medications in ways shown to be effective. Instead, he was referred back to AA.

Had I held a crystal ball up for the last "addiction specialist" he saw, revealing that healthy-looking, sober, smiling Randy would be dead two months later after a protracted binge, would that doctor have taken the disease seriously enough to prescribe the medications and support that Randy asked for?

I'll never know and I guess it doesn't matter anymore, other than to fuel me to want to help other people get the help that Randy couldn't get.

I talked to him about this book. I wanted him to know that his life and experiences weren't a waste—they could help people we would never meet. He told me to tell his story. It's in Part 5 if you'd like to read it.

I hope (as he did) that you can learn from him, and I hope his death will remind you of the deadly serious nature of alcoholism. This disease can kill you or your loved one too. It's no joke.

During my friendship with him, I saw how Randy was treated by the medical and healthcare community; how he was eventually shunned by members of his family; how many of his experiences in fighting a medical illness were so demeaning. Eventually the system just abandoned him. There was no solution for him that they could offer.

Randy's life was an example of a person being processed through a broken system and coming out dead on the other end.

So it's not just that I want medication, or better yet—Medication Assisted Treatment—to be available to people who need it. I want the whole system to be better. I want this book to help change the way we treat and look at alcoholics.

Because there but for the grace of God, or genes, or fate, or whatever you believe, go I. Or you.

03 | YESTERDAY & TODAY

*"A complex brain disease requires many approaches, the
addiction field needs to bring the best of these together, not
fight over who's right."*

–Hazelton Doctor Marvin Seppala

HEADLINES

And as new discoveries have emerged, so has evidence showing that alcoholism can be treated safely and effectively with medication–like any other illness.

But unfortunately, in the last twenty years, little of the scientific body of work supporting medication for alcohol addiction treatment has translated into readily available treatment options for those suffering from the disease.

There is a profound gap between what we know and the treatment people receive.

Good, FDA-approved medications to treat alcoholism have been available for many years, but until recently 'alcohol culture' wasn't ready for them.

But we are now at a tipping point.

If a tipping point could have a name, this one would be called Matt.

Or actually–MAT–which is short for "Medication Assisted Treatment".

It's a new phrase that is emerging, used by clever spin-doctors in the US government, peppered into reports from the country's top health, drug and addiction organizations, and finding its way into newspaper articles and addiction websites.

The first surprising headlines of change started in 2012.

A long-time-stronghold of 12-step treatment–Hazelton–shocked the recovery community when it introduced anti-addiction medication into their recovery programs for the first time in history.

Time Magazine quoted Dr. Marvin Sepala, Hazelton's Chief Medical Officer saying, "This is a huge shift in our culture and organization... we believe it's the responsible thing to do."[24]

Shortly afterward, in Europe in 2013, pharmaceutical company Lundbeck made headlines when it launched the first drug approved in over a decade (nalmefene) for alcohol-dependent patients with high-risk drinking levels.[25]

Then in 2014, under a swell of pressure from advocates and alcoholics, French health authorities gave the green light to doctors to formally prescribe a drug called baclofen to treat people with an addiction to alcohol.[26]

Recently, in the US in February 2015, Obama's government made a historic appointment, which kicked off a tidal wave of change.

The Washington Post headline screamed out: "Drug Czar Approaches Challenge from a Different Angle: As a Recovering Alcoholic." Instead of another militant leader to fight the war on drugs, the US brought in someone with his own criminal record.

Obama had appointed Michael Botticelli–a recovering alcoholic with a DUI on file.

Sober for over 26 years, and despite his strong ties to 'anti-medication' AA, Botticelli is fighting for evidence-based treatment (which means medication) for substance abuse treatment.[27]

The Drug Czar appointment was followed up quickly with two more government announcements in February and March.

The first was from The Substance Abuse and Mental Health Services Administration about the new use of penalties for judges that order addicts (including alcoholics) off of medically assisted treatment:

> *"Drug courts that receive federal dollars will no longer be allowed to ban the kinds of medication-assisted treatments that doctors and scientists view as the most effective care…. We've made that clear: If they want our federal dollars, they cannot do that."*[28]

The second was an announcement that for the first time in the United States, the Affordable Care Act would legislate that substance abuse must be treated like any other illness:

"These rules are...a sea change in the way that health plans approach the coverage of mental health and substance abuse disorder benefits ... Essentially, President Obama's health care act enshrines in federal law that substance abuse is a medical issue—not the result of poor morals, and not a criminal justice problem."[28]

However, as we'll see later in this book, all the government legislation in the world makes no difference to the use of medication if pharmaceutical companies cannot be profitable in making it and doctors won't prescribe it.

But for the first time in North America in 2015, a medication that can be used for the treatment of opioid and alcohol dependence saw profitability.

In October 2015, Alkermes Pharmaceutical's historic press release announced that they were improving their financial expectations for the remainder of the year, driven by the accelerating growth in net sales of their naltrexone injection product Vivitrol, which had experienced an unprecedented sales increase of 72%.

Around the world, pharmaceutical company CEOs turned their heads and tipped their hats at Alkermes. It was a clear signal that a category of medication once avoided and practically hidden from shareholders could now be profitable.[29]

And finally, most recently, in October 2015, in front of President Obama, Botticelli, senators and a crowd of people in Charleston West Virginia, Secretary of Health and Human Services, Sylvia Burwell spoke of their new priorities around substance abuse, saying:

"Number one is changing prescribing practices... and second is working on medication assisted treatment."[30]

Finally... MAT might end up on your doctor's prescription pad.

Times they are a'changin. And not a moment too soon.

So Overdue

These events are overdue—woefully overdue.

The state of treatment for people with alcoholism is shameful.

Nowhere in the field of modern medicine is treatment more antiquated than in the area of alcohol addiction treatment, where time has stood still since AA's Big Book was published in 1939.[15]

In the last 25 years, cancer death rates have gone down by 22% while in the same period addiction overdose death rates have tripled.[31]

A 2012, exceptionally well-written report from the National Center on Addiction and Substance Abuse (Entitled '*Addiction Medicine: Closing the Gap Between Science & Practice*') compared the current state of addiction medicine to general medicine in the early 1900s.

The report said: "The vast majority of people in need of addiction treatment do not receive anything that approximates evidence-based care."[3]

Markus Heilig, an internationally respected addiction researcher, and doctor, recently wrote:

> "*People with addictive disorders continue to be offered, with great certitude and frequently at great cost, "treatments" that are unsubstantiated by data or already known to be without beneficial effects.*
>
> *Meanwhile, advances that may be modest but have solid scientific support are arrogantly rejected by treatment providers in ways that would cause an uproar in other areas of medicine.*"[4]

FDA-approved drugs exist which may be even more effective at battling alcoholism than widely prescribed drugs such as cholesterol-lowering statins are at fighting heart disease.[14]

Yet in the US, of the approximately 19 million patients meeting criteria for alcohol dependence, less than 150,000 are treated with FDA-approved pharmacotherapy.[32]

However, most shockingly, the medications proven most effective and life changing for alcoholics have been researched and FDA-approved for decades.

•••

I don't remember the day that I went to my computer and started the Googling that led me to the research that ultimately led to writing this book.

But I do know that the more I read, the more I wondered how it was possible that in the year 2015, an area of medicine for a major disease could be so backward.

And I also noticed that unlike most major illnesses, where government, pharmaceutical companies, not-for-profits and medical institutions play the leading roles in educating consumers about medical treatment, many of these stakeholders were strangely quiet when it came to this particular illness.

There was a curious void of information about medical treatment from the usual suspects.

In fact, there seemed to be only two groups of people who were sharing information about medical solutions: uber geeks and advocate alcoholics.

The uber geeks (okay–'scientific researchers') were slogging away in labs and at conferences, speaking in strange tongues, working hard despite growing frustration that their discoveries were not reaching the critical mass of people they should be helping.

And as good as they are at research and report writing, they seem in equal parts weak or uninterested in translating their work into plain English and making it accessible to alcoholics and their treatment providers.

On the other hand, the advocate alcoholics were a passionate, outspoken and interesting bunch.

For the small group of people who have been lucky enough to learn about these medications, it is the advocate alcoholics that are mostly to thank.

This group includes recovering doctors who walked away from careers, outing their own alcoholism to write about medication that saved their lives; public figures who abandoned anonymity in the face of heavy stigma to push for more public awareness, and hundreds of recovering alcoholics from all walks of life who reached out online (both anonymously and publicly) to help others discover and access these medications.

Most of the material written in plain English in book form and online that currently exists and is related to this area of medicine comes from this group.

Highlighting the void of information from the usual sources is this: one of the best (and only) documentaries on one of these medications–*One Little Pill*–comes not from any government organization or pharmaceutical company, but was crowd-funded and produced by one of these advocate alcoholics I speak of. This advocate also started an organization with branches in the US and Europe to help alcoholics access the medication that helped her.

I'm speaking of Claudia Christian here. She's an intelligent and courageous woman, who also happens to be an actress from Babylon 5 and a former Playboy model who was Dodi Al Fayed's love interest before Princess Diana was. I don't make this stuff up folks.

But as much as I respect Christian, I had to ask myself, what are the agendas at work here, when a lady I can watch on TV in an episode of Criminal Minds is also my primary source of information for medical treatment options for a significant medical illness? I imagine she probably wonders this herself.

I also came to the conclusion that the group that I had thought were the knights in white armor when it came to addiction–namely AA–has sadly been part of the problem–a big part.

Instead of taking a page out of the playbooks of other not-for-profits like the Heart and Stroke Foundation or the Susan G Koman Breast Cancer Foundation, AA sticks to its own 1930s playbook–the 'Big Book'–and refuses to acknowledge any medical treatment that didn't exist in 1939.

And evil pharma? They aren't evil in this story–they've mostly stayed away from the wholly unprofitable mess, waiting for AA-thinking to loosen its hold and doctors to decide to start treating alcoholism like any other illness.

So now you know a little about what's new today, the state we are in, and some of the players that got us to where we are today.

Next, I'll back up some of my claims about the effectiveness of the medication and the research behind it.

04 | SIX SAD TRUTHS

"I'm not trying to predict the future. I'm trying to let us see the present."

−William Gibson

JUST THE FACTS

As I read research report after research report about medications that can treat alcoholism, these facts became apparent:

1. There is an abundance of high-quality research that shows the effectiveness of medications for alcoholism.

2. Many of the medications are safe and FDA-approved, and as effective in alcoholism as other widely prescribed drugs are for other illnesses.

3. Research backing some of the medications has been in existence, and growing, for over a decade—if not longer.

4. Despite the lack of other effective treatments, the vast majority of alcoholics are not told about or prescribed these medications, even when they seek help.

5. The failure of medical professionals to prescribe drugs to alcoholics who need them has caused negative repercussions for future treatment innovations.

6. These issues have slowed down medical development—something which will have repercussions well into the next decade.

The first three points are good news for alcoholics and their families—there is hope—there is something you may not have tried.

But that fourth fact—that so many people are suffering and dying, and not being told about these options—is simply unacceptable.

The fifth and sixth statements—about negative repercussions—are something I'll delve into near the end of this chapter. But in a nutshell: when pharmaceutical companies can't sell good medications to those who need them, they stop developing them.

I'd like to back up those statements with data now, so let's look at some of the medications that you'll find more information about later in this book. Let's look at these five:

1. Acamprosate

2. Baclofen

3. Naltrexone

4. Topiramate

5. Gabapentin

These are five of the medications that are grouped into the A-List (Most Important Medications for Today), later in the book, where extensive detail is provided on each one.

FDA-APPROVAL

To achieve FDA-approval, a medication has to go through extensive testing. Safety is one of the many things tested.

These five medications are all FDA-approved—which means they have been shown to be safe in humans, and they are currently prescribed by physicians.

Some of them are FDA-approved for alcohol addictions, and some achieved FDA-approval for a different illness.

All five in my list above have been FDA-approved for over a decade.

Here are the years in which they were approved and made available to doctors and patients:

• Acamprosate—11+ years of FDA approval (since 2004)

• Baclofen—38+ years of FDA approval (since 1977)

• Naltrexone—21+ years of FDA approval (since 1994)

• Topiramate—21+ years of FDA approval (since 1994)

• Gabapentin—13+ years of FDA approval (since 2002)

Years of Research for Alcohol Treatment

Of course, research into medications takes years before drugs reach the point of gaining FDA-approval.

When a drug is very new, with few years of research behind it, it is possible that there may be surprises around some of a medication's effects that have yet to be seen. That's why newer drugs deserve more caution than older ones.

But all five of the drugs we are examining here have been researched for years, again—over a decade even for the newest.

Here are the years when research began for each ones' effectiveness in alcoholism:

- Acamprosate: 30+ years of research (since 1985)

- Baclofen: 39+ years of research (since 1976)

- Naltrexone: 23+ years of research (since 1992)

- Topiramate: 12+ years of research (since 2003)

- Gabapentin: 15+ years of research (since 2000)

Number Needed to Treat (NNT)

An important term to know when evaluating the effectiveness of a medication is the medication's NNT—the Number Needed to Treat.

The NNT is the number of people that need to receive the medication before one individual is helped. So, for example, if a medication has an NNT of 10, it means that one in ten people treated with the drug is helped; or that the medication is effective 10% of the time.

The lower the NNT, the more people the medication is effective for.

To give you an idea of the relative effectiveness of medications for alcoholism it may be helpful to understand the NNTs for other common drugs.

Many medications commonly prescribed for depression have an NNT of around 5-10[1].

This means they help one out of every 5-10 people who take them. (And these are for the most effective anti-depressants–less often prescribed ones can have much higher NNTs).

Here are the NNTs for other often-prescribed drugs:[33]

- Antibiotics for sinusitis–1 in 15 were helped (an NNT of 15)

- Nicotine replacement to quit smoking–1 in 15 quit smoking (an NNT of 15)

- Antiplatelet agents (blood thinners) for stroke–1 in 79 were helped (an NNT of 79)

- Blood pressure medications (anti-hypertensives) to prevent death, heart attacks, and stroke–1 in 125 prevented death; 1 in 67 prevented stroke; 1 in 100 prevented heart attack (an NNT from 67-125)

- Daily aspirin to prevent first heart attack or stroke–1 in 1667 were helped (an NNT of 1667)

In comparison, the NNT numbers for the medications we're examining here for alcoholism have been found in research to be significantly lower (which means better):

- Acamprosate NNT: 1 in 7-12 were helped to reduce drinking or maintain abstinence (an NNT of 7-12)[134]

- Baclofen NNT: 1 in 3 were helped to reduce drinking or maintain abstinence (an NNT of 3)[35]

- Topiramate NNT: Unknown NNT

- Naltrexone NNT: 1 in 7-10 were helped to reduce drinking or maintain abstinence (an NNT of 7-10)[36]

- Gabapentin NNT: 1 in 5-8 were helped to reduce drinking or maintain abstinence (an NNT of 5-8)[37]

These NNT numbers are excellent—and not just for one of these drugs—all four of the drugs with known NNT numbers are the same or better than those of commonly prescribed medications doled out in doctors' offices every day.

Who gives medications their NNT numbers?

Scientists learn these numbers through repetitive research.

If you look at the small endnote numbers I've added as references you can trace them back to the bibliography at the end of this document and see the names of researchers, their research, and where the research was published.

You can then go to a search engine such as Google Scholar (scholar.google.com), search for the name and read it yourself.

QUALITY AND QUANTITY OF THE BODY OF RESEARCH

For research to be deemed credible, one research paper isn't enough.

There has to be a 'body of research' for a medication to be considered credible.

So in other words, many well-published researchers, in many well-run research studies need to be able to consistently duplicate positive results for research to be considered highly credible and a medication to be regarded as effective.

Some individual studies can be so extensive and well-run that they carry a lot of weight by themselves, but usually a single study with new findings is of little significance until it can be reproduced by others.

There are also studies called 'Research Reviews' and 'Meta-analysis' which are useful too because these are 'studies of studies' which look at numerous individual studies of a particular drug to determine whether the entire body of research is conclusive.

Reviews and Meta-analysis are the aggregators of information in the world of research, and should be important sources of information for medical practitioners.

Many of the medications have such a body of research.

Here are statements from just a few of the papers:

For Acamprosate:

- There are "more than 450 published original investigations and clinical trials and 1.5 million treated patients which together has resulted in a convincing body of knowledge around acamprosate as an effective treatment for alcohol dependence."[38]

- The effectiveness of acamprosate is "robustly documented in meta-analyses of available studies…the latter of these was a meta-analysis of 17 studies which included 4087 individuals."[1]

- Acamprosate was found to be superior to placebo in the maintenance of abstinence in a 2015 study in patients with alcohol dependence. The 2015 report cited that "these findings concur with 11 randomized, blinded, placebo-controlled clinical trials conducted in Europe."[39]

- A 2012 analysis included 1317 women and 4794 men from 22 studies within 18 countries and found that acamprosate had "significant beneficial effect across 4 efficacy endpoints–percentage of abstinent days, the percentage of no heavy drinking days, the rate of complete abstinence and rate of no heavy drinking. Acamprosate also had a high rate of treatment completion and medication compliance.[40]

- A meta-analysis of data from 11 European clinical trials that included over 3000 showed that "acamprosate nearly doubled the likelihood of preventing relapse to drinking and increased the probability that patients would remain in treatment by nearly one-third."[41]

- In addition, acamprosate is available in at least 30 countries, including the United States, most of Europe, China, Singapore, and Australia, as well as Central and South American countries. It has been prescribed to over "1.5 million persons with alcohol abuse or dependence in those countries with no apparent pattern of serious side effects. European data indicate that the drug has no potential for abuse or rebound effect after discontinuation. European data have also indicated that the drug effectively reduces craving for alcohol and can help maintain abstinence in dependent patients."[42]

You don't have to be a rocket scientist to understand from those quotes that acamprosate should be on every doctor's radar.

Here are some research quotes for the others.

For baclofen:

- "The majority of clinical surveys conducted to date–including case reports, retrospective chart reviews, and randomized placebo-controlled studies–suggest the ability of baclofen to suppress alcohol consumption, craving for alcohol, and alcohol withdrawal symptomatology in alcohol-dependent patients."[43]

- "The constancy of improvement over the 2-years was remarkable...ninety-two percentage of patients reported that they experienced the craving-suppressing effect of baclofen."[44]

For topiramate:

- "There is now solid clinical evidence to support the efficacy of topiramate for the treatment of alcohol dependence."[45]

For naltrexone:

- "Meta-analyses of available trials, even when the negative study is included in the analysis, unequivocally support NTX [Naltrexone] efficacy"[1].

- "There is abundant evidence supporting the use of naltrexone for the treatment of alcohol dependence (Level A)."[41]

- As early as 2002, one report showed that up to 2001 there had already been 14 trials assessing the effectiveness of naltrexone compared with placebo for treating alcoholism, enrolling 2127 subjects, in five countries. It stated, "there is strong evidence that naltrexone significantly reduces alcohol relapses to heavy drinking, the frequency and quantity of alcohol consumption in those who do drink, and alcohol craving."[46]

- "Naltrexone is one of the most evaluated medications in clinical research for reducing craving. It was superior to placebo in lessening craving, preventing relapse to heavy drinking, and in increasing the percentage of abstinent days."[47]

- "Oral and long-acting injectable naltrexone... are approved for treatment of alcohol dependence. Their availability and consideration of their use in treatment are now standards of high-quality care."[48]

And for gabapentin:

- In a review of six randomized controlled clinical trials lasting at least 4 weeks, the four largest trials showed "beneficial effects of gabapentin on at least one alcohol-related outcome measure."[49]

- A large, well-managed 6-year study found Gabapentin significantly improved rates of abstinence and no heavy drinking. Abstinence rate was 4.1% in the placebo group ... and 17.0% in the 1800-mg group. The no heavy drinking rate was 22.5% in the placebo group ... and 44.7% in the 1800-mg group.[37]

- "Gabapentin's effect on drinking outcomes is at least as large or greater than those of existing FDA approved treatments...plus it's the only medication shown to improve sleep and mood in people who are quitting or reducing their drinking, and it's already widely used in primary care."[50]

RESEARCHER CREDENTIALS

On the internet anyone can come across a lot of questionable 'research', written by a lot of questionable 'researchers.' Snake-oil salespeople are in abundance online, unfortunately.

But the researchers who wrote the above statements, and who found and stand behind the NTT numbers are some of the most educated, most published, most respected scientists in the field of addiction research in the world at this time.

They work at the most respected institutions in the world and those statements have been published in the top scientific addiction and medicine journals. And less than 20 researchers were quoted. There are hundreds more, highly credible scientists who are on the research teams for these studies, as well as contributing to other research cited in this book.

A few of the individuals (whose names are also in the endnotes at the back of the book), and who led the research just cited include:

- Dr. Rainer Spanagel, Director of the Central Institute of Psychopharmacology at the University of Heidelberg

- Dr. Markus Heilig, M.D., Ph.D., Head of Neuroscientific Research, Linkoping University (former Chief of the Laboratory of Clinical Studies, and Clinical Director of the United States National Institute of Alcohol Abuse (NIAAA) Division of Intramural Clinical and Biological Research)

- Dr. Mark Egli, Program Officer, Division of Neuroscience and Behavior, National Institute on Alcohol Abuse and Alcoholism

- Dr. Susumu Higuchi, MD, Ph.D., Director, National Hospital Organization, Kurihama Medical and Addiction Center, Japan

- Dr. Barbara Mason, Director, Laboratory of Clinical Psychopharmacology and Pearson Center for Alcoholism and Addiction Research

- Dr. Phillippe Lehert, Senior Consulting Statistician at United Nations, University of Melbourne

- Dr. M. Soyka, Head of the Department of Forensic Psychiatry of the Psychiatric Hospital of the LMU Munich

- Dr. Roberta Agabio, Head of the Centre for the Study of Adolescent Alcohol Dependence, Italy

- Dr. Renaud de Beaurepaire, Psychiatrist and neurobiologist, head of Psychiatry at the Paul Guiraud Hospital

- Dr. Bankole Johnson, Chair of the Department of Psychiatry, University of Maryland School of Medicine

- Dr. Nassima Ait Daoud Tiouririne, MD, Associate Professor in the Department of Psychiatry and Neurobehavioral Science and director of the Center for Addictions Research and Education, UVA

- Dr. Stewart Leavitt, MA, Ph.D., Addiction Treatment Forum Researcher/Editor

- Dr. Carolina L Haass-Koffler, Postdoctoral Fellow, Center for Alcohol and Addiction Studies, Brown University

- Dr. Adron Harris, Director of the University of Texas Waggoner Center for Alcohol and Addiction Research

- Dr. Morgan D. Greutman (Pharm D.) Southwestern Oklahoma State University

- Dr. Lorenzo Leggio, M.D., Ph.D., M.Sc., Chief of Clinical Psychoneuroendocrinology and Neuropsychopharmacology, NIAAA/NIDA

- Dr. George A. Kenna, assistant professor, Psychiatry, Center for Alcohol and Addiction Studies, Brown University, and a senior scientific advisor, Tufts Health Care Institute Program on Opioid Risk Management

If my life was at stake, that is a list of people that I would trust. And I'd want my doctor to trust them too.

How about you?

PUBLICATION QUALITY

Lending even more credibility to the researcher findings are the peer–reviewed journals where their work is published.

The statements and NNTs quoted above were published in highly respected, peer-reviewed journals, including these ones: Neuropsychopharmacology, Pharmacology and Therapeutics, American Psychiatric Association Journal, The Journal of Clinical Psychiatry, Alcoholism: Clinical and Experimental Research, World Federation of Societies of Biological Psychiatry, Frontiers in Neuroscience, Frontiers in Psychiatry, Current Pharmaceutical Design, CNS Drugs, Alcoholism:

Clinical and Experimental Research, Journal of Pharmacy Technology, and JAMA (Journal of the American Medical Association).

I hope that briefly these sections have helped to illustrate my points about the quality of the body of research that has developed supporting the use of these medications for alcohol addiction treatment.

And that's just a small sampling–a *minute* sampling–of the much larger body of research that exists.

LACK OF OTHER EFFECTIVE
TREATMENT

There are other kinds of (non-pharmaceutical) treatments available for alcoholics. The best known of these other approaches is Alcoholics Anonymous, which is discussed extensively later.

But this book is about 'evidence-based medicine'. Or, in other words, treatments that have a substantial body of research backing them.

Evidence-based medicine is the foundation of modern medicine and the only kind of medicine that should matter to licensed doctors who wish to avoid malpractice suits.

Some treatments certainly have an incredibly extensive body of *anecdotal* support (both for and against them), but judged in terms of raw, scientific data, other treatments have very little conclusive scientific support.

When we look at evidence-based medicine, there are no other treatments for alcoholism that have as strong a body of research backing them as do the medications I identified above.

Other treatments–which consist of either 12-step programs or behavioral therapy, have a 70-90% relapse rate.[51]

One of the most highly respected organizations in the world when it comes to meta-analysis' discussed earlier is an organization called Cochrane. Cochrane reviews are trusted worldwide for their credibility, impartiality and extremely high quality.

There have been several reports and reviews published by Cochrane that support many of the medications discussed in the book. However, they also concluded in a 2006 review of studies going back to the 1960s that:

> *"No experimental studies unequivocally demonstrated the effectiveness of AA or [12-step] approaches for reducing alcohol dependence."*[5]

The report explicitly stated:

> *"People considering attending AA or TSF [Twelve Step] programmes should be made aware that there is a lack of experimental evidence on the effectiveness of such programmes."*[5]

The fact is, these treatments fail—for most people, most of the time.

Because of the lack of published data supporting other approaches, the US government has publicly backed Medication Assisted Treatment.

The US Government's Center for Substance Abuse Treatment, Substance Abuse and Mental Health Services Administration (SAMHSA) published a guide written for physicians and healthcare professionals in 2013, stating:

> *"Medication-assisted treatment has shown much promise in reducing alcohol use and promoting abstinence in patients diagnosed with alcohol use disorder.*
>
> *Considerable research evidence and consensus among experts support the use of pharmacologic treatments... A number of FDA-approved medications have been shown to be important elements of such treatment."*
>
> *"Although some patients do not benefit from medication-assisted treatment, most do.*
>
> *For each patient deemed an appropriate candidate for medication-assisted treatment, multiple pharmacologic agents offer a variety of options so that treatment can be tailored to each patient's needs and circumstances."*[7]

A Decade Ago, Alcoholics Weren't Told

Earlier I discussed how many years the most important medications have been researched for, and how long they have been FDA-approved.

So it should be quite clear that none of the most important drugs I have identified in this chapter are new.

And while there is new research every day, which builds the case for their effectiveness, there was already abundant evidence of the efficacy of some of them many years ago.

Not only did evidence exist over a decade ago of their effectiveness, but it was also red-flagged by prominent researchers ten years ago that effective medications were not making it to the people who needed them most.

For example, nearly a decade ago, Mark Heilig and Markus Egli wrote a paper on behalf of the National Institute of Alcohol Abuse and Alcoholism (NIAAA) identifying the fact that even addiction medicine specialists were failing to prescribe drugs, such as naltrexone, that could help alcoholics.

It was clear that alcoholics just weren't receiving prescriptions for the life-saving medications they were researching.

For example, in 2007, in the United States, only about 720,000 prescriptions were written for alcohol treatment medications, representing approximately 78 million dollars in sales.

Compare that to the sales volume for the antidepressant Lexapro, generating 1.7 billion dollars in 2004, even though the number of US adults suffering from major depression is similar to those suffering from alcohol use disorder.[52]

Stepping beyond their usual clinical scientific demeanor, of naltrexone, the two highly respected scientists wrote:

"It is highly disturbing that this drug is not made available to the patients that need it."[1]

They echoed the sentiments stated the year before, in 2005, when the American Council on Alcoholism pointed out:

"In other areas of medicine, it is highly probable that the development of such efficacious medication would prompt physicians to use it readily," but that in the area of addiction medicine, patients were not being treated with the efficacious medications that already existed.[53]

TODAY, ALCOHOLICS STILL AREN'T TOLD ABOUT MEDICATIONS

Today, alcoholics *still* aren't being prescribed these safe, effective drugs that could save their lives.

We learned earlier that the NTT numbers for the most important medications today are similar to the NTT for most antidepressants.

The prevalence of depression and anxiety disorders is two or three times that of alcohol dependence. However, antidepressants are prescribed 100 to 200 times as often as medications for alcohol dependence.[54]

SAMHSA's guide, referred to above stated:

"Although many experts in addiction believe that patients with moderate or severe alcohol-related problems should be offered medication-assisted treatment (MAT) on a routine basis, considerable resistance to the use of MAT persists..."[7]

The resistance of health-care professionals to prescribe them has resulted in dismal numbers: multiple sources support numbers ranging from only 3-11% of those who need it receiving any kind of treatment.

One important 2012 study found:

> *"Analysis indicates that only one in 10 (10.9 percent, 2.5 million) of those in need of addiction treatment (excluding nicotine) receive it, leaving a treatment gap of 20.7 million individuals."*[3]

And the same report attacked the medical system, saying,

> *"There simply is no other disease where appropriate medical treatment is not provided by the health care system and where patients instead must turn to a broad range of practitioners largely exempt from medical standards."*[3]

Addiction medicine is simply the ugly sister of the world of medicine.

Dr. Shelly Greenfield, Director at the Harvard Medical School, has singled this out, stating of the existing treatments:

> *"There is no other comparable example in medicine where you have evidence-based treatments that are not available.*[3]

A 2014 report published in the American Journal of Psychiatry confirmed the 2012 report's points, stating explicitly that "a recent study of Veterans Health Administration facilities showed that nationally, only 3% of Veterans Health Administration patients with alcohol use disorder received treatment medications."[2]

The authors echoed earlier sentiments once again, stating:

> *"There is an enormous gap between the number of alcohol use disorder patients who would potentially benefit from medications and the number of patients who actually receive medications."*[2]

Elsewhere in the world, treatment seeking alcoholics are little better off.

In the United Kingdom, the vast majority (80-95%) receive no treatment[55], and the few medications that are most often prescribed are limited to only three early medications–disulfiram, acamprosate, naltrexone–instead of the wider options now shown to be effective.

In comparison with other kinds of mental illness, alcohol addiction has the broadest treatment gap of all mental disorders:

82% of people with schizophrenia, 60% of people with bipolar disorder and 55% of people with major depression receive treatment versus the dismal 8% of people with alcohol dependence that need and receive treatment. [5556]

So clearly, my fourth point—that despite the lack of other effective treatments, the vast majority of alcoholics are not told about or prescribed these medications, even when they seek help—is clear.

And that sums up the situation we are in today: Alcoholism—the world's most deadly disease[8] can be treated with lots of life-saving, promising, safe, FDA-approved medications…but nobody is getting them.

A LOST DECADE FOR DRUG DEVELOPMENT

If that isn't bad enough, it gets worse.

When promising, well-supported medications are researched, known about for over a decade, and then never make it into the hands of the patients that need them, there are negative repercussions: research and development 'get stuck.'

In 2006, Heilig wrote a roadmap for the next generation of development for drugs to fight alcohol addiction.

In it, he identified three waves of pharmacological treatments.

The first wave, already heavily researched and FDA-approved by 2006, included disulfiram, naltrexone, and acamprosate.

He predicted a second wave of drugs that would improve efficacy and allow more tailored treatment, taking genetic makeup into account. The second wave would include drugs like ondansetron, baclofen, and topiramate.

The third wave would target systems in the brain already identified as holding much potential for treatment using new, yet-to-be-named medications.[1]

Heilig's three waves may have seemed overly optimistic—but they weren't. His roadmap merely represented the great promise that existed (and still exists) for the treatment of alcohol addiction.

Heilig was correct in his predictions about which drugs and targets would be important in the coming years.

But today, unfortunately, the government is still trying to get the medical community on board to prescribe even the very first wave of drugs.

And the appetite of pharmaceutical companies to shepherd the second and third waves through expensive clinical trials, is weak at best.

When pharmaceutical companies can't sell effective drugs they have spent millions of dollars developing—like naltrexone for example—they stop investing (or they fail to start in the first place). After all, why would a pharmaceutical company risk investment in new drugs, when the old, proven ones, sat on shelves?

So instead of the second and third wave of medications getting pushed through to the FDA-approval stage, only the first wave got over that hump.

The second wave is FDA-approved—but for other illnesses.

And the third wave is having difficulty getting out of the pre-clinical research stage.

It's been a lost decade in research and development for addictions.

DRUG PIPELINE IS DRY

We can see the impact of this lost decade in the drug pipeline, which is the name for the process that drugs follow to get from discovery to FDA-approval.

In the drug pipeline is the set of substances that pharmaceutical companies have in discovery or development at any given time.

On average each year in the United States, 25 drugs finish their journey through the pipeline and are given FDA approval.

It can take 10-15 years and millions of dollars in investment for a drug to progress from the beginning through to the end of the drug pipeline.

The drug development cycle is so long that if there is a period of a decade when the drug pipeline slows down, that slowdown will negatively impact drug development well into the future.

Last year in the United States, a bumper crop of 41 new drugs made it through to attain approval.

Several (four) of these were for type 2 diabetes, four were antibiotics and five were for cancer treatment.

And over 40 percent—or 17 of the new drugs were for rare diseases— diseases that affect 200,000 or fewer Americans.[57]

If each of these rare diseases affected 200,000 Americans, it would mean that at most 3.4 million Americans could now be treated with these new drugs.

But at least five times the number of Americans (18 million)[14] suffer from alcohol dependence—and not a single drug was approved last year to treat these Americans.

Nor the year before, nor the year before.

Despite the great work researchers have done in understanding the illness, and the enormous need for medical treatment, not a single drug has been approved for the treatment of alcohol dependence in the United States for over 10 years.

Nor is it likely that this trend will change soon.

In April 2014, there were 113 substances registered in human clinical trials for the treatment of any type of mental illness.

Of these 113, only four were in human trials specifically for the treatment of alcohol dependence.

Only 20% of drugs going through clinical trials ever progress to FDA Approval, so for the odds to work in their favor, at least 23 of the drugs in clinical trials right now would have to be targeted to alcohol dependence for one of them to achieve FDA approval.

With only four at that level right now, the chances are small that we will see a new drug for alcohol dependence in the next five years.

And those, my friend, are the sad truths about medications for the treatment of alcoholism.

05 | THE PLAYERS

"If you have hypertension and it flares up, you go to a specialist. The specialist doesn't discharge you to a church basement.
If he did, we would call it malpractice."[58]

—Psychologist Thomas McLellan, University of Pennsylvania

ALCOHOLISM CULTURE

If you are reading this book, the chances are that you, like me, live in a first world country.

I used to naively presume that one of the benefits of such privilege was that drugs that work would automatically be channeled to the people that needed them. That isn't the case with alcoholism though.

To understand why, we need to look at a broad, amorphous collection of issues and groups which I lump into a category I call 'alcoholism culture'.

All major diseases have their own unique culture. Look at the Google image search results when you search for the name of a disease and you'll see a visual depiction of that culture.

For example, breast cancer culture is defined by the pink ribbon, and imagery of 'survival.' The face of breast cancer is predominantly female. Imagery and copy carries a tone of hope, conquer, walking for the cure! And power in numbers! (And excessive use of enthusiastic exclamation marks!)

In contrast, alcoholism culture appears in shadows and dark colors. It's more masculine. There are images of handcuffs and alcohol and people sitting in shadows and garbage. The tone is overwhelmingly that of desperation and a loss of dignity.

Every disease culture has its issues. Documentarian Ravida Din looked at breast cancer culture and made a movie about its dark side (Pink Ribbons Inc.).

Her work highlighted how some major corporations use the pink ribbon on products to increase sales while donating only a tiny fraction to the cause. The movie illustrated how women are encouraged to participate in cheerful pink pep rallies instead of tackling harder issues.

Din says, "the question I was intrigued by was, 'How did we get to this kind of breast cancer culture that privileges shopping [as a solution] as opposed to getting angry and asking for change?"[59]

We might take a page out of Din's book and ask, "How did we get to this kind of alcoholism culture where doctors send patients to a religion-based program that fails 90% of the time, as opposed to getting angry and asking for change?"

Din says, "I want people to learn to ask questions…I want to change the discourse which has been the same for decades, and to see what we can do to be more efficient to counter this terrible disease."[59]

We have to ask the same question about alcoholism.

Because if how we are tackling breast cancer is *'inefficient'*, how we tackle alcoholism is downright backwater inept.

And we can't improve on the system we have unless we find its weaknesses.

Din looked at the key groups involved to find their inefficiencies. And that's where we need to look too.

This chapter looks at alcoholism culture's stakeholders and the roles they play.

If, as Din says, 'we need to learn to ask questions', then it's these groups those questions need to be directed to.

ALCOHOLICS ANONYMOUS

AA is a community of individuals who are struggling with a devastating, lonely, isolating disease. To its members AA offers companionship, friendship, support, love, the opportunity to grow through helping others, and a system for living a moral, positive lifestyle.

The support provided to alcoholics by fellow AA members can be overwhelmingly positive, and for those individuals who are assisted in overcoming addiction by relying on that support and the AA system, AA can be nothing short of miraculous and life altering.

But as great as AA is in many ways, it is also a problem.

In fact, it's the biggest problem.

It's this single stakeholder that has been the most influential and detrimental to the advancement of medical treatment for alcoholism.

It spreads mistruths and myths that block our understanding of what science now holds to be true.

Its influence is behemoth.

Its viewpoints form the cultural backbone of alcohol addiction treatment throughout the world.

It has profoundly influenced the medical profession and become the basis of expensive treatments at a plethora of treatment centers and rehab programs.

And it doesn't even work.

Its turnover rate is massive, and its failure rate is estimated around 90%.

•••

AA's originator—Bill Wilson—died over 40 years ago in 1971. His death occurred more than a decade *before* the first medications for the treatment of alcoholism were first discovered and more than twenty years before ideas about evidence-based medical treatment began to appear.

To say AA is a unique organization is an understatement. It has a culture unto itself and it has been pointed out by many critics that it shares characteristics similar to cults.

But that doesn't really matter, because that's not the issue.

If it were a cult that actually was a statistically proven, effective treatment for addiction and encouraged the advancement of effective medical treatment, then I'd probably applaud it.

EVIDENCE-BASED MEDICINE

"The wisdom to know the difference."

—Last line of the Serenity Prayer

In the fall of 1974, a doctor named Dr. David M. Eddy was asked to give a talk about how physicians make decisions.

Eddy decided to write about diagnostic mammography. He thought he would find "strong evidence, good numbers, and sound reasoning."

But to his amazement he found "very few numbers, no formal rationale, and blatant errors in reasoning."[60]

So he decided to look at another treatment, one that had been used for more than 75 years for ocular hypertension.

"Tens of millions of people were receiving it; surely there would be solid trials to support those decisions."

But to Eddy's dismay, he found just the opposite—only eight controlled trials had been conducted—all small and poorly designed.

"But perhaps the most startling, six of the eight trials showed that patients got worse with treatment, not better."[60]

Eddy tried to look at yet a third medical treatment but experts he consulted told him there wasn't enough evidence or data to do an analysis.

Wrote Eddy, "that clinched it. If there wasn't sufficient information to develop a decision tree, what in the world were physicians basing their decisions on? I then realized that medical decision making was not built on a bedrock of evidence or formal analysis, but was standing on Jell-O.[60]

Eddy spent much of the rest of his career contributing to an area now called 'Evidence-Based Medicine.'

Evidence-Based Medicine is the philosophy that says that doctor's treatment choices need to be based on solid proven data about the potential outcomes of those choices.

It is now widely recognized by medical associations, educators, physicians and insurance companies as the gold standard for determining what is and is not solid, defendable medical care.

In just 40 years, this approach has changed the way decisions are made about treatment in every single field of medicine.

Every single field of medicine that is, except the treatment of alcoholism.

•••

When it comes to addiction medicine, the majority of physicians, hospitals, treatments centers and other caregivers advise patients to pursue an 80-year old treatment which has never had any quantitative research evidence to support it.

And even worse, instead of helping alcoholics get proper medical care, Alcoholics Anonymous participants dissuade fellow members from taking medications that can help them treat their alcoholism.

In his recent book, *The Sober Truth: Debunking the Bad Science Behind 12-Step Programs and the Rehab Industry*, Dr. Lance Dodes, a retired psychiatry professor from Harvard Medical School, used data from more than 50 studies[6] to show AA's success rate is probably somewhere between 5 and 8 percent.[61]

In 2006, the Cochrane Collaboration, a health-care research group that produces some of the most respected meta-studies in medicine today, reviewed studies going back to the 1960s. They found that "no experimental studies unequivocally demonstrated the effectiveness of AA or [12-step] approaches for reducing alcohol dependence or problems."[5]

But a decade later, doctors are still sending patients there. And that's dangerous.

NO DATA

"With no other affliction, and with no other disadvantaged group, would such a pathetic outcome be deemed a success."[11]

—Dr. Peter Ferentzy, Addiction Scientist

Despite the lack of evidence for AA, members continue to support it.

They do so vigorously, emphatically, passionately, with great loyalty, sometimes angrily, but with no supporting empirical data whatsoever.

AA does not track the success of its members.

AA could take some of their book royalties and fund a major, international, scientifically-run research study, run by respected third party scientists, from respected institutions, that unequivocally shows that it is helping people.

By helping its supporters with credible data, AA could help more alcoholics.

But AA has not done this and has shown no interest in doing so.

To justify why no transparent, credible data is produced for outside critics, its members rely on the tenth tradition that instructs, AA "has no opinion on outside issues; hence the A.A. name ought never be drawn into public controversy."

But lack of credible data achieves just the opposite—AA supporters passionately and publicly advocate for the program while falling back on research shown to be flawed and biased.

It creates a heated and meaningless dialogue and pulls the AA name into controversy, whether they like it or not.

For example, take a 2013 Huffington Post article written by author and AA advocate Anna D.

She stated, "words like 'evidence-based' treatment are thrown around, and that certainly sounds like something wise and logical, especially when measured against an anonymous organization that has never and does not plan to track its membership numbers or the success of those members."

But then, despite her criticism of the idea of evidence-based treatment, Anna D. goes on to reference a 2005 study that was according to her "the largest study ever done on the topic, out of Stanford…" The study "reported that there were 33 percent higher success rates for AA participants than non-AA participants at the 16-year follow-up mark."

Unfortunately, the "largest study ever" cited by Anna D. was conducted by a researcher that critics have called a 'professional propagandist for the 12-Step treatment industry.'

Five years before Anna D.'s 2013 article, a report was published in the *International Journal of Mental Health and Addiction* which reviewed other pro-AA 'studies' including five studies by the author of the study that Anna D. cited.

It thoroughly discredited the research, stating that it was "based on studies lacking a no-treatment control … infused with extraneous and discordant conceptual elements."

It said, "this design could not constitute a legitimate evaluation of the effectiveness…clearly there was no scientifically valid evaluation."[62]

In less scientific terms, according to one critic, the research was "invalid, erroneous, badly done, and downright deceptive and faked."[63]

Even if the study Anna D. cited was meticulously run, the author's credibility had already been destroyed. So why even quote him?

Because even a Huffington Post author couldn't find anything better.

The example of Anna D. and the flawed study is not a unique one. It is illustrative of the quality of the emotion-laden debate that rages on between AAs' loyal supporters and those who are less supportive.

So instead of focusing on solutions, while people die, mudslinging triumphs.

It's like watching children at a debate.

Did it work for Anna D? Do you think AA works? Do I think it works? Do we know people it worked for? Does my doctor like it? Has he been recommending it for years? Does it make you feel good? Did it help your mom? Do I like it? Do you like it?

If there's no quantitative research supporting it, then it doesn't matter what you or I think, because the practice of medicine is no longer based on subjective opinion in this century.

No data, no can do.

The bottom line is that if one of the world's most highly respected research review organizations, the Cochrane Collaboration, can't find evidence to support its efficacy, then any doctor claiming to practice good medicine should not be recommending it.

End of discussion.

IS AA DANGEROUS?

How is AA dangerous?

Dodes put it so succinctly:

> *"I'm not trying to eliminate AA...I'm just saying it should be prescribed to that tiny group who can make use of it.*
>
> *It's terribly harmful when you send 90 percent of the people for the wrong treatment advice."*[6]

So perhaps there is no research data proving AA is helpful. But can it really be dangerous?

Yes—it really is 'terribly harmful'.

One reason it is harmful is because it actively deters, even shames members who wish to take medication to treat their addiction. And that's deadly.

To underline this point, let's go back to Anna D.'s article again.

IT'S HARMFUL

The topic of Anna D.'s original article was her outrage over the partnering of Hazelden (a treatment organization rooted in 12-steps that recently adopted medication assisted treatment), and the Betty Ford clinic (an treatment organization that had not).

These two organizations were the two most respected, best-known names in the private recovery-business before they merged.

She wrote, "if the recent news results in a conglomerate that owns both Betty Ford and Hazelden and supports medication-assisted treatment, that would be a *tragedy of unspeakable proportions*."

Or in other words, she was expressing her view that treatment for addicts that includes medication is a tragedy worth getting really angry about. Her view underlines the view of many AA members and supporters.

Two years later, in January 2015, another article was published in the Huffington Post–an article by Jason Cherkis called, 'Dying to be Free.'[64]

This time, HuffPost carefully examined the treatment histories of 93 people who died of drug overdoses after treatment.

They found that the majority of the dead had participated in 12-step programs that dissuaded them from taking FDA-approved medications that would help them manage cravings for drugs.

The newly clean addicts graduated from treatment, committed to drug and medication-free abstinence.

But soon their addictions caught up with them, and with nothing to fall back on to help them control the cravings that are symptomatic of addiction, they overdosed, and died.

Cherkis concluded that the philosophy of the 12-step abstinence approach directly contributed to the deaths of the 93 addicts.[28]

Had they been taking medication, many of the deaths may not have occurred.

Instead of arguing (as had Anna D.) that treatment with medication was an 'unspeakable tragedy,' Cherkis argued that *12-step treatment, without medication,* had *caused* an unspeakable tragedy.

•••

AA was once a convenient, even romantic (and highly romanticized) idea.

We've been seeing this romanticized, clichéd view of AA for years in movies and on TV. I can't watch a crime drama without seeing the scene where the cop with the secret addiction attends the program after a stressful day on the job.

And in one of those paradoxical moments that occur in life from time to time, even actress and the naltrexone advocate mentioned earlier (Claudia Christian) once starred in a movie featuring AA.

She played a young addict in the major Hollywood blockbuster '*Clean and Sober*' alongside Michael Keaton and Morgan Freeman.

According to the description of the movie (I suggest you say this out loud in that deep announcer voice for full effect), "a hustling drug addict checks himself into rehab to escape trouble with the law, and realizes that it's *exactly what he needs.*"

We love the idea of AA and have long been happy to send alcoholics there without question. It's *exactly what they need,* isn't it?

But now, as we saw with the deaths of the 93 freshly sober addicts, AA's philosophies are clearly *interfering* with–not operating in tandem with–medical treatment.

OPIATES AND ALCOHOLISM: A CLARIFICATION

Yes, it is true that the Cherkis story was about deaths from drug overdose; and yes, this is not the same as alcohol abuse.

And much of the brand new approach we are now seeing around addiction treatment led by the Obama administration is being driven not by the epidemic of alcoholism, but by rising numbers of deaths of drug addicts (which evidence shows are helped more effectively by medication than by 12-step programs.)

Couldn't it be argued that drug addiction and alcohol addiction are two completely different things?

There isn't as much of a distinction here as you might think.

All chemical addictions—whether from a pill, an injection, or a bottle—are fundamentally the same—they create a chemically-triggered series of adaptations in the brain that erode critical circuits.

And 12-step programs—whether for drug or alcohol addiction—are also fundamentally the same: they are religion-based programs that encourage an abstinence philosophy that dissuades participants from using medication to assist them in sobriety.

The only difference is that when 12-step programs don't work for drug addicts, the outcome is faster and more jarring than the outcome for alcoholics.

Drug addicts can seem healthy, hopeful and promising one day as they walk out of 12-step programs clutching their 12-step literature.

And then they die abruptly with a needle in their arms the next.

The tragic demise of young drug addicts (like Glee star Cory Monteith, dead a few months after leaving rehab in 2013) is devastating and dramatic, and when it happens in great enough numbers (as it is now in the United States), it begs attention and investigation.

But when alcoholics die (after 12-step programs fail them too, sometimes over and over again), there is rarely a swift death (except suicide, which carries its own secretive stigma).

Alcoholics die slowly, agonizingly, quietly.

By the time they die, they no longer hold the promising, hopeful glow that clean young drug addicts carry. Like scrubbed birds, they lick their wounds and die quietly, alone.

The connection between the failure of the AA program they attended, and their eventual deaths is blurred by time and age.

THE SHIFT

The headlines I wrote about near the beginning of this book illustrate society's evolution toward medically assisted treatment, and away from our love affair with 12-step programs.

And in two short years, these Huffington Post articles—and their strongly diverging viewpoints from the same publication—show the same shift.

A third article—an October 2015 piece in Huffington Post—further crystallizes this change.

It reported:

> *"The treatment industry overwhelmingly resists a medication-assisted model based on decades-old beliefs about sobriety that have been passed down by those in recovery, but have never been rigorously tested.*[28]

It stated that for decades treatment had "ignored the scientific consensus that the best approach involved medications approved by the Food and Drug Administration, coupled with counseling."

It reported that "instead, the treatment industry insisted on a model known as 'abstinence,' in which any prescription medication aimed at addressing a patient's opioid use disorder was forbidden."[28]

That article shows a change of direction, but one of the most telling phrases—the one that jumps out at me—is this: "a model known as 'abstinence'."

There is something about this new phrase that sticks out like a sore thumb in the subtle way it creates distance and doubt between proper medical treatment and the 12-step approach.

Instead of Anna D.'s loving reference to AA programs as the 'gold standard of care'… for the first time, abstinence isn't the only way—it's simply 'a model'.

And not only that—but it's one that 'ignores scientific consensus' too.

Roots of AA

Back to the Beginning

Today, AA is large and powerful. The organization estimated in January 2012 that there were nearly 64,000 groups with 1.4 million members in the United States and Canada.

Worldwide, it's estimated there are more than 114,000 groups and 2.1 million members.[65] And AA's extremely high attrition rate means millions more have cycled through the doors of AA.

But that's just the tip of the iceberg for the number of people who have experienced AA's model, since AA's numbers don't include other 12-step based programs (which are essentially AA programs, without the AA name).

Twelve step programs, modelled on AA are the programs most recommended by doctors to patients with addiction. Even physicians with addiction receive 12-step based treatment for addiction 95% of the time.[66]

AA's influence is monolithic.

To understand how it got that way, we have to go back to the beginning.

•••

Bill Wilson was the genius behind AA. He systematized the recovery method that worked for him in 1935, and by doing so AA (and all other 12-step programs, including AA's family programs Alanon and Alateen) were born.

He and his cronies developed the 12 Steps, 12 Traditions and many more fundamental elements of the program and its unique, networked, ground-up organizational structure. It is a testament to his genius that it is still a thriving organization 44+ years after his death in 1971.

Yet while this iron infrastructure he built for the organization kept it strong for decades, it also capsulized a fatal flaw: its complete inability to change and evolve.

There are very few things that are the same today, as they were in 1935. But one of the things that is very much the same is AA, and many AA members like it that way.

There is not only comfort in consistency and repetition, but the thinking is that since we don't really know what the 'magic sauce' is that supposedly helps so many people, changing any aspect might just change the program's potential for success—and nobody in AA wants that to happen.

Unfortunately, unknown to many AA members, Wilson did not want the organization to stop evolving.

The one element that even the visionary Wilson was unable to impart into AA's DNA was the ability for the organization to evolve and progress. And by the time he realized this, he had already lost control of the organization to its own strangely-networked structure.

AA COMMANDEERS THE MEDICAL COMMUNITY

One of the ways that Wilson shared the idea of AA with other alcoholics was through the medical community.

He and his fellow AA-members realized that if they reached just one doctor, that doctor would be able to contribute credibility as well as reaching many more alcoholics. Endorsement of AA by the medical community was crucial to its growth (as crucial back then as it is today).

Wilson (a brilliant salesman—but not a doctor) sold doctors on AA so well that if he were still alive today, he could teach classes to New York PR agencies.

He coddled them, he stroked their egos, he bowed down to them all, humbling himself, while selling them on AA.

He sold physicians of the day so hard that he practically made them believe the whole thing was their own great idea.

He called himself a 'drunk' and worshiped at their feet.

It was great salesmanship—not data—that sold the medical community on Alcoholics Anonymous.

He spoke around the world to doctors, and transcripts of those speeches still exist.

In one, he said:

> *"Now we come to the specialist, usually the psychiatrist. I'm glad to say that psychiatrists in great numbers are referring alcoholics to A.A. — even psychiatrists who more or less specialize on alcoholics. Their understanding of alcoholics is now great. Their patience and their tolerance of us, and of A.A., have been monumental.*
>
> *In 1949, for example, the American Psychiatric Association allowed me to read a paper on A.A. before a section of its Annual Meeting. As these doctors specialize in emotional disorders — and alcoholism is certainly one of them — this act of theirs has always seemed to me a wonderful example of fine humility and generosity. The reprints of even that one paper have had a vast effect, worldwide. I'm sure that we A.A.'s have never been sufficiently appreciative of all of this."*

And he said,

> *"It is very gratifying to know that today the subject of alcoholism is being taught in many of our medical schools. In any case, the facts about alcoholism are easy to obtain. Organizations like the National Council on Alcoholism, the Yale School of Alcoholic Studies, plus innumerable state rehabilitation and clinical efforts, are ready sources of helpful knowledge. So armed, the family physician can — as we say in A.A. — "soften up" the drunk so that he will be willing to take a look at our Fellowship. Or, if he balks at A.A., he may be directed to a clinic, a psychiatrist, or an understanding pastor. At this stage, the main thing is that he recognize his illness and that he start to do something about it."*
>
> *"If the family physician's job is carefully done, the results are often immediate. If the first attempt doesn't work, the chances are better than even that persistent and successive approaches will bring results. These simple procedures do not rob the family physician of much time, nor will they be necessarily hard on the patient's pocketbook. A concerted*

effort of this sort by family physicians everywhere could not fail to achieve immense results. In fact, the effect of the family physician's work of this sort has already been great. And for this, I would like to set on our record the very special thanks of A.A. to them."[67]

Wilson's selling job came from the heart. He, like many people in the area of addictions who see people suffer from the disease, was compassionate and simply trying to help others in the best way he knew how.

The results of Wilson's selling job? His incredible influence on the medical community is still seen today.

It is estimated that 40% of members are referred by a doctor or other health care professional.[65]

And the medical community has invested itself in AA's 12-step approach so much, in fact, that it is the gold standard of care when it comes to treating their own.

Most Physician Health Programs (PHPs), which are attended by doctors with addiction problems, operate under the principles espoused by AA. Virtually all physicians are expected to attend AA or other 12-step meetings.[66]

One study looked at nearly 1000 physicians in PHP programs in the United States. It found that "regardless of setting or duration, essentially all treatment provided to these physicians (95%) was 12-step oriented, with a goal of total abstinence from any use of alcohol and other drugs of abuse and included the expectation of continued participation in AA or other 12-step oriented post-treatment support."[66]

In contrast, the study found that medication for the treatment of alcoholism was prescribed for only 5% of physicians.[66]

WILSON WANTED MEDICAL ADVANCEMENT

Wilson didn't want AA to become 'anti-medication'. But something happened over time.

Wilson knew AA was not the final solution for many alcoholics.

He wanted the medical community to buy into AA, but he also wanted the medical and research community to continue to look for treatments for alcoholics, and he wanted AA to support these efforts. This is something AA has conveniently forgotten.

He said in one speech:

> *"I would like to make a pledge to the whole medical fraternity that A.A. will always stand ready to cooperate, that A.A. will never trespass upon medicine, that our members who feel the call will increasingly help in those great enterprises of education, rehabilitation, and research which are now going forward with such promise."*[67]

He was well aware that AA wasn't a solution for everyone.

In 1961, he wrote, "It would be a product of false pride to claim that AA is a cure-all, even for alcoholism."[68]

In 1965, he even wrote a letter encouraging the "Dear Physicians of AA," to consider investigating niacinamide as a treatment for alcoholics.[69]

But the horse had already left the barn.

It's hard to sell the idea that AA is 'the solution' on one hand while encouraging science to seek better solutions on the other.

The founder of AA himself couldn't get anyone to listen. Wilson was as successful in his ability to influence the medical community as he was unsuccessful in influencing those in AA to support the medical and scientific advancement of addiction treatment.

Despite his pledge that AA would "stand ready to cooperate" in "those great enterprises of education, rehabilitation and research," the program was set in stone, and would continue to be for another eight decades.

And in practice, then, and today, other than integrating 12-step methodology firmly into most rehabilitation and treatment centers, there was no cooperation in the enterprises of education, rehabilitation and research.

Don't Mention Medicine

Despite Wilson's own wishes, today in the AA fellowship nobody talks about the implications of biochemistry on treatment. And nobody applauds the success of any other method than AA.

See for yourself: stand up in an AA meeting one day and talk about all of the advances in medical science when it comes to the treatment of alcoholism and see the response you receive.

Wilson might actually have applauded this, but most AA members don't know this, and certainly won't applaud you. You'll be rewarded with nasty looks, and pulled aside for 'a talking to' by old timers after the show.

Within AA, discussion of medical advances in the treatment of alcoholism is not allowed.

Now, those in AA will bristle at the use of the term 'not allowed'–you can talk about anything at AA–there are no written rules.

But the unwritten ones are numerous and conformity to them is heavily protected by a currency that is like lifeblood to isolated alcoholics–social inclusion.

Conformity means inclusion and non-conformity carries with it the risk of social rejection.

And it's well implanted in the heads of AA members that rejection from the group carries with it the risk of death.

I'm not over-exaggerating or making that up.

Death appears over and over again in AA's core tome (the Alcoholics Anonymous Big Book), and in another favorite book, 'Twelve Steps and Twelve Traditions (12 & 12)'.

It appears in phrases like: "unless each AA member follows to the best of his ability our suggested Twelve Steps of recovery, he almost certainly signs his own death warrant."

So any AA member talking about or recommending a pharmacological alternative to another alcoholic is quickly shunned and even excluded from the community–at great cost to the alcoholic, since AA may sometimes contain the only friends an alcoholic may have in the world.

STEP ONE IS NARCISSISM?

AA's complete lack of support of any kind of medical or research advancement is also very clearly seen in what it does not do: AA–the most powerful alcohol-treatment community in the world–has donated not one penny to medical research for the advancement of treatments for alcoholism.

It says so in the traditions: "An A.A. group ought never endorse, finance, or lend the A.A. name to any related outside facility or outside enterprise."

AA doesn't put money into prevention; it doesn't put money into medical research; it doesn't put money into the search for a cure or better treatment options. There's no pink ribbon for AA.

This is worth repeating again because it is a shameful truth of AA.

In 80+ years, AA has neither contributed nor endorsed the contribution of a single dollar to medical research. Not a dime. I hope someone will prove me wrong on this fact, because if you can, then that would be a wonderful precedent for AA to begin to do more.

In comparison, imagine if a group of cancer survivors refused to donate to cancer research, or the families of ALS sufferers declined to fundraise for ALS research.

In avoiding financial contribution, the message from AA is: the treatment we have is perfect; neither our fellow sufferers nor we need anything else.

That's unacceptable.

I have attended many AA meetings where at some point near the beginning, a somber announcement was made that an alcoholic–usually a young man–had died of alcoholism.

In any other community–people would ask, 'What can we do to help? How can we stop this from happening again and again? If so many people are dying, is what we have now really enough?!'

But at the end of the AA meeting, the chairs will be folded, the coffee pot washed, the ashtrays emptied, and everyone will go home.

AA collects money from its own members to keep the meetings going, and funds are generated through book sales, but no money is ever donated to the cause.

It begs the question: when an organization becomes as powerful as AA has become, is there not a *fundamental moral responsibility* to look at the role it plays in a wider community?

AA is a big black hole of alcoholics that do not contribute to finding medical solutions to their own disease.

How sad, how shameful, that such an influential organization has not used the strength of its membership to look for other ways to help its own.

If they had, perhaps this book would have been written 30 years ago and alcohol addiction would be something of the past.

THE AA EFFECT

Can a single non-medical organization like AA unintentionally change the way medical treatment for a disease has developed for decades?

Yes—for lack of a better term, I call it the AA Effect.

It works like this—

AA's influence extends outward to members, family, and friends. Eighty-year-old beliefs filtrate out to this wider circle. These beliefs define society's perspective of 'what is wrong with alcoholics' and how best to treat them.

The dominance of this influence on doctors, treatment programs, pharmaceutical companies and other key players in health care means other potential treatments and solutions aren't supported or funded.

The absence of endorsement is rejection; and so scientific and medical advancement starves, only inching along, instead of thriving.

And the direction of AA's influence is one-way only. There is no reverse osmosis. AA is impervious of and protected from influence from the opposite direction.

It achieves this insularity since anyone trying to change the group from within becomes a threat. Anyone who wants change is accused of wanting it because AA isn't working for them. But the message from the group is: 'If AA can't help you, there's no flaw in the system or change required. The flaw is in you and your weakness in following the program. Work harder.'

If an individual continues to push change, they are ostracized from the group. And because of this insularity and the non-emergence of any other viable alternative, the system remains strong and carries on.

Without knowing or intending to, AA has become a stifling force of nature deterring the kind of advancements in addiction medicine we've seen in the last 80 years in virtually every other area of medicine.

THE AA EFFECT AND MEDICATION

The full AA Effect can be seen playing out within the launch of one of the most important medications in this book–naltrexone.

Naltrexone is a medication that performed well in clinical trials, and then hit barrier upon barrier once released into the market.

It was originally synthesized in 1963 and patented in 1967 as 'Endo 1639A' by Endo Laboratories, a small pharmaceutical company in New York.

In 1969, DuPont purchased Endo Labs, and in 1972 the Special Action Office for Drug Abuse Prevention (SAODAP) was created by President Nixon. Director Jerome Taffe saw the development of naltrexone as one of his top priorities.

DuPont marketed the drug under the name 'ReVia'[70] after it obtained FDA approval in 1995 to market it for use in alcoholism.

The biggest barrier to marketing success is usually poor results in clinical trials. But in this case, clinical trials were successful. Data showed that the drug could work. (And in fact this is the very same drug that today– in a monthly-injection format–is finally getting market traction).

DuPont's problems began when they tried to market the medication to the medical and treatment community.

That's when they hit a wall.

Many doctors and alcohol addiction specialists were focused on AA as the only solution to alcoholism and wouldn't prescribe it.

DuPont faced an uphill battle just trying to convince providers that it was appropriate to treat addiction with a pharmacotherapy.[70]

DuPont failed.

Sales were dismal, and eventually The American Council on Alcoholism reportedly published the following scathingly worded statement on their website in 2005:

> *"Many physicians and non-physicians in treatment programs are unaware of the usefulness of naltrexone or how to use it.*
>
> *In other areas of medicine, it is highly probable that the development of such an efficacious medication would prompt physicians to use it readily.*
>
> *The biggest obstacle to using naltrexone for the treatment of alcoholism is the 'pharmacophobia' of many alcoholism-treatment professionals.*
>
> *This near-hysterical resistance to medication for treating alcoholism (or other substance-abuse disorders) has deep and tangled roots. Many recovering professionals learned in their recoveries that MDs and their prescription pads were evil purveyors of pharmacological lies and temptations.*
>
> *This attitude is often accompanied by a deeply rooted and strongly held belief that recovery has only one successful formula (usually the 12-step program) and that any modification to that approach is unethical.*
>
> *Scientific evidence is irrelevant to these individuals.*
>
> *They believe they have the 'truth' about recovery and don't want to be bothered with other points of view."*[70]

In 1997, ReVia's market exclusivity ended.

Other companies (Barr Laboratories and Bristol-Myers Squibb for example) began to sell generic naltrexone, but now, without the potential of high profitability, any pharmaceutical company producing it became very unlikely to market and promote it to a widespread audience.[53]

And today, not much has changed. Naltrexone (the pill form anyway) faces the same barriers.

Without profit potential, there is no naltrexone pill advertising campaign, no pharma sales reps talking to doctors about naltrexone; no free samples which doctors can stock and provide to patients; no information sessions or conferences about naltrexone for health care professionals.

It also means that in markets where drug companies choose to make it available, prices can be extremely high for those wishing to purchase it.

And this is why you will never see an ad for one of the most effective drugs to ever fight alcoholism in a TV commercial or on a poster in your doctor's office. This is why Claudia Christian is the person you are most likely to hear about naltrexone from.

Even worse, not only did AA-fueled medical resistance to evidence-based treatment of alcoholism cause naltrexone's launch to flop, but it cast a much wider shadow which would stunt research and development for decades.

Dupont's naltrexone flop taught pharmaceutical companies that doctors would not prescribe medication—even clinically-proven medication—as part of a treatment plan for alcoholics.

Pharmaceutical companies learned very well that the medical community, with its 'pharmacophobia' was sold on AA and only AA.

It is this lesson that has severely hampered pharmaceutical company investment in the business of alcohol addiction medicine ever since it was first learned.

Why would any pharmaceutical executive risk his or her career following in Dupont's footsteps to invest in or market any other alcohol addiction medication—even an incredibly effective one—when medical specialists and the sufferers of so many *other* diseases are crying out for new treatments?

That's why pharmaceutical company investment in the alcohol addiction pipeline has been nothing but a trickle for decades: And that's the AA Effect in action.

THE USUAL CLICHÉS AND STIGMA

FROM AA TO OUR LIVING ROOM

Peter Ferentzy is an outspoken research scientist at CAMH (the Canadian Association for Mental Health). He is also a historian of addiction, a recovering alcoholic and drug addict and the author of *'Dealing with Addiction—Why the 20th Century was Wrong'*. His views are controversial, and right on the mark.

Ferentzy writes, "I'm sick of seeing people suffer needlessly and die needlessly. The assumptions upon which the North American approach to addiction is built… are mistaken, nasty, and stupid."[11]

A lot of these assumptions simply ooze right out of AA. It's like a wormhole from 1937 straight to our living rooms.

Without realizing it, they define our perspectives and our assumptions about what is wrong with alcoholics and how best to treat them.

Some of them pass through the rooms of AA into everyday language and become part of the zeitgeist-part of 'what we know' about alcoholics. Others are so questionable and strange that they haven't made it into society's vernacular.

•••

What we believe as a society is often held up to us in the mirror of pop culture, on TV shows and movies.

One of the reasons that the hit show *'Mad Men'* is so effective is because it reflects back to us beliefs held about men and women's roles in the 60s. The beliefs of the time jar so intriguingly with what we hold to be true today that it makes for a great backdrop to drama.

Society's beliefs around alcoholism and alcoholics, fed to us from AA, filter through via television and movies too.

Often we see the guy at the podium speaking humbly: "I needed an *attitude adjustment*. I finally *surrendered to my higher power* and *let go and let God*. I woke up at *rock bottom*, in a gutter and I decided to change."

These lines could slide easily into any TV drama. Yet they are incredibly damaging–and maybe in 20 years they will seem jarringly out of place too–as they should.

They are damaging because they imply that alcoholism is a moral failing and a shameful personality disorder, that requires severe punishment before it can be resolved.

Some of the clichés heard in AA rooms (what Ferentzy calls "powerful, culturally induced myths") include:

- "It's a spiritual malady."

- "Recovery from alcoholism requires a spiritual awakening from a higher power."

- "Rarely have we seen a person fail who has thoroughly followed our path."

- "The only solution to alcoholism is complete abstinence."

- "You've got to hit rock bottom."

Yet there is no medical or scientific data in existence that indicates that any of those myths are true.

Alcoholism is not caused by a bad attitude or planted in us by God. It is not the only illness in the world that is actually removable through a spiritual awakening. It is not something that requires the complete loss of dignity and surrender to recover from. It is not something that requires you to 'hit rock bottom' before you can recover.

Alcoholism is a mental illness. A brain disease. There are about a thousand papers in the uber-geeks' filing cabinets that say so. If only someone would read them.

This section delves further into a few of these myths.

THE ALLERGY MYTH

One of the most ridiculous myths–well known and believed in AA, but not as often heard outside their doors–is the idea that alcoholism is an allergy.

Ask an AA alcoholic why they drink like they do and it's likely they will tell you they have an allergy to alcohol.

This big whopper is symbolic of all the other more subtle, more believable, equally outdated fallacies taught to alcoholics at AA.

In the 30s, when the big book was written, Bill Wilson's doctor, W.D Silkworth, explained to Wilson that alcoholism was an allergy.

He was not using the term as a metaphor. He was trying instead to use terminology to position alcoholism as an illness and explain its mechanism of action.

At the time, little more was known about allergies than was known about alcoholism. So the 'allergy explanation' was included in the AA Big Book and has remained there ever since—undisputed and uncorrected.[71]

Even the most recent 2001 edition supports the theory, stating: "As ex-problem drinkers, we can say that his explanation makes good sense."[72]

The Spiritual Malady Myth

AA members say their program is 'spiritual, not religious.'

Religious or not, whatever you want to label it, God is a significant part of the program, mentioned by name in four out of the 12 steps.

God in AA can be traced back at least to the early 1900s.

AA's early development was heavily influenced by an organization called The Oxford Group, which was an evangelical Christian movement that emerged in the 20s, growing up under the leadership of a Lutheran minister.

Bill Wilson always acknowledged that AA's spiritual and working principles came from this group.

The religious roots are reflected today in many elements of AA's approach. It appears not only in the phrase "spiritual malady", but also the belief that a "spiritual awakening" must occur before abstinence is granted or made possible by one's "higher power".

AA describes alcoholism as a 'threefold disease' that combines the alcohol 'allergy', a mental obsession, and a "spiritual malady."

AA teaches that when all three aspects are adequately addressed, addiction will 'lift'.

Alcoholics do have a mental obsession.

But they have a 'spiritual malady' that causes alcoholism, just about as much as they have an allergy.

CHARACTER DEFECTS & SHAME

The phrase 'spiritual malady' is often tied to another common AA concept and phrase—the idea that alcoholics are rife with 'character defects'.

AA teaches us: 'character defects' must be identified and remedied and where they have emerged at their worst, amends to others must be made.

Alcoholism is a medical illness. Yes, it has enormous repercussions to those with the disease—some of which emerge as what could be termed as character defects.

But character defects are by no means exclusive to alcoholics, nor do they cause alcoholism.

This misconception is damaging.

It leads to shame and stigma for the alcoholic and their family. It keeps our focus on alcoholics as the black sheep, instead of the ill family member.

As Markus Heilig wrote in a 2006 scientific journal:

"A medical approach to alcoholism treatment offers an established framework for developing and implementing evidence-based, rather than opinion-based treatment strategies.

An additional appeal of this approach is that it offers an alternative to moralizing and confrontational approaches, which are neither effective nor ethically attractive."[1]

ENABLING

AA and its sister organization for family and friends (Alanon) teach us that enabling is bad–that ALL negative consequences of drinking should be borne in full by the alcoholic.

In the 12-step world, any help you give to an addict that they wouldn't have needed if they didn't have an addiction in the first place is defined as enabling.

So, if an alcoholic needs ten dollars to buy another drink, and you give it to them, you are enabling.

If they need $50 to help cover their rent, and you give it to them, it is enabling.

If you give them a ride to detox, it is enabling. If they lost their license and need a ride to come join the family for Christmas dinner, it is enabling.

We don't want to be enablers, so we don't give them the drink money, the rent money, the ride to detox or the ride to the family dinner.

And they go into withdrawal seizures, lose their apartment, hawk the watch that grandpa gave them to get a motel room for a night, and end up alone, sick, lonely, homeless and broken on Christmas day.

Merry Christmas.

The problem is that condemning all enabling behavior ignores the fact that people with addictions are human beings that are suffering and need connection, love and help, to get better.

It re-enforces the idea of rock bottom: that the more the person with an addiction is left to suffer and stew in their own mess, the more likely they will be to recover.

And this is not based on any kind of factual understanding of what might actually help someone begin to recover.

Sometimes, just the opposite is needed. In fact, when people recover without professional help, it is often a lot to do with the support they receive from family and friends.[11]

The three best predictors of success in recovery are[11]:

- Social support from family and friends

- Social standing—the things that give you esteem and dignity—like your job and your home

- Cognitive functioning—how well your brain continues to function

Notably, the first two elements—social support and social standing—are sometimes the two things that are taken away when we stop enabling.

And isn't it only a matter of time, for anyone, that when your social support and social standing are gone, your cognitive functioning starts to slip? Who can think rationally when they are lonely, cold, tired, degraded and sick?

Researchers say:

> *"Among alcoholics the recovery rates for one year are about 60 to 80% if you have both intact family and intact job. If you were missing one of those, it dropped in half to 30 to 40% after one year. If you were missing both, it drops in half again to 15 to 20%."*[73]

ROCK BOTTOM

The idea that an alcoholic must experience severe pain ('rock bottom') before they can recover is especially damaging.

Ferentzy writes of the ignorance of this perspective, saying:

> *"With no other medical condition—not even mental illness or neurosis—is the governing idea that the disease must be allowed to cause a great deal of damage in order to prepare someone for help"*[13]

He goes on to say:

> *"And this one stupid lie has—by means of treatment practice, social policy, societal attitudes, and even "wars" waged by politicians all over the world against drug users— killed millions and caused many more to suffer needlessly."*[13]

Friends of alcoholics are told not to create a crisis for the alcoholic—but not to avert one either. In other words, don't stand in the way of an alcoholic finally hitting rock bottom.

Well, many families wait and wait for that rock bottom to occur… and 3.3 million alcoholics every year finally hit rock bottom on the day they die from alcoholism.

For those that can't quit (that seem to bump along from rock to rock, unable to 'change'), including the one I once loved, many finally experience rock bottom at the end of a noose.

For very few, perhaps rock bottom does come with such massive pain that they are able to harness the last vestiges of control and mental focus they maintain.

But that massive pain can come in the form of killing someone while drunk driving, watching the faces of their children as child services take them away, spending Christmas alone with nobody and nothing… the lives that severe alcoholics live, while they wait for 'rock bottom' can be immensely painful.

Compassion For Addiction is an organization that was started by Vicky Dulai after her brother passed away.

She says, "Compassion and understanding when offering support must be constant. Addicts need not be punished, for they are already punishing themselves."

She also agrees that we must challenge the notion of 'rock bottom,' because "in my experience, rock bottom means death."[74]

Rock Bottom in the Medical System

Outside the family dynamic, we see 'rock bottom' formalized in the medical system.

Doctors, nurses, health care workers, the emergency room staff, detox center workers, police–the behaviors of many of the people that the alcoholic may need help from after relapse–are tainted with the notion that the alcoholic needs a measure of punishment upon discontinuation of drinking.

They may be doing their best; they may be caring, compassionate individuals; but sadly they are practicing an outdated, dangerous approach.

One place we see this is in detoxification facilities.

They are often unpleasant places where recovering alcoholics are treated more like naughty children or inmates than people with an illness.

Whereas other medical facilities help provide comfort to those in pain and discomfort, detox facilities are rarely equipped to provide, for example, medications which can lessen the intense physical discomfort felt by someone with an addiction. The more misery an alcoholic goes through when they detox, the better, it seems.

Medical care for people with alcoholism follows a different code. It's one that is silently, wordlessly justified by the myth of 'rock bottom.'

PURE ABSTINENCE

In a recent Newsweek article about medications for alcoholism, one longtime AA member was quoted as saying, "I'm not judging others, but for myself, using something like Vivitrol [naltrexone injection] or Campral [acamprosate] feels like a crutch ... It's not *true sobriety*."[58]

In alcoholism culture, you are either substance free, and counting your progress one day at a time, or you are failing.

And abstinence for AA–"true sobriety" does not include any of the medications in this book.

Oh, but remember: they aren't "judging others."

Abstinence or nothing is a very binary, black and white view of life. You are winning or you are failing—there's really no in-between.

But such black and white thinking is a set-up for failure. It doesn't work for most human beings.

One of the things 'all or nothing abstinence' leads to, is something called the 'Abstinence Violation Effect'—a dangerous phenomena.

The Abstinence Violation Effect was a term coined in 1980 by researchers Marlatt and Gordon. They noticed that a long-term relapse starts with just one drink.

That first drink (or small bout of drinking) was what they called a 'lapse.'

And they saw that whether the drinker continued from that first lapse to a full blown binge (a 'relapse') was highly dependent upon their emotional response to the initial lapse.[75]

Someone taught to believe that a lapse is a complete and utter personal failure, is likely to experience guilt and negative emotions that lead to increased drinking as a further attempt to avoid or escape their feelings and thoughts.

However, someone taught that a lapse is not a failure—just an opportunity to learn from one's mistakes—might not continue into full blown relapse.

It's the difference between blowing your diet for the next three weeks because you slipped up on one meal, or identifying that slip-up as a learning opportunity and applying the lesson to the next meal.

In contrast to other mental illness, one researcher says:

> *"We no longer blame people for sliding back into depressive states. We used to and were wrong to do so. Now, instead, we work within the depressive relapse to make it as painless as possible. That's the right approach. We must turn in that direction with addictions as well."*[11]

●●●

Alcoholism culture is built around so many damaging notions: it's an allergy, you have a spiritual malady; you have a character flaw; relapse is failure; medication is weakness; punishment is helpful; if the program doesn't work for you, it's your fault; abstinence is the only way.

Perhaps many of these ideas were common outside AA in the thirties when the program first started. But as thinking around many other social issues changed with the times, these notions, incubated from change by AA, remained unquestioned.

And they continue to filter, year after year, into our zeitgeist.

We can't continue this way.

I don't pretend to know all the answers, and I'm well aware that alcoholism is a complex disease.

But I can tell you that we need to start questioning all of these stagnant beliefs and approaches.

If we continue to see alcoholism as a character failing, use incorrect and outdated medical terminology, and allow dangerous clichés to slip into our language, people will continue to die from it.

Babies will continue to be born with fetal alcohol syndrome, children will continue to be abused and neglected by alcoholic family members, drunk driving alcoholics will kill innocent people, relationships and lives will continue to be destroyed.

Let's used an evidence-based approach. It's good enough for every other disease.

I believe that a hundred years from now, just as we look back at the ridiculous medical notions and practices of people before us, future generations will look at ours and think how primitive we ever were for thinking about and treating addictions in the way we currently do.

What kind of culture sends people with an illness to a religion-based program that fails 90% of the time?

Ours does.

THE MEDICAL COMMUNITY

"It is highly disturbing that this drug is not made available to the patients that need it."[1]

—*Dr. Heilig and Egli, 2006*

When I started reading about this topic and realized that AA was not helping (and possibly even harming) most people who arrived at their doors with alcoholism, I felt angry at AAers.

But after a while I realized that people in AA are people with an illness who are just trying to keep themselves healthy and help others with the same illness to do so too.

They see people die around them and they cling, terrified, to the only life raft that someone has passed them—whether it has a hole in it or not.

Their hearts are in the right place even if their methods are questionable and dangerous.

But people in AA come from the general population: usually it's not their job to look after the health of others.

But it *is* the medical community's job to look after others, by using evidence-based medicine as a guide for their decision-making.

It's their job to *do no harm*. But when it comes to alcoholism, they aren't doing a very good job.

It's a convenient and comfortable solution for doctors and others in the medical system to send people with addictions to free 12-step based programs.

It costs the system nothing, the doctor's time is not further 'wasted', and if the program fails to be effective, then the blame for its failure is always placed on the person with the addiction.

It's really the perfect business—if it doesn't work, it's not the *doctor's* fault now, is it?

The financial burden of subsequent illnesses as the alcoholic's health falls apart (triggering one or more of the 200+ diseases as mentioned earlier in the book) is never formally linked to the failure of the system to address the problem properly in the first place.

•••

I have a good friend who is a respected doctor.

When I first told her I was writing a book about pharmaceutical options for the treatment of alcohol dependence she laughed and asked me if my book was a work of fiction.

I'm not the first (nor will I be the last) to wonder why, (now that the facts and research are available—even to laypeople like myself), the medical community is not *leading* this approach to providing better treatment to people with alcoholism.

Doctors and other health care professionals can be wonderful, caring people. The good ones know how little they know; and that they can learn as much from their patients as from a textbook.

But developing a big ego is an occupational hazard for those in the medical profession.

Without enormous confidence, how else could you make life and death decisions?

And in our extremely hierarchical medical care system—where everyone knows the pecking order and there is no such thing as a flat structure—arrogance is encouraged and incubated.

Dr. Oliver Amiesen—a cardiologist, and the man who discovered the use of high-dose baclofen to treat his own alcoholism—wrote about the inability of his colleagues to admit flaws in their approach to treating alcoholics.

In his case, as he wrote, he,

"Spent countless hours via email and telephone answering questions about baclofen and advising people on how to speak to their physicians about it.

In almost all cases, sadly, they could not convince their doctors to prescribe an unfamiliar medication off-label."[22]

Amiesen blamed their ignorance on 'dogma'. He wrote that it "led me to wonder if people in addiction medicine and research might not be able to see beyond the dogma of their field–something that is common in every medical specialty, not to mention being a familiar fact of human nature."[22]

I looked up dogma. It means, "a belief or set of beliefs that is accepted by the members of a group without being questioned or doubted.'" That sounds right.

There is another term I looked up.

Its definition is "a dereliction of professional duty or a failure to exercise an ordinary degree of professional skill or learning by one (as a physician) rendering professional services which result in injury, loss, or damage."

That's malpractice. And somehow that sounds right too.

EGO, DOGMA, AND STIGMA, OH MY

Is it ego? Is it dogma? Or is it something else: stigma.

There is another reason why medical professionals don't respond to alcohol dependence with medical skills.

And that is because many of them don't think addiction is a medical illness.

In one national study, US doctors were asked what proportion of alcoholism is a disease and what proportion is a personal weakness. The average proportion thought to be a personal weakness was 31%.

In another study of physicians, only 25 percent actually believed alcoholism to be a disease.[76]

In *Managing Alcoholism as a Disease*, the author wrote, "based on my experiences working in the addiction field for the past 10 years, I believe many, if not most, health care professionals still view alcohol addiction as a willpower or conduct problem."[77]

A survey of doctors at an annual conference of the International Doctors in Alcoholics Anonymous reported that 80 percent believe that alcoholism is merely bad behavior instead of a disease.[77]

In his 2014 JAMA article, researcher Edward Nunes suggested that to get medications more routinely utilized, doctors needed more training, but more importantly what is needed is "an embrace by all physicians, particularly those in primary care specialties, of the mandate to recognize and treat alcoholism and other addictions."[78]

Let me repeat that—he is simply asking doctors to "recognize and treat."

The 2012 report *Addiction Medicine: Closing the Gap Between Science & Practice* stated:

> *"This profound gap between the science of addiction and current practice related to prevention and treatment is a result of decades of marginalizing addiction as a social problem rather than treating it as a medical condition."*[3]

Despite the massive evidence found in scientific literature to the contrary, people with substance dependence don't receive medical treatment.

Compared with people suffering from other mental disorders that are not substance related[79] alcohol dependent people are much less frequently regarded as mentally ill, held much more responsible for their condition and their inability to change it themselves.[79]

In *The Deadly Stigma of Addiction*, Dr. Richard Juman writes:

"The idea that those with addictive disorders are weak, deserving of their fate and less worthy of care is so inextricably tied to our zeitgeist that it's impossible to separate addiction from shame and guilt.

Addiction comes with a second punch in the gut: the burden of being treated like a second-class citizen and expected to act accordingly."[80]

The definition of the word 'stigma' is "a mark of disgrace," and it is this black mark which clouds the lens through which the healthcare provider often views an alcoholic.

The Surgeon General has stated that stigma attached to mental illness constitutes the "primary barrier" to treatment and recovery.

Stigma is an insidious animal that only seems ridiculously out of place years after it has faded.

Years ago, long before breast cancer was pinkwashed, there was a great deal of stigma around it too. Its culture also contained a heavy element of shame and secrecy.

Some women weren't even told they had breast cancer. Others who were diagnosed with it kept it a secret or lied about what they had. Obituaries simply noted a 'long illness.'

At one time, even the New York Times refused an advertisement for a breast cancer support group.[81]

Today that sounds ridiculous. But stigma always looks that way in hindsight. It's like a retrospective stigma litmus test.

Dr. Juman says the "system is hard-wired to prolong stigmatization, and stigma contributes to addiction's lethality."[80] He gives several reasons why stigma in healthcare is lethal:

- People fail to seek treatment

- Medical professionals fail to treat addicts properly

- People with addiction are ostracized

- People in treatment are always under suspicion

- People in treatment are confronted with roadblocks constantly

- Stigmatization can contribute to poor treatment outcomes

That's all consistent with my experience.

For many people hearing about the state of alcoholism treatment, it reminds them of how depression was once treated and stigmatized.

Instead of diagnosing depression, doctors would describe patients with negatively charged terms like 'lazy' and 'slovenly.' Health care professionals looked at symptoms of depression through a warped moral lens.[79]

But a study that looked at changing perceptions over the last 10 years concluded that as more people came to understand the neurobiological underpinnings of mental illness, the more the social and moral judgments dropped.

Unfortunately, while that has helped destigmatize depression, the study showed that was not the case for alcoholism, where misconceptions were unchanged and the use of stigmatized labels actually grew by 16%.[82]

What changed for stigma around depression was that the medical community realized that medication could be used to treat it.

They started to prescribe early medications like Prozac and saw changes in their patients' functioning. And they realized that if a medication can be used to treat it, it might just be an illness, not a character defect after all.

One day that will be obvious for alcoholism too.

I'm not sure what it will take to get doctors to start doing their jobs.

But I hope that if enough patients bring enough research to enough doctors and make enough convincing arguments, that we'll nudge them into the 21st century for this disease too.

TREATMENT & THE REHAB INDUSTRY

"There simply is no other disease where appropriate medical treatment is not provided by the health care system and where patients instead must turn to a broad range of practitioners largely exempt from medical standards."[3]

— 2012 Report: Addiction Medicine: Closing the Gap Between Science & Practice

Before Amy Winehouse died of alcoholism she wrote a famous song about rehab and how she said "No, no, no."

It may have been a heartbreaking decision for her family. But had she spent a year in rehab, it may not have saved Amy anyways.

Families and loved ones of alcoholics will pin our hopes and dreams on anything when we see someone we love circling the drain. That, and the fact that the medical system is failing alcoholics, is what the private treatment industry feeds on.

A public system that fails consistently plays right into the coffers of private care.

A critical 2012 report on medical treatment for those with addictions linked the emergence of an ineffective private treatment industry to the failures of a neglectful medical system:

"This neglect by the medical system has led to the creation of a separate and unrelated system of addiction care that struggles to treat the disease without the resources or the knowledge base to keep pace with science and medicine."[3]

Private addiction treatment is a money maker in the United States—a staggering $35 billion a year industry—and growing.[83]

It is also an industry that is mostly privately managed, not regulated by the government and run by unlicensed individuals where being 'in recovery' oneself is often the only line needed on a resume to justify an approach and become a treatment provider.

Marketing claims of fabricated success rates go unchallenged, and the families of sufferers become burdened with debt, remortgaging homes and maxing out credit cards to pay for expensive residential programs.

And of course, the basis of most private treatment is 12-step programs, which if offered by AA would be free, and which, as mentioned earlier, has no evidence of success anyway.[83]

If the treatments offered by most rehab centers don't work, though, why does the industry remain so profitable?

Here's why: Because there's nowhere else to turn.

When your loved one is staggering around on your front lawn as your children head off to school in the morning, what else is a loving family to do but *whatever they possibly can* to help their alcoholic.

And if helping that alcoholic means sending them away somewhere for 30 days to the only 'help' that is offered, so be it.

It may seem to be the only solution, and so families will send their alcoholics off to treatment until the bank won't lend them another dime, in the hope that 'one will take' or the alcoholic will finally 'smarten up'.

It's really the perfect business—if it doesn't work, it's not the *treatment center's* fault now, is it?

We watch these systems fail our loved ones.

It's agonizing and painful.

Some people survive.

A lot of them don't. It's born out in stories like this one:

> *"I lost my son to addiction and ultimately suicide.*
>
> *From the time I knew he had a problem until the day he died, I tried everything at my disposal to help him get quality care. He went to eight different programs and they all had a different approach; many offered conflicting advice …*
>
> *In the last weeks of his life, Brian was suffering from severe depression. On the day before he died, his aftercare program made the decision, without consulting Brian's therapist, or his parents, to terminate their relationship with him.*
>
> *At the time Brian most needed help, he was left alone.*
>
> *And so was I."*[3]

THE PHARMACEUTICAL INDUSTRY

There is an excellent article called *'Targeting Addiction'* that focusses on one scientist's (Dr. Bankole Johnson) groundbreaking research into the medication topiramate.[84]

The work—and the results—are impressive.

But not impressive enough for one comment-poster.

Shortly after the article was published, in 2010, commenter 'Heisenberg' summed up his perspective on the 21-page article this way:

> *"It's all hogwash supplemented I'm sure by the drug companies."*

His comment remains there today (as I write this book anyways). An ugly postscript to the last sentence of the article.

Aaaahh…. the Internet, where, in one dismissive sentence, anyone hiding behind a fake name can insult your integrity and your life's work, for all the world to see, pretty much permanently.

But the comment begs the question, was Heisenberg right?

While it's an easy and common conclusion to jump to if one distrusts big pharma, in this case, he couldn't have been farther from the truth.

In topiramate's defense, it is a medication with a wealth of data supporting its use in alcoholism treatment. (In other words—not hogwash).

But aside from that, topiramate (like the majority of medications that treat alcoholism) has several black marks against it which cause pharmaceutical companies to stay away.

First, there's a double whammy: Topiramate is both generic and off-label (as are many treatments for alcoholism).

So not only is there no money to be made for pharmaceutical companies in the marketing of topiramate, but they could face hefty fines if they do.

And next, all medications for addiction have an element that serves as a barrier to pharmaceutical company development and backing. And that is stigma.

Addiction medicine is a line of business that still carries with it a negative stigma that many in big pharma would prefer not be associated with.

And finally, up until recently, it's been difficult, if not impossible to be profitable with any medication that treats alcoholism. (Due to the AA effect described earlier).

None of these black marks—loss of marketing protection; off-label approval legislation; stigma or lack of profitability are realities that big pharma created. But they certainly do form a significant roadblock for them.

Before I go any further, in case Heisenberg wishes to come along and label my writing as pharma-supplemented hogwash, I'd just like to note— I am writing this entire book without any funding or endorsement from any company or organization—and that includes any pharmaceutical company.

Addiction may be an enormous market with vast potential, and pharmaceutical companies may be powerful money-hungry corporations on the look-out for the next Viagra. But medication for the treatment of alcoholism hasn't been good business for them so far.

Maybe Alkermes' strong profit announcement with Vivitrol will be just the signal that they need to begin to increase investment. But I suspect they will need to see some strong success with nalmefene in Europe, or another strong signal of change before a true turnaround begins.

And until that day comes, investments will remain small, researchers will continue to rely heavily on government funds and drug discoveries will fall consistently into the Valley of Death.

THE VALLEY OF DEATH

There is another factor that is compounding the lack of forward momentum in the further development of medications for alcoholism. And this is something that industry and government call 'The Valley of Death.'

(Is it just me, or is it strange that an industry that is so tied to human life and death uses a phrase like 'The Valley of Death', to describe a place where drugs go when the business case doesn't work out?)

The 'Valley of Death' is the black hole that medications can fall into between the point where a drug's potential is first discovered, and when a doctor uses that drug to treat a patient. Or to use an industry phrase— between the pathway from 'bench to bed'.

The vast majority of promising molecular discoveries by scientists fall into a couple of gaps in that valley, and never climb back out. Those gaps exist:

1) Between lab discovery and human clinical trial testing; and

2) Between human clinical testing and the doctor's office.

This valley exists for every area of medicine right now. It's a deep and growing chasm that industry leaders all over North America and Europe are struggling with.[85]

But because medications for alcoholism have not had a good track record of profitability, molecular discoveries that show promise for the treatment of alcohol addiction are far more likely to fall into that valley than medications that show promise for nearly any other major illness.

On one side of the divide are biomedical researchers and scientists who, at a cost of about $30 billion per year in the United States (NIH's budget for medical research), focus on understanding how diseases work and how they can be fought.

That's a relatively small feeder industry if you compare it to the other side of the valley where the health care system resides. It's a massive industry, with annual healthcare spending in the US costing over $3.8 trillion.

There used to be a system that bridged the gap between the two sides, but that bridge no longer works.

•••

In the fifties and sixties, medical research was often done by doctors.

Doctors were also scientists who spent time both in the lab and treating patients. There was no gap between discovery and treatment because doctors themselves bridged this gap.[85] Doctors didn't rely on pharmaceutical companies or the government to share medical knowledge with them to the same extent they do today.

Today, most research is done by highly specialized Ph.D. scientists.

So now, even if medications make it beyond the lab, most doctors don't learn about new discoveries.

And exacerbating the problem is the fact that the cost of getting a drug from discovery through to the end of clinical trials costs more and more every year. So pharmaceutical companies are that much more careful about which drugs they choose to shepherd through the process.

And then, once a drug is approved, even if research showed that the drug is useful for other illnesses, there are strict (million and billion dollar) fines applied to pharmaceutical companies that mention other applications for the drug in anything that can be construed as marketing.

So doctors never learn about other scientifically-backed uses for the medication.

Every single area of medical research is facing the same problem right now. Whether its cancer treatment, Alzheimer's or ALS, there are gaps in progress caused by the Valley of Death problem.

But medical research for people with addictions has more black marks to contend with than any area of medicine.

The lack of advancement in the medical community regarding addiction, the lack of support from AA, the stigma issue and no track record of profitability for alcohol addiction medicine means that no other area of medical research faces the same hurdles to drug development as this one. That's why the ones we already have—the ones that work—are truly precious.

Pharma and Existing Medications

Earlier, topiramate was identified as having two issues that make it unattractive for pharmaceutical companies—it's generic, and off-label.

Generic medications that are on-label treatments for alcoholism (meaning they were FDA-approved specifically for alcoholism, not other illnesses), like naltrexone and acamprosate, are no longer protected by patent.

Any pharmaceutical company can make and sell them, and because generic medications are a commodity, there is much less profit in them, and drug companies usually discontinue marketing efforts around them.

Off-label drugs are those which have been found to be effective treatments for alcoholism, but were not officially approved for that medical treatment, like baclofen and gabapentin for example, which were approved for other medical purposes.

For off-label drugs, governments have put strict rules in place about pharmaceutical marketing, which bar pharmaceutical companies from marketing a drug for an off-label purpose.

Some pharmaceutical companies have received crippling fines for crossing the line.

In recent years for example, fines have been doled out in the billions for this practice: Johnson and Johnson ($1.391 billion), Glaxo Smith Kline ($1.043 billion), Pfizer ($2.3 billion) and Ely Lilly ($1.415 billion) all received massive fines for off-label marketing that would have bankrupt most companies.[86]

Topiramate was actually one of the drugs that resulted in a large fine for Ortho-McNeil Pharmaceutical and Ortho-McNeil-Janssen Pharmaceuticals, Inc. in 2010: both were fined for their role in promoting topiramate to psychiatrists for purposes it had not received approval for.

So why don't drug companies just take the off-label drug through the approval process so that it can be used for that purpose on-label?

Because it takes a lot of time and money to complete the studies and testing and other regulatory requirements involved in drug approval, and the drug would move closer to generic status each year that they invested in the approval process.

So, as highly respected addiction researcher Barbara Mason put it in a 2014 presentation about gabapentin, there is "no industry support for FDA approval of a new use for a generic drug that has shown promise for treating CNS disorders," even ones with few other treatment options.[87]

The reality is that in the pipeline at the moment numerous drugs have shown initial signs that they may be helpful in the treatment of alcoholism. But very few of these are being developed for the treatment of alcoholism.

If they are in a drug company's development pipeline, with the exception of only a handful of medicines, they are being developed (and could eventually be FDA-approved), for another purpose–not for alcohol dependence. (So they would be off-label, and unmarketable).

So the treatment of alcohol dependence with medication will continue to rely predominantly on off-label drugs.

This means that the general public and medical system will likely not learn about these medicines' ability to target alcoholism via any communication channel funded by pharmaceutical companies.

This bears repeating: even when researchers prove that a drug can help alcoholics; and even though that drug may have already been proven safe in humans; it is unlikely to be supported or marketed by a pharmaceutical company because of legislation that works against it.

Gabapentin, and several others, for example, are safe, affordable, readily available and effective.

They can save many lives. But they are not marketed and can't be marketed for alcohol dependence.

Does it Matter if a Pharmaceutical Company Doesn't Market a Drug?

Does it matter if a pharmaceutical company can't market a drug? Yes– very much so.

It's a sad fact of our system that it is extremely critical to patient care whether a pharmaceutical company sees enough profit in a medication to market it to doctors and patients. It doesn't seem like our health should be dependent upon profit potential, but it is.

Many drugs are extremely well known and established, and for those that have been incorporated into routine medical care, it doesn't matter as much if the drug is no longer marketed to doctors. Doctors are likely to be aware of it and prescribe it anyways.

But if a medication is not well known either for its on-label or off-label capabilities, and it is not an established part of routine medical care (and nearly every important drug in this book falls into this zone), then it matters very much that a pharmaceutical company isn't marketing it.

Because your doctor is unlikely to hear about it and is therefore much less likely to prescribe it to you even if you bring it to their attention.

Medication that is marketed to doctors by pharmaceutical companies brings credibility. Medication that is marketed to doctors by patients is typically ignored.

While the pharmaceutical industry can be very heavily regulated by government healthcare arms, the government does not market medication.

It relies on the business dynamics of the pharma industry to promote the medication that you and your doctor need to know about. But if this communication system that relies so heavily on pharmaceutical marketing breaks down in some way (as it has with medications for alcoholism), there is no 'plan b' that makes sure you get the right medications.

This peculiar weakness of the system leads pharmaceutical companies (at least those in health-care areas with profit potential) to do a ridiculously wasteful, time-consuming dance.

They look for ways around the system by developing variations ('biosimilars') of successful medications, which can be patented, win regulatory approval and which will then enjoy marketing protection.

In other words—they spend millions of dollars and decades of research, trying to discover drugs that have already been discovered.

SELINCRO LAUNCH IN EUROPE

With all of these barriers that pharmaceutical companies have experienced in developing medications for alcoholism, the nalmefene (Selincro) launch mentioned earlier in Europe is critical. It could change the entire face of alcohol addiction treatment.

Not only has Lundbeck launched a new product, but they are lobbying for approvals, endorsement and financial subsidization from influential governmental health groups across Europe; marketing to an army of doctors; and attempting to educate an entire health care system on hard-to-grasp concepts which includes two revolutionary 'new' concepts, which are:

(a) reduced drinking is just as important a goal as abstinence; and

(b) that alcoholism can be moderated, managed or even eliminated through medication.

It's an enormous challenge that they have taken on.

I have no affiliation with any pharmaceutical company, but I hope that Selincro sales go through the roof. I applaud Lundbeck, and CEO Ulf Wiinberg, for their work in improving conditions for people suffering from brain disorders, including addiction.

Lundbeck's 2015 Q2 report showed sales of DKK 51 M for the quarter and indicated that sales were being driven by the French market and showed "continued solid growth" in France, with slower growth in other areas.[88]

Nalmefene itself may not be a slam-dunk (the jury is still out), but the changes Lundbeck are introducing are critical. It's important that other pharmaceutical companies see that medication for the treatment of alcoholism can finally be effective *and* profitable.

STIGMA AND PHARMA IMAGE

Bell Canada is a Canadian telecom company that runs a campaign called 'Let's Talk'. Well-known athletes and celebrities are highlighted by the brand, speaking up about their own struggles. It's a positive example of a major corporation leveraging its brand to help reduce stigma around mental illness. The company encourages Canadians to talk and text about mental illness.

This campaign contrasts heavily with the approach some pharmaceutical companies take. In a 2008 Newsweek article, Alan Leshner, the former head of the National Institute of Drug Abuse (NIDA) said, "companies with billion-dollar stakes in selling drugs for osteoporosis or cholesterol don't want their names on a product used by heroin addicts.[58]

Seven years later, the perception that ties addiction medication to the stigma attached to the people suffering from them seems not to have changed much.

In an informal review of the worlds' major pharmaceutical companies, very few of them (even those known to be investing funds and supporting research in the area), openly indicate addiction medicine as a research focus on their corporate websites. It's like addiction research is still a dirty little secret.

Profit potential can change all that, though.

Steven Paul, while he was the head of research at Eli Lilly, said there used to be a stigma attached to depression too, but Prozac put an end to it.

"Anything that has a large unmet need," says Paul, "is ultimately going to succeed commercially."[58]

DECLINE IN CNS INVESTMENT

There is yet another pharma industry issue hampering the development of new medications for alcohol addiction.

It's an issue which has professionals in all areas of mental health—not just addictions—worried. Development of CNS drugs (for Central Nervous System illnesses—of which alcoholism is one) is amongst the most expensive, highest risk area in medicine.

As pharmaceutical companies have come to realize the perils involved in CNS drug development, research and development in the field of mental health concerns has lost ground across the board.

One report, written by the Director of the US National Institute of Mental Health and Steven Hyman of Harvard University said that "Despite high prevalence and unmet medical need, major pharmaceutical companies are de-emphasizing or exiting psychiatry, thus removing significant capacity from efforts to discover new medicines."

The report pointed to the problems lying in "stringent regulations and approval processes for mental health drugs…as well as difficulty with developing medications that can be proven to actually combat mental illness."[89]

Since 2011, major companies—Glaxo Smith Kline, AstraZeneca, and Novartis closed neuroscience divisions globally. And those significantly downsizing operations include Pfizer, Sanofi, Janssen and Merck.[90]

Pharma shareholders don't like to see companies they have invested in spend millions on new drugs only to have them fail before they make it to approval. There are only so many stock price drops senior executives will tolerate before the risk of further failure and loss leads them to reinvest in less risky areas of development.

The economics of neuropsychiatric drug development just aren't positive at the moment.

It takes 1.9 years on average to get regulatory approval (compared with an average of 1.2 years for all drugs). And human testing takes on average 8.1 years (two years longer than the average for all drugs). So counting the 6 to 10 years of preclinical research, drugs for CNS (Central Nervous System) illnesses take about 18 years to reach approval.[91]

When was the last time that you wanted to invest in anything that lost money for 18 years in a row before it had a chance to make a single dollar?

The harsh environment for CNS drugs means that only about 8.2 percent of those that begin human testing reach the marketplace, compared to 15 percent of drugs overall.[91]

CNS drugs are nearly twice as likely to fail as all drugs on average. And when CNS drugs fail, they fail at the most expensive, high-profile phase in the pipeline–in phase 3 trials. Only 46 percent succeed at this point (compared with 66 percent on average for all drugs).[91]

Recently, Pfizer, Johnson & Johnson, Eli Lilly and Baxter all experienced high profile failures in large phase 3 clinical trials for Alzheimer's while biotech Satori Pharma had to completely shut down operations after the poor performance of their Alzheimer's compound.[90]

If that's not a bleak picture of mental health drug development, I don't know what is.

And keep in mind that those numbers are for CNS drugs across the board–which include areas of intense interest such as Alzheimer's. The numbers are far more dismal for any drug related to addiction disorders.

A NEW WAY

However, companies with the stomach to stay in the CNS drug development game will benefit in some ways too.

If a company can develop drugs and remain profitable in the CNS drug development game, it's earned the chops to be profitable in any area of drug development.

These companies are developing new ways of doing business that the enterprises that exit the arena won't develop. And these new ways of doing business will serve the companies that learn them and help them in every area of development, giving them a competitive advantage against competitors who couldn't stomach or survive the risk.

The companies that are staying with CNS drug development are taking a hard look at how drugs have always been developed and changing things. In the past, drug development has been secretive, soloed and fraught with proprietary secrets. Information sharing across pharmaceutical companies was grounds for termination.

Now, there is much more innovation and collaboration. Instead of failing at enormous cost individually, competitors are minimizing risk and maximizing brain power by working together.

In an article in Scientific American called *A Dearth of New Meds*, the author writes that "ultimately, making new CNS medicines may depend on a networked approach to innovation, in which many organizations share in the risks and the rewards. It is clear that the challenges of developing new neuropsychiatric medicines are greater than any one company, institution or organization can bear alone."[91]

Pharmaceutical companies are working it out. Today, it is reported that the "vast majority of neuropharmaceutical development is being conducted in a partnership or collaboration basis. Most commonly, a smaller biotech's trials will receive 50-100% of the funding from one or more big pharma players, on conditions of key milestones being met."

This means that if trials flop, the big pharma partner can cut their losses, and a failure in a small partner's trial won't look as bad to shareholders as the same failure occurring from the company's own trial.[90]

Whereas once, small biotech players may not have had the resources to develop essential drugs, today the role they play in the CNS drug pipeline has become critical.

Companies like Merck, Roche, Glaxo Smith Kline and AstraZeneca are also investing in genetic research—a critical area since more and more mental illnesses have been shown to have a strong genetic biomarker component. (Alcohol dependence is no exception to this—many of the effective medications for alcoholism have been found to work best for individuals with very specific genetic markers and gene clusters).

By identifying genetic biomarkers, pharma can change how patients are selected for drug trials, significantly improving trial outcomes, perhaps even with previously failed drugs.

ADVANCEMENTS

There are exciting twinkles of hope for alcohol addiction medicine within small pockets of the pharmaceutical industry. And there are a few things that larger companies can take away from the firms that are making headway. Here are what some companies are doing in the area of alcohol addiction medication development.

RECKITT BENCKISER & INVIDIOR

Powerhouse Reckitt Benckiser is one of a handful of companies making strategic business moves in the space.

Its spin-off, Invidior, has been developing and marketing drugs for the treatment of opioid addiction for over ten years. In 2014, it made its first foray into a medication for alcohol addiction when it entered into a global licensing agreement with XenoPort Inc. to develop and market arbaclofen placarbil for the treatment of alcohol use disorder.

Invidior's CEO Shaun Thaxter says that arbaclofen placarbil is the company's biggest commercial opportunity and that they will be actively looking for opportunities to further expand their pipeline in the addiction arena.[92] Their press release stated that "there is a tremendous need for more effective, well-tolerated treatment options among the growing patient population with alcohol use disorders."[93]

The Invidior website is bold, forward thinking and has an inspiring message about addiction medicine which other pharma companies should take note of. It says:

"Our goal is to help remove the stigma of addiction, expand treatment access infrastructure, and to help patients take the first step in their journey—empowering them to act before the moment of readiness is gone.

Together, we are making considerable progress in the U.S. and Australia, with the drug policy and regulatory environment moving towards recognizing addiction as a normal, legitimate disease, creating shifts in public perception, and allowing broader access to mainstream medical treatment models, similar to other chronic diseases.

Globally, a movement is underway, with the EU also making strides to move away from a harm reduction environment towards a medicalized, recovery model like other chronic diseases.

We intend to transform addiction from a global human crisis to a recognized and treated disease worldwide."[94]

Is it marketing copy for shareholders? Sure. Did I drink the Koolaid? Yes, I did.

But it's also a step forward. Good on you Invidior.

ALKERMES

Alkermes may be the first pharmaceutical company in the alcohol dependence space that is seeing a substantial return on their investments—proving that profitability in this space is now possible—even with a new take on an old generic medication.

In July of 2015, Alkermes announced that they were improving the company's 2015 financial expectations driven by accelerating financial performance of Vivitrol, Alkermes' injectable naltrexone product for opiate and alcohol dependence.

Commented James Frates, Chief Financial Officer of Alkermes, "driven by the accelerating quarterly growth in net sales of Vivitrol, our long-acting injectable medication for the treatment of opioid dependence and alcohol dependence…net sales of Vivitrol were $37.2 million, compared to $21.6 million for the same period in the prior year, representing an increase of approximately 72%."[29]

But Vivitrol won't be a one-hit-wonder for Alkermes. They are translating their learnings and earnings from the naltrexone injectable into new treatments for alcohol dependence. They seem to have more compounds for the treatment of alcohol dependence in clinical trials right now than any other company.

Several compounds have performed well. Samidorphan, which has been reported to have similar efficacy to naltrexone but possibly with reduced side-effects[95], and ALKS-3831, an olanzapine/samidorphan combination targeted to patients with schizophrenia and alcohol use disorders both look promising.

A third drug, ALKS-5461, a buprenorphine/samidorphan combination is also in clinical testing. And another Alkermes CNS drug, Aristada, was recently approved for treatment of schizophrenia.

Partnership and collaboration are a key strategy for Alkermes and they have successful partnerships with AstraZeneca, Janssen Pharmaceuticals, Acorda and Acceleron Pharma.

ASTRAZENECA

The AstraZeneca corporate website says, "The best science doesn't happen in isolation." And their extensive approach to partnering and collaboration has resulted in a few deals that hold promise. They have made strategic investments in two biotechs with promising addiction products (Eolas Therapeutics and Heptares).

Both have orexin-1 receptor antagonists in development which may be promising for addictions. They have also partnered with NIDA (National Institute of Drug Abuse) to explore Neuroscience iMed's (AstraZeneca branch) drug AZD8529, for smoking cessation. AZD8529 may also treat other substance abuse.[96]

And unlike so many pharmaceutical companies, they are not afraid to publicly mention addiction disorders[96] on their website as an area of focus.

They also have a core focus on personalized healthcare (medications driven and tested with the benefit of genetic research), and according to them, 80% of their programs benefit from this approach.

LUNDBECK

Lundbeck is a crucial player in the alcohol dependence space right now, fighting on many fronts for Selincro's success in Europe and elsewhere.

In addition to their outstanding work with Selincro, Lundbeck is not afraid to stand up to mental health stigma.

In October 2015, Lundbeck celebrated World Mental Health Day, promoting dignity in mental health treatment. Their primary research and product focus is brain diseases, with alcohol dependence appearing prominently, listed first on their website.

OTHERS

Other inspiring work by other pharmaceuticals includes the following:

- Adial Pharmaceuticals (focused on addiction and founded by Dr. Bankole Johnson) is making steady progress with alcohol dependence medication AD04.[97]

- Addex Pharmaceutics' focus on collaboration with patient advocacy groups, academic institutions and governmental organizations including NIAAA (National Institute on Alcohol Abuse and Alcoholism) is paying off with progress for promising pre-clinical compounds as well as ADX71441.[98]

- XenoPort Pharmaceuticals is collaborating with the NIAAA in the development of their medication Horizant, as a potential treatment for AUD. The patent on Horizant (gabapentin encarbil) runs until at least 2026.[99] They've also been granted exclusive worldwide rights for the development and commercialization of carbaclofen placarbil, another promising medication.[100]

- Eolas is a specialty company committed to treating the disease of addiction. It recently signed a global licensing and partnership agreement with AstraZeneca for the development of a drug designed to block a neuropeptide associated with addiction to nicotine and stimulants such as cocaine, opiates, and alcohol.[101]

AstraZeneca's website states, "The collaboration is a great example of our unique approach to Neuroscience drug discovery and development, partnering to advance the most exciting scientific opportunities in areas of high unmet medical need."[96]

- Japan's Sosei Group Corporation purchased a smaller biotech–Heptares–in February 2015. Heptares has an orexin receptor antagonist in development which they hope will target the treatment of addiction and compulsive disorders.[102]

- France's D&A Pharma has several exciting projects to treat alcohol addiction in development. GHB has long been used in Europe effectively to help alcohol addictions but has several drawbacks, including its own addictive qualities. D&A Pharma have developed two variations on the drug–one is an immediate-release formulation which has been redesigned with lower abuse potential, and the second is an even more exciting variation, which has a longer duration of action.[103]

- Italy's Laboratorio Farmaceutico CT Srl has many years of experience in the study of new and innovative drugs for alcohol addiction. Laboratorio Farmaceutico initially developed the product Alcover (which is now being extended by D&A) and is currently developing a highly promising new medication called GET73 which is in the clinical study phase in the US.[104]

GOVERNMENT

Barry's father moved back to the US in 1971, running away from a third broken marriage. Barry and his siblings knew his father could be a violent and abusive man, so the breakup of the marriage was no surprise.

His dad had no job and a car accident had left him severely injured. So he stayed with Barry for a short time in Hawaii to regroup, and then returned home.

At home, a second car crash cost him his legs and then a third one cost him his life.

As with the previous accidents, he had been drunk at the time, and behind the wheel.

Barry is–of course–Barack Obama, the President of the United States. And he knows something about alcoholism, because his father, Barack Obama Sr. was an alcoholic.

•••

In October 2015, President Obama, the Secretary of Health and Human Services, Sylvia Burwell, and the new czar, Michael Botticelli, spoke at a US town that had been hit hard by opioid addiction.

Between 2002 and 2013, heroin-related deaths in America nearly quadrupled. In 2013, 37,000 Americans died of drug overdose.

This shocking, hockey-stick shaped increase in overdose death is as good a visual depiction as any of the disaster that the war on drugs has turned out to be.

But there is a silver lining to this epidemic. It's the impetus for change that just might be needed to pave the way for a new approach.

And that new approach will change the way alcoholics are treated too.

Because after all, alcohol is a drug. Addictive drugs of abuse–whether cocaine, heroin, alcohol (or even, some might argue, tobacco)–all do the same thing–they hijack parts of brain. Some just kill more slowly than others.

The government's focus on MAT clears a path for all substance addictions. If MAT is supported, funded and legislated for one kind of substance addiction, it must be supported for all.

•••

Earlier in the book we covered some of the moves made by the Obama administration which will impact treatment made available to people with alcoholism.

There is a surprisingly long list of promising moves that the US government can be applauded for. They include:

- Appointing as a figurehead for this movement, a new Drug Czar who is a recovering alcoholic with strong ties to AA groups.

  The new Czar has publicly stated that "we have highly effective medications, when combined with other behavioral supports, that are the standard of care...[28]

- Introducing the term 'MAT' (Medication Assisted Treatment) into public vernacular; and publicly announcing support for this approach–and only this approach.[105]

- Taking the focus off of criminalization and onto medical treatment.[30]

  Obama has said, "rather than spending billions of dollars — taxpayer dollars — on long prison sentences for nonviolent drug offenders, we could save money and get better outcomes by getting treatment to those who need it."[30]

- Removing funding from judges who 'practice medicine from the bench' by removing federal funding from those courts barring addicts from receiving MAT.[28][106]

- Providing funding through the appropriations bill for medications like naltrexone and ensuring that substance abuse disorder is treated on par with other mental illness (which must be treated on par with other illness–period.)

  Obama has stated, "I've made this a priority for my administration ... And under the Affordable Care Act, more health plans have to cover substance abuse disorders. The budget that I sent Congress would invest in things like ... expanding medication assisted treatment programs."[30]

- Directing federal agencies with health care responsibilities 90 days to identify barriers to MAT and to come up with ways to remove them.[28]

•••

At the October 2015 event, the president and his team spoke about what they are doing to curb this overdose epidemic.

Burwell spoke about her top priorities. She said:

> *"Number one is changing prescribing practices...Second is working on medication assisted treatment."*

This is incredible news and such a promising announcement for proponents of MAT.

But let's step back for a moment and put this in perspective.

The drug overdose numbers sound bad–37,000 American deaths in 2013. But the number of people dying of drug overdose each year is *dwarfed* by the number of people that die in the US of alcoholism each year–88,000 people.[14]

And the epidemic of alcohol-related deaths has been going on much much longer.

But at the October event, alcoholism was not mentioned.

Given that it was an event focused on addiction, and as far as drugs go, it's alcohol–not opiates—that kills the biggest number of Americans, is there something wrong with this picture?

Yes.

But it's also a step forward.

Nobody seems to be screaming at the American government about all the dying alcoholics–so they aren't a priority.

And Obama, Botticelli and Burwell know that while an announcement by a political leader promoting medication for the treatment of alcoholism would not go over well, the 12-step movement was never as ingrained in the psyches of doctors and society for drug addiction as deeply as it was, and still is, for alcoholism.

It's easier politically–especially with the parents of many dead overdose victims in the audience from failed 12-step programs–for Obama to focus on tackling drug addiction with medication.

But while it may never be publicly stated, I would like to believe that for Obama and Burwell, MAT is as much about getting proper medical treatment for alcoholics as it is about getting medical care to opiate-users.

I believe this for two reasons.

First, you can see the names of medication for alcoholism beginning to show up in government directives that list medications for opiate dependence.

And second, just as it is for me, for Obama and Burwell, it's personal.

First–look at, as an example–one of SAMHSA's recent announcements:

> *"Recognizing that Medication-Assisted Treatment (MAT) may be an important part of a comprehensive treatment plan, SAMHSA Treatment Drug Court grantees are encouraged to use up to 20 percent of the annual grant award to pay for FDA-approved medications (e.g., methadone, injectable naltrexone, noninjectable naltrexone, disulfiram, acamprosate calcium, buprenorphine, etc.) when the client has no other source of funds to do so."*[106]

If there's any doubt that the government's new approach is strictly for opiate users, the list at the end of that order confirms otherwise.

Six drugs were mentioned in the announcement. Four of the six are treatments for alcoholism. And two of the six–disulfiram and acamprosate–are *exclusively* for the treatment of alcoholism.

There are no other addictions that those two medications are used to treat.

So if Obama's approach isn't just as much about alcoholism as it is about opiate overdose, those medications would never have made it into that list.

As for the 'it's personal' part, it's clear. As the earlier story showed, Obama had a father who died from alcoholism. The President was the child of an alcoholic and as such was deeply affected by this disease. Perhaps he struggles with it himself. Perhaps he worries that one of his children will inherit it.

And Botticelli (the Drug Czar) is of course the recovering alcoholic who endorses medication assisted treatment.

Both of them have seen and experienced enough heartbreak from alcoholism to know that if there is a medical solution, it needs to get to alcoholics–even if doing so involves some extremely strategic stepping.

LINCHPINS

"The linchpin sees the world very differently…The linchpin feels the fear, acknowledges it, then proceeds."
–Seth Godin[107]

The late artist François de Kresz drew a picture of a vast plain of sheep, all walking passively in the same direction together.

There's one little black sheep heading against the stream, politely saying 'excuse moi…. excuse moi… excuse moi…', as he heads away from the edge of a cliff–off of which the rest of the passive white beasts plummet.

That little black sheep is a linchpin–a term coined by author Seth Godin.

A linchpin is an ordinary person who does extraordinary things. Sometimes at great personal risk they defy the status quo and conformity. They head in their own direction, sometimes singularly; and their ideas and actions can create great change.

I've always admired linchpins, and in this story there are several. This chapter says thank-you to a few of them.

•••

As I write this book, there are no other books available that provide a single resource to alcoholics, their families or medical professionals that cover the range of available pharmaceutical options now available.

This resource–while much needed–just does not exist–either in book format or online.

Why governments of the world have funded billions of dollars in research to discover substances that help fight alcohol addiction, and then not spent a few thousand writing a book or building a website to let the general public know about them is a puzzle I don't have an answer for.

The discovery of research findings is important, but the translation of those findings into plain English is critical. Until scientific research is translated into plain English, it's lost on the majority of people that need it.

The majority of the information available on the topic of medications for alcoholism that is available in plain English was created not by science, medicine or government, by a colorful collection of individuals—some highly credible in a traditional sense, and others unfortunately not.

To help others discover what they had already found, they published memoirs, personal case studies in medical journals, wrote Internet postings, launched websites, and crowd-funded a documentary.

And because of alcoholism's stigma and the AA effect, these people shared their discoveries at great cost to their careers, privacy, and reputations.

•••

The second 'A' in AA is not there by accident. Regardless of the danger some may present to those around them, maintaining anonymity for alcoholics and their families means that they don't fall further victim to stigma.

By maintaining anonymity, they avoid losing jobs and careers or facing lawsuits and the public humiliation and anger they would experience if they were outed.

Obama's Drug Czar Michael Botticelli himself said that it was much harder for him to come out as someone with an addiction, than as a gay man.

If you have not attended AA or one of the support groups, you may not realize who the people are around you that struggle with addiction.

There are alcoholics that teach grade three, while drinking gin from a coffee cup all day long; there are alcoholics who perform intricate surgeries, then binge themselves to oblivion on their days off; there are alcoholics who experience heavy withdrawal symptoms, as they drive massive 4-wheelers down the highway, there are alcoholics sipping from a hidden mickey before clocking in for their shifts in the nuclear power plant up the street. You've met them, I've met them.

Sadly, alcoholism is a disease that can cause great harm to those without it.

For an alcoholic to stand up and speak about their alcoholism and argue for the use of medication in treatment, they must be comfortable in outing themselves and their loved ones and transforming their private desperation into a public affair.

So when anyone steps forward and publicly declares themselves an alcoholic to advocate for other medical options, they are often putting their careers, licenses, and lives in jeopardy in ways we might not immediately see.

Even non-alcoholics—doctors and writers like Gabrielle Glaser for example—who stand up against the status quo, are exposing themselves to threat.

Sharing information without the shield of anonymity, discussing their own alcoholism publicly, sharing non-conventional medical approaches, or standing up under harsh public scrutiny from the public and the powerful AA and rehab groups is not without significant risk.

Despite this, a handful of people have gone public and shared information without the security of anonymity.

Among others, these pioneering individuals include:

- The late Dr. Olivier Amiesen, a French-American cardiologist who died of a heart attack in 2013 after publishing a book and series of medical articles on the medical cure he discovered for his own severe alcoholism;

- The late Dr. David Sinclair, a quirky American neuroscientist who made his home in Helsinki and was the grandfather of addiction research in 'as needed' methods of treatment.

Other notable linchpins, some of whom I'll tell you more about, include Claudia Christian, Dr. Roy Eskapa, Dr. Fred Levin, the late R. Evan Picard, Dr. Linda Garcia and Dr. Phillip E. Thomas.

DOCTORS, WRITERS & ALCOHOLICS

DR. OLIVIER AMEISEN

When I think of the handful of people who have risked their careers to help alcoholics find medical treatment, the face that always immediately comes to mind is that of French-American cardiologist Dr. Olivier Ameisen, posing for a May 2010 article in *The Guardian* about his work in the field.

In the photo, at the age of 56, Ameisen looked tired and gaunt, but determined. Written on his face perhaps one can read the years of work and study that put him at the top of his field; the debilitating anxiety he medicated with alcohol; the years spent struggling with devastating alcoholism, and the effort of the fight he began once he cured his own alcoholism with baclofen, to let others in the medical community know of his discovery.

Sadly Dr. Ameisen died on July 18, 2013, but during the final decade of his life he left an incredible legacy. This cardiologist and symphony-level pianist did more to advance the treatment of alcoholism with medication in a single decade than most addiction physicians do in their lifetimes.

In the late 90s and early 2000s, desperate to find a medication to treat his own severe, debilitating alcoholism, Ameisen never gave up trying treatments and medications. After tireless research and self-experimentation, he finally treated himself with high doses of baclofen. One day, amazingly, he realized that he was "completely and effortlessly indifferent" to alcohol.[22]

Knowing that his discovery could save the lives of thousands of other alcoholics, Ameisen spent the rest of his life trying to get the medical community to take notice.

Publicly 'outing' himself as an alcoholic, he bravely wrote his experience as a 'self-case report.' It was published in December 2004 in the journal Alcohol and Alcoholism, published by the Oxford University Press.

As Amiesen wrote in his excellent 2008 book, 'The End of My Addiction':

"A deafening silence ensued. Except for Giovanni Addolorato and a few of his colleagues in Italy, no one inside or outside the field of addiction research and treatment seemed to have any interest in the first peer-reviewed report of complete suppression of the deadly disease of alcoholism with the alleviation of comorbid anxiety."[22]

And in the entire year after the paper was published, only two people in the medical and research community contacted him.

Because of Amiesen's journal publication, the subsequent publication of his book (which circumvented the dogmatic medical community and was written for those suffering from alcoholism and their families) and his tireless work until his untimely death, Amiesen helped thousands of people find a way out of alcoholism.

After reading Ameisen's book, another doctor–Dr. Phillip E. Thomas began to take baclofen himself, completely suppressing his own cravings for alcohol and allowing him to have an occasional drink in a social setting.

Inspired by Amiesen's bravery, Thomas also bravely published his own self-case report in the journal *Progress in Neurology and Psychiatry*.[108]

Due to Ameisen's efforts, in June 2014, the French government became the first government to recognize the importance of baclofen in the treatment of alcoholism by publicly announcing that it would reimburse patients for the cost of baclofen when used in connection with the treatment of alcoholism.

In the United States, what Ameisen accomplished would be the equivalent of gaining both FDA approval *and* public health care insurance reimbursement for the treatment of alcoholism with baclofen–something unlikely to happen for many years.

FATHER OF ADDICTION RESEARCH DR. DAVID SINCLAIR

Dr. David Sinclair was a kindly and quirky American-born research scientist who spent much of his life's work in Finland, focused on addiction medicine.

His contributions to the field were groundbreaking and extremely relevant even today. Thousands of people whose lives have been saved by naltrexone and the 'as needed' method developed by Sinclair can credit him with saving their lives.

Sinclair passed away in April 2015. And at the end of his obituary, it states, "In honor of David's life, his family requests that you learn about The Sinclair Method of alcohol treatment and then help others become educated about it."[109]

Despite his impactful work, recognition of Sinclair's contributions (aside from the many citations and references to his research publications in science and medical journals) seems strangely absent in North America.

Perhaps because Sinclair's discoveries and hypothesis' were so far ahead of his time, the world of addiction research and medicine looked at him more like an outlier than as the innovator he has proven to be.

There are only a few medications that have gained FDA-approval or European medical approval specifically for their use in alcoholism (others are effective for alcoholism, but have gained their FDA approval for the treatment of other, non-related illnesses).

In Europe, one of a handful of drugs specifically approved for the treatment of alcoholism is nalmefene, which is currently patented and marketed by Lundbeck[110111]. However, it was Dr. Sinclair who first patented nalmefene[112] in 1992.

And in the United States and Canada, one of the few FDA-approved (and Health Canada approved) medications is naltrexone, which also was first patented by Dr. Sinclair,[113] in 1989.

Sinclair also demonstrated and conducted very early research into the Alcohol Deprivation Effect (ADE), which is the addiction/detox/binge behavior seen in lab rats and which has been researched and observed by other scientists many times since.

Very early on, Sinclair also wrote extensively about the Pharmacological Extinction Hypothesis, which is a now often-cited theory used to explain the effectiveness of naltrexone and nalmefene when taken by alcoholics as needed.

Based on his understanding of alcoholism and naltrexone, Sinclair developed a method of taking naltrexone–the 'as needed' method, which was coined TSM–or The Sinclair Method.

In 2012, Dr. Roy Eskapa, a clinical psychologist who had worked with Dr. Sinclair wrote a book (with a foreword written by Dr. Sinclair) about treatment with naltrexone using TSM.

The book, (*The Cure for Alcoholism: The Medically Proven Way to Eliminate Alcohol Addiction*') is an excellent resource and defacto 'how to guide' for taking naltrexone in the manner that Sinclair developed. (Though if naltrexone does not turn out to be the cure for you–remember there are many other effective medications available).

ACTRESS AND ADVOCATE CLAUDIA CHRISTIAN

Claudia Christian is a beautiful American actress who may be best known for her starring role in the 90s sci-fi hit Babylon 5, creating a cult-following with the Comic-Con crowd.

In the late 90's late-onset alcoholism began to wrap its tendrils around Christian. She started drinking too much, too often, binging and detoxing her way into addiction and desperation.

One day, in a detox center she came across a pamphlet on the monthly naltrexone injection, Vivitrol. The pamphlet led her to research naltrexone and come across the book written by Dr. Roy Eskapa based on addiction research pioneer Dr. David Sinclair's method for taking naltrexone.

Just as Baclofen had worked astonishingly well for Dr. Olivier, Christian was one of the lucky ones when it came to naltrexone. She wrote about her amazing recovering from alcoholism in her excellent 2012 book *Babylon Confidential–A Memoir of Love, Sex, and Addiction.*[114]

Christian became heavily committed to helping other alcoholics recover using naltrexone as she did. She started an organization (cthreefoundation.org) and released an outstanding documentary she produced and appeared in called '*One Little Pill.*'

The documentary provides excellent insight into naltrexone for alcoholism. (Though abstinent individuals who are very reactive to alcohol imagery cues may wish to avoid watching the documentary as it could trigger intense cravings.)

Still a working actress (recently appearing in the Mentalist, Castle, and Criminal Minds), Christian is one of the dominant forces that have allowed naltrexone to become more widely known, saving many lives.

And despite her fame, Christian still works at a grass-roots level. I'll always be grateful to Christian: once when I was still very early in learning about alcoholism medications, she reached out privately by email to me, encouraging me to continue my work.

COURAGEOUS DR. FRED LEVIN & THE LATE R. EVAN PICARD

One of the most difficult barriers for alcoholics to overcome is simply to find a doctor who will prescribe medication like baclofen and naltrexone to them and who will support them in their treatment.

However there are individual doctors who, after prescribing medication successfully to some of their patients, realized the desperate need for doctors who would write the right prescriptions and support the medical treatment of alcoholics.

After treating 40 patients successfully with baclofen and following Dr. Amiesen's work closely, Dr. Fred Levin made it known online that he was willing to advise those who would otherwise treat themselves, over the phone, out of hours, so that they could take Baclofen safely with medical support.

Levin helped hundreds of alcoholics who couldn't find help elsewhere to obtain both medication and medical supervision.

Baclofen is a safe, FDA-approved medication. But if someone discontinues the drug suddenly it can result in serious depression. Levin not only gave alcoholics access to baclofen, but he provided them with the medical support to ensure that they took it (or reduced from it) safely.

In August 2013, Levin, who was an associate professor in the department of psychiatry at Northwestern University Feinberg School of Medicine, and at the Chicago Institute for Psychoanalysis where he taught neuro psychoanalysis for 10 years, was sanctioned by the state of Illinois.

He was charged by the Illinois medical board with "unprofessional conduct, improper prescribing of controlled substances and failure to establish and maintain medical records."

The respected physician, 71-years old at the time, was fined $10,000 and his license was placed on probation indefinitely.

The message boards used by so many of the people that Levin had helped lit up. Individuals whose lives Levin had saved defended him.

One individual—the late Evan Picard (known as Lo0p—whose life Levin had saved, and who had gone on to help hundreds more find help with baclofen), broke his anonymity to start a letter writing campaign. Many of the comments published on the board speak for themselves.

•••

This is all just so, so, so sad.

He sacrificed his career for us. He didn't ask for much money…he believed so strongly in the medication that he was willing to go out on a limb to help alcoholics. He was so kind. I know that what he was doing was legally questionable, but he was a believer. I give him full credit for saving my life back in late 2010 when I was hopeless and lost. I am so sad he can't continue helping more lost souls who need his help.

•••

I'd be honored to write a letter for Dr. Levin. He believed in me when I was lost and almost beyond hope. He helped me find my way out. I'm forever grateful.

•••

Dr. Levin has selflessly provided his services to myself and other alcoholics like me, asking virtually nothing in return. Several times, I found myself asking him about compensating him for his services because he never even billed me for it. It seemed as if he was doing it, simply to be of service and help those in need.

He also made himself available via phone, at ANY time, if I needed to discuss my treatment or had any questions, concerns or problems. Dr. Levin is anything but a "mail-order Doc", who is just shelling out prescriptions to anyone with a checkbook.

•••

I humbly ask that you please reinstate his medical license and allow him to continue his invaluable treatment to me and many others who have been freed from the hells of alcoholism. Without his care, I will be forced to stop taking baclofen and return to a life of alcoholic misery.

He is a passionate and caring doctor who dedicated himself to helping those in need and should not be punished for it.

I was destitute when I approached him. He said: "If you can send me a check for $10, do that."

So I did. He filled my baclofen prescriptions for 2 years, for $10. He also made himself available to me whenever I needed him. For $10.

•••

It was Dr. Levin who had the courage back in 2011 to prescribe baclofen for my son when he really needed it...and it made all the difference. It broke the cycle of anxiety and craving and gave my son space to get his life back together. I will be forever grateful.

Dr. Fred Levin prescribed baclofen off-label to alcoholics nationwide at a reasonable cost. He has saved the lives of hundreds as a result. Countless others have benefited from knowing he was there as a resource, and from his emerging prominence as an advocate for baclofen, an FDA-approved medication.

OUTSPOKEN AUTHORS

In addition to the alcoholics, doctors and researchers I've cited here, several authors stand out for their controversial and outspoken work criticizing the AA approach extensively.

They include:

- Dr. Lance Dodes, author of *'The Sober Truth: Debunking the Bad Science Behind 12-Step Programs and the Rehab Industry.'*[61]

- Gabrielle Glasser, author of both *'Her Best-Kept Secret: Why Women Drink-And How They Can Regain Control'*[115] and more recently a scathing but on-the-mark article for *The Atlantic* entitled, *'The Irrationality of Alcoholics Anonymous'*.[15]

- Dr. Peter Ferentzy, outspoken author of *'Dealing with Addiction: Why the 20th Century was Wrong.'*[11]

- Terrance Hodgins, the author of *The Orange Papers*, an extensive collection of essays that will make you rethink AA, found at orange-papers.org.

- Roberta Jewel & Dr. Linda Garcia, authors of the first self-account of recovery from alcoholism using topiramate. The book ('*My Way Out…*', spawned a forum on the mywayout.org website that is a lifeline for many alcoholics looking for an alternative to AA.

- Kenneth Anderson, author and advocate for evidence-based strategies. He founded the HAMS Harm Reduction Network (hamsnetwork.org) and published '*How to Change your Drinking*' in 2010 that provides treatment alternatives to AA.

THE ANONYMOUS

There are many hundreds of people who quietly and anonymously help alcoholics and their families discover medical options for the treatment of alcoholism.

They are active on forums—encouraging, cheering on successes, translating research and helping pick up the pieces when things don't go well.

I invite you to meet them by reading through the forum sites I have mentioned in this book (thesinclairmethod.net or mywayout.org/forum are two examples).

RESEARCHERS

"If I have seen a little further it is by standing on the shoulders of Giants."
Isaac Newton

In my research I have read the work of doctors, researchers, and scientists who have spent their lives seeking funding in a severely under-funded space, conducting research and slogging away in the trenches of science to further addiction medicine.

For every one of the hundreds of research reports I read, these scientists and others spent thousands and thousands of thankless hours working meticulously in offices and basement labs.

I imagine that one might start to seriously question their life's work and career choices in the middle of the night in an empty lab surrounded by drunken rats. But these are scientists who stuck with their research nonetheless.

I wanted to list some of them, but I realized that for every one that I list I'll probably be excluding five more that should be listed too. However many of their names appear throughout the book, as well as in the bibliography at the end.

For all the poignant and touching real life stories of alcoholics whose lives were saved by the medications written about in this book, these are the men and women that saved those lives.

06 | THE BOTTOM LINE

"In homes, doctors' offices, hospitals, schools, prisons, jails and communities across America, misperceptions about addiction are undermining medical care.
Although advances in neuroscience, brain imaging and behavioral research clearly show that addiction is a complex brain disease, today the disease of addiction is still often misunderstood as a moral failing, a lack of willpower, a subject of shame and disgust."
–Dr. Drew E. Altman, CASA Columbia National Advisory Commission on Addiction Treatment

PRESCRIBING PRACTICES MUST CHANGE

Fundamentally, (naively?), I believe that the number one thing that has to change is how doctors treat alcoholics.

Regardless of all of the issues around AA, the treatment industry and the pharmaceutical industry, the one group that can change this entire picture are doctors.

When doctors start treating patients with evidence-based care for their alcohol addictions, other stakeholders will fall in line, or simply get walked over.

If more doctors prescribe evidence-based treatments, more people suffering from alcohol dependence will regain control and begin to lead happy healthy lives again.

Others will see these changes and request medications from doctors, which will reinforce evidence-based prescribing habits.

As happened with other heavily stigmatized mental illnesses like depression, as people see that alcoholism can be treated medically, it will become more widely understood that it is a disease, and less stigmatized.

Doctors will seek information and solutions from pharmaceutical reps, and pharmaceutical companies will be financially-motivated to further market medications and fund research into new medication.

Researchers will be motivated to continue researching and will be better supported by government and big pharma.

Treatment centers will start, as they already have, to incorporate evidence-based treatment into their programs, as a matter of survival.

Is this a pretty and naïve picture I am painting? No. All of this is starting to happen on a small scale already.

This book is a little cog in the wheel of that larger change.

So doctors, please—the lives of so many people with alcoholism depend on you.

- Read the scientific studies referred to in this book with an open mind.

- Read the free study—'*Addiction Medicine: Closing the Gap Between Science and Practice*'[3] It's thorough, free, on the mark and with many recommendations on how to change the way we do things.

- Start integrating Medication Assisted Treatment and evidence-based practices into your work.

•••

And for the rest of us:

Write a letter.

Have a conversation.

File a complaint.

Give this book to someone.

Set up a meeting with a doctor.

Build a website.

Share your story.

2

PART 2: HOW ALCOHOLISM WORKS

07 | DISEASE THEORY

"The history of addiction as a brain disease looks a lot like the history of atoms or germs, insofar as these were all older and controversial ideas for which scientific confirmation later became available."

–Dr. David T. Courtwright, University of North Florida[3]

WHEN A DISEASE NEEDS A THEORY

Much of this book relies on what some people call the 'Disease Theory' of alcoholism.

We don't hear the phrase 'Disease Theory of Diabetes', or 'Disease Theory of Heart Disease' or 'Disease Theory of Alzheimer's,' because the use of the term 'theory' indicates that there is some doubt as to whether it is a disease at all.

Maybe it has to do with how little credit we give to the organ in our own heads.

Judy Cameron's beautifully written article *'Brainfacts'*, describes this wondrous piece of biological engineering:

> *"The human brain — a spongy, three-pound mass of tissue — is the most complex living structure in the universe.*
>
> *With the capacity to create a network of connections that far surpasses any social network and stores more information than a supercomputer, the brain has enabled humans to achieve breathtaking milestones — walking on the moon, mapping the human genome, and composing masterpieces of literature, art, and music.*
>
> *What's more, scientists still have not uncovered the extent of what the brain can do.*
>
> *This single organ controls every aspect of our body, ranging from heart rate and sexual activity to emotion, learning, and memory. The brain controls the immune system's response to disease, and determines, in part, how well people respond to medical treatments.*
>
> *Ultimately, it shapes our thoughts, hopes, dreams, and imaginations. It is the ability of the brain to perform all of these functions that make us human."*[116]

Is alcoholism a disease or a choice?

Is it a brain disease or a personality disorder?

The brain is so incredibly complex, and has such unbelievably vast capabilities, why *wouldn't it* malfunction in complex and unpredictable ways too?

But there seems to be little agreement about this. And it's a polarizing debate that encourages stigma while clouding and distracting from the larger issue, which is simply to find effective treatments.

As a friend said to me, 'Does it really matter?'

Yes–it matters a lot. Here is why.

IF IT'S A CHOICE

The term 'choice' implies free will–the notion that if I just decided to behave differently, I could.

It implies that biologically we are basically the same. And therefore, if one person can simply decide to stop drinking, anyone can.

And if *I* choose not to stop, then *you* can be justified in your anger at me; you can put me last in the treatment line in the emergency room; you can stop inviting me to Christmas dinner; you can punish me for my choices until I smarten up.

If drinking is a choice, then I might feel I deserve that treatment, and worse.

And if drinking is a choice, then when I seek help, my psychologist will try to understand the origins of these bad choices I make. My treatment will involve looking at my 'demons', and attempting to wrestle them to the ground (whatever that means).

BUT, IF IT'S A DISEASE

The term 'disease' implies that there is a biological process going on in my body that I cannot control and which is making me feel things that otherwise I wouldn't feel.

If I have a disease, my body behaves in ways that are beyond my control.

If I have an illness that is beyond my control, then others' anger at me is not as justifiable; putting me last in the treatment line is unconscionable' and not inviting me to Christmas dinner is cruel.

Punishing me for something I can't control is abusive. And looking back into my childhood for 'deep rooted issues' seems like an exercise in futility.

So you may see that depending upon what this is, and what you believe it to be, the outcomes—but most importantly the treatment—for someone with it can be very different.

As one scientist wrote:

> "Understanding the psychological mechanisms and the underlying neurobiology of relapse behavior is essential for improving the treatment situation."[117]

•••

If you begin to understand the neurobiology of addiction, perspectives change.

For example, a 2009 Addiction Biology journal article explained relapse like this:

> "Relapse in alcohol-dependent patients does not seem to reflect "bad intentions" or "weak willpower." Rather ... imaging studies point to an increased sensitivity of brain areas to alcohol-associated stimuli, which may be in part genetically influenced."

> "Cue-induced brain activation predicts the relapse risk of alcohol-dependent patients better than conscious craving, which is not surprising given that activation of some brain areas such as the striatum is hardly associated with conscious experiences.

> Therefore, it seems plausible that patients often relapse "against their own [conscious] will" and they should be treated with the same respect as any other patient in the health care system."[118]

To gain a new perspective and truly help someone suffering from alcoholism, I believe we need to understand alcoholism in a medical sense.

IF IT'S A DISEASE OF CHOICE

'Disease' or 'choice' represent the two very polarizing views that impact the treatment we receive from others.

But what if alcohol addiction combines both—disease AND choice?

What if alcoholism were a disease that alters my ability to choose well and robs me of the capability of exerting my freedom of will in healthy, non-destructive, ways?

Could a brain possibly malfunction in such a way? Yes.

The *ability to choose* is tied inextricably to a biological system. *Choosing* is a function of brain matter. 'Choosing behavior' occurs inside our brains. Healthy neural circuitry enables healthy choosing.

Our hearts beat and pump; our kidneys filter; our brains choose. It's not magic. It's biology.

•••

Addiction is a disease that "erodes the neuronal circuits in our brains that enable us to exert free will."[119]

Or in other words, our choosers are broken.

In a recent presentation Dr. Nora Volkow, who is the Director of the National Institute of Drugs, characterized addiction as a chronic disease where "the most fundamental circuits, that enable us to do something that we take for granted—make a decision and follow it through" have been disrupted.[120]

Volkow and Koob (Director of the NIAA), have written that alcohol (and, in fact, all drugs of abuse), increase dopamine in the brain in an unusual way.

Its release is more prolonged and unregulated when triggered by chemicals that are not native to the brain, than when dopamine is naturally triggered in the brain.

This results in changes in the brain that undermine the way our brains normally learn habits and automated responses.

The changes cause a form of habit-learning that becomes stubbornly persistent even in the face of significantly adverse consequences.[121]

A habit that is unlearnable—or 'terminal'—is a frightening concept. And that's addiction.

Images of the brains of addicts confirm many of Volkow and Koob's hypothesis. They show alterations in regions crucial to judgment, decision-making and behavioral control.[122]

Free-will, self-control, choice. As Volkow says, we take them for granted.

It's almost impossible for most people to believe that biology and chemistry determine the extent to which we are capable of exercising free will, self-control, and choice. And it's even harder to understand the actual mechanisms at work.

To say that the mechanisms behind alcoholism are complex is a massive understatement.

But just because it's hard to understand and imagine, does not mean that they don't exist. Biological causes and mechanism exist in alcoholism, just as they do in every other disease.

There are those that disagree with Volkow and Koob though.

I received an email the other day from a highly respected doctor whose help I was seeking in writing this book.

His thoughts were this:

> "I feel very confident that addiction is primarily a psychological symptom, a compulsion... I am even more certain that the "chronic brain disease" idea that arose from research with rats by a few neuroscience researchers at the National Institute of Drug Addiction in Washington is completely wrong."

The doctor's perspective just 'did not compute' for me for many days as I thought about it. And finally, I realize why. His perspective (and the crux of most arguments against the 'brain disease' notion), is one that separates biology from psychology.

I don't know how that is possible, though.

Our psychologies (how we act, think, feel), come from a chunk of spongy tissue inside our skulls. There isn't one place where compulsive behaviors come from, and another place called the brain.

How is it possible to separate one from the other?

Is it such a leap of logic to believe (especially based on the genetic heritability of alcoholism and what scientists have now seen inside the brains of people with addictions) that compulsive behaviors come from brains that aren't functioning properly in a biological sense?

Most people would probably like to believe that there is no biology behind choosing and exercising free will.

We like to believe that everything we do, feel and think is within our control. As the Nike ad says, we just..... do it!

But that's not the case. In our brains, every thought, feeling, decision and choice are the end result of a complex series of chemical and electrical processes. In addiction, the processes are broken.

Imagine it this way: When other organs in our bodies stop functioning properly, they alert us to illness by causing us pain, causing vomiting, creating a feeling of sickness, generating bruising, producing swelling, reacting with an irregular heartbeat.

In other words, the organs in our bodies keep being organs, but they 'act out' in the way that only each organ uniquely can.

When the most complex organ–the brain, stops functioning properly, it alerts us to illness in some similar ways as other organs–pain and swelling for example.

But the brain has far more capability than the slab of meat that is your kidney.

It has other ways of acting out to alert us to an illness that your kidney does not.

We recognize bleeding and swelling as red flags of illness. But as a society we don't immediately recognize the ways that the *brain* alerts us to illness and it's about time we did.

Here are the things that the brain does when it is ill–when chemical and electrical processes aren't working as they should:

It obsesses, hoards, tells us to wash our hands despite the skin peeling off, tells us to stop leaving the house–ever, makes us binge on food, creates feelings of paralyzing anxiety, motivates us to steal compulsively, drives us to eat obsessively and then vomit it up; encourages us to cut ourselves, lets us hear voices that aren't our own, makes us feel hopeless, generates manic energy, tells us to jump in front of a train, makes us lose all ability to focus, forgets things, drives us to purchase compulsively, engages us in watching porn for hours, removes all motivation to get out of bed. And it tells us we must have another drink, no matter what.

Our sick brains generate a whole lot of disturbing behavior that alerts us to the fact that its biology is malfunctioning. It's a far more capable organ than a kidney or heart in the ways it alerts us to illness if we would just see these symptoms for what they are. All of these behaviors, thoughts, feelings, urges are manifestations–symptoms–of a malfunctioning brain.

But there's a catch. When our kidney malfunctions, our brain can still behave in a healthy manner. For example, our brain can still make the rational decision to take us to a hospital for dialysis once a week.

But when our brain malfunctions, unfortunately, we have a sick organ inside our heads that we, and others wish would act like a healthy organ.

And not only this, but others expect us to use it in a way that fixes a biological problem that lies inside.

It's a conundrum: It's like expecting you to use your kidney to fix your kidney.

But how about the alcoholics that *can* and *do* stop drinking?

Some people–for example, people who are able to stop drinking for the rest of their lives–are able to use the control that they may still retain to abstain from drinking, even though part of their brain is telling them to keep drinking.

But that doesn't mean that the illness has necessarily resolved (though sometimes it can, all by itself, just as other illnesses can).

An alcoholic who is sober for 30 years, who begins to drink again will binge just as if they never stopped drinking in the first place.

That's because abstinence (and all the counseling in the world) doesn't change the fundamental issues within the brain's biology.

That's also why sometimes when an alcohol stops drinking, they start a different compulsive behavior. Like binge eating, or obsessive house cleaning, or hoarding. Again, the behaviors are just symptoms of brain biology that is not working the way that it should.

Do We Hurt Alcoholics When We Treat it Like a Disease?

Some critics argue that by calling alcoholism a disease it somehow gives the addict an excuse, taking some responsibility off of them and placing it more on the healthcare system, including, of course, doctors.

They think that calling it a disease somehow gives the person with an addiction permission not to try to use the abilities that they have left to get better.

That's very possible. But it doesn't make it any less of a disease.

(And I'd also argue that the opposite has been true–by avoiding treating it like other illnesses, we've given people around alcoholics an excuse not to apply compassion, fairness and evidence-based medicine for far too long).

It doesn't matter what illness you have, it's the role of the person with it to advocate for their own healthcare and make an effort to do what they can to get better. (And it's the role of the medical system to use the tools and knowledge that they have to help that individual).

Maybe in the 1950s labeling something as a disease took all responsibility away from the sufferer, and placed it on the caregiver. My parents were brought up in a time when you did what your doctor told you to do and asked no questions.

But times have changed.

Today it is widely accepted that patients must participate in and commit to their own recovery, regardless of the illness.

Many parallels can be drawn between alcoholism and other diseases. For example, let's compare diabetes with alcoholism.

In both diseases:

- Patients need to take responsibility and manage their illness: take their medication, eat a healthy diet, reach out for support, and look after their physical and mental health;

- There are both environmental and genetic contributors to their development;

- There are nearly identical rates of noncompliance and relapse in both—between 30 and 40 percent of each group failed to follow even half their doctor's instructions. (This is also the case in asthma and hypertension).[58]

It strikes me however that there is one significant difference between the two: when people with diabetes relapse (for example, slipping into a diabetic coma), very rarely are they made to feel so much shame for doing so that they kill themselves. Whereas in alcoholism, that is not uncommon.

08 | WHAT IS ALCOHOLISM

"Addiction [is] a chronic disease where drugs have disrupted the most fundamental circuits, that enable us to do something that we take for granted—make a decision and follow it through."

—Dr. Nora Volkow, Director of the National Institute on Drug Abuse

A COMPLEX BRAIN DISEASE

So, if alcoholism is a disease, what kind of disease is it?

Most definitions only scratch the surface, specifying the symptoms, not the causes:

- "Alcohol dependence is typically characterized by someone having at least three of the following symptoms within the preceding 12 months: tolerance to drinking large amounts, withdrawal reactions when drinking is discontinued, loss of control over use of alcohol, efforts to stop or cut down, a great deal of time spent on drinking, giving up other activities to make way for drinking, and continued use despite resulting physical or psychological problems."[123]

- Webster's defines an alcoholic as "a person who is dependent on alcohol and who drinks compulsively and in such a way that his drinking is damaging to himself, to his way of life and to those about him."

- AA defines alcoholism as a "physical compulsion, coupled with a mental obsession."

Scientists tend to describe it more in relation to the organ it involves, than to its external symptoms.

For example, scientists Gilpin and Koob say that "Alcoholism is a chronic relapsing brain disease."[124]

And other scientists call it "a complex brain disease with significant behavioral characteristics."[3]

ALCOHOLISM 101

One of the (many) fascinating things about alcoholism is that it affects so many people, but very few of us can do anything but explain the outward symptoms of the disease.

For example, most people with diabetes know enough about their disease to say: 'my pancreas isn't fully functioning; my body doesn't make enough insulin so it can't process glucose properly and this can make my blood sugar levels too high.'

But ask an alcoholic what is going on inside their body and they probably won't be able to tell you what's going on with any accuracy at all.

If we are going to treat this as a disease then we need to think about it and understand it and be able to talk about it as one.

If I were an alcoholic, with one kind of alcoholism (there are probably many variations), I might try to explain this complex disease in a simple way, like this:

> *Early on, when I drank and alcohol entered my brain, my brain—through the dopamine and opioid systems—would reinforce the effects of the alcohol differently than yours.*
>
> *I felt alcohol more profoundly. Alcohol may have been to me more like a stronger drug would have been to you. This probably led me to drink more and drink more often than you.*
>
> *When we drink, our brains respond to alcohol by rebalancing chemicals such as GABA, glutamate, and dopamine. And then when alcohol leaves our brains, it readjusts those chemicals to normal levels.*
>
> *Eventually, maybe due to differences in my genes that affect how my brain can adapt and how it reacts to alcohol, my brain stopped going back 'to normal' after I stop drinking.*
>
> *For my brain, 'normal' became having alcohol in it.*
>
> *Now, when alcohol isn't in my brain, the balance of all of those natural chemicals is wrong. I have lower levels of some chemicals and higher levels of other chemicals than you.*
>
> *The number of receptors in my brain is increased in some areas and decreased in others. When I experience some things, electrical impulses light up parts of my brain, which would not light up in your brain, and vice versa.*

After many years of alcoholism, if you were to be able to see into my brain, you'd see visible gaps. My brain will be missing areas that your brain still has.

Because the balance of chemicals is wrong, I have high tolerance—my brain does not react as sensitively to alcohol as your brain does, and, therefore, I must drink far more to feel the effects of it now. This imbalance will worsen each time I drink.

All of this rewiring of my brain means that I am more impulsive and not as good at stopping impulses; I am more reactive to stress; I can't feel as calm as others; I feel less pleasure and interest in other things; I crave and think about and focus on alcohol; I don't interpret the weight of consequences in the same way other people do; I am less able to override the decision to drink than you are.

My brain has less ability to make choices that move me away from alcohol than yours does. When alcohol isn't in my brain, my brain makes me feel like I need it to feel normal.

ALCOHOLISM: A FOUR STAGE DISEASE

The above summary is a very simplistic description of alcoholism. The next few chapters delve further into research that explains more about the process of alcoholism in the human brain.

The progression of alcoholism follows four stages, and the final stage–addiction–is chronic, cyclical and progressive, worsening with every cycle.[125]

The stages are:

1) Stage 1–Initiation of substance use

2) Stage 2–Experimental use

3) Stage 3–Established use

4) Stage 4–Addiction

Within the fourth stage—Addiction—a continuous, vicious loop begins to cycle over and over again.

Like spokes on a wheel, this loop consists of the three 'sub-phases' of addiction, which are known as:

1)   Sub-phase 1: Withdrawal (and Negative Affect)

2)   Sub-phase 2: Preoccupation (and Anticipation & Craving)

3)   Sub-phase 3: Binge (and Intoxication)

Each of these sub-phases involves chemical interactions that trigger behaviors and motivators that are related to different areas of the brain:

1)   Withdrawal: extended amygdala

2)   Preoccupation: orbitofrontal cortex-dorsal striatum, prefrontal cortex, basolateral amygdala, hippocampus, insula

3)   Binge: ventral tegmental area and ventral striatum; cingulate gyrus, dorsolateral

Stages 1, 2 & 3: Awakening the Sleeping Giant

The first three stages of alcoholism may not look like anything out of the ordinary.

In these stages, drinking begins, alcohol is experimented with and ultimately drinking becomes established and routine.

In some people, routine drinking never crosses the line into uncontrollable drinking—and these three stages are benign.

But for others, the pathway through these stages awakens a sleeping giant.

There are several different factors that start to combine forces during the first three stages.

These factors include existing environmental and genetic vulnerabilities; as well as the hijacking of two of the brain's unique capabilities, called neuroplasticity and homeostasis.

Let's look at environmental and genetic vulnerabilities first. Then we'll move on to neuroplasticity and homeostasis.

Environmental and Genetic Vulnerabilities

Why do some individuals develop an addiction, while others do not?

The answer to that lies in a combination of environmental and genetic factors that create vulnerabilities in some people, making addiction more likely.[123]

And while environmental factors come into play early in the progression of the disease, genetic factors are important both in the early progression, and also contribute to maintaining the dependent state in some individuals.[1]

Let's look at the environment part first.

If you plant two identical, healthy seeds, you can grow two very different plants—depending upon the environment you plant them in.

Whereas a healthy environment is more likely to result in a healthy plant, an environment starved of nutrients, sunshine and water is more likely to result in an unhealthy plant that is vulnerable to further disease.

The same is true for humans.

If you'd like to turn a healthy baby into an addict, then abuse them, traumatize them and make alcohol an available outlet to salve their wounds from an early age.

Researchers have found that in environments where alcohol is more available and affordable, and where drinking can be initiated at a young age, vulnerability to alcoholism is increased.

They have also found an increased risk for individuals in families where both parents abuse alcohol and other drugs; where the parents' alcohol abuse is severe; where an alcoholic parent suffers from other mental illness; or in families where conflicts lead to aggression and violence in the family."[126]

Dr. Gabor Mate is an addiction specialist who has worked with addicts in some of the most addiction-riddled communities in Canada.

In his book, 'In the Realm of Hungry Ghosts: Close Encounters with Addiction', Mate writes about the severe impact troubled childhoods have on later problems with addiction.

In working with these communities, he consistently found that individuals with severe addiction had experienced "extraordinarily high percentages of childhood trauma of various sorts, including physical, sexual and emotional abuse."[127]

So, even with no apparent genetic predisposition, some individuals, if raised in environments that make them vulnerable, eventually struggle with addiction.

But what of those individuals who already have a genetic predisposition to alcoholism?

In this case, the environment can still be critical to the outcome in reducing or exaggerating existing genetic vulnerabilities.

For example, studies have found that "environments that exert more social control (e.g., higher parental monitoring, less migratory neighborhoods, etc.) tend to reduce genetic influences, whereas other conditions allow greater opportunity to express genetic predispositions, such as those characterized by more deviant peers and greater alcohol availability."[128]

The individual with the greatest potential for a less than optimal outcome is the one both genetically predisposed to illness, and who is raised in an environment that allows the genetic vulnerability to flourish. A child with a strong family background of alcoholism, and raised in a toxic environment is fighting some very high odds.

But what if environmental factors are removed? This is where we see the strong impact of genes.

Regardless of any environmental influence at all, children of alcoholics (even when not raised by the alcoholic), are four times more likely than the general population to develop alcohol problems.

And hinting at the relationship between clusters of genes related to a range of mental health issues, children of alcoholics (even when not raised by the alcoholic) also have a higher risk for many other emotional and behavioral problems.[126]

With a perfect upbringing an individual with a genetic pre-disposition to alcoholism can still emerge as an alcoholic because the disease is simply part of their DNA.

Genetic Processes

Genes influence many mechanisms in our body—from the way our senses interpret stimuli, to the amount of reinforcement our brains generate when we do something pleasureful.

Specific genes are tied to an array of processes: how much we desire reward, relief, excitement, to be soothed; to feel good; our levels of risk taking, impulsivity, how things taste to us—all of these things and many more that are related to drinking behavior not only increase our risk of developing dependence but are also heavily influenced by our genes.

Alcohol disorders cluster in families, as do other brain diseases with strong genetic elements, such as mood and anxiety disorders.[123]

Because the illness can appear over and over again in successive generations, studies of families affected by alcoholism have given scientists a way to learn some of its mysteries.

The Collaborative Study on the Genetics of Alcoholism (COGA) is a study that looked at alcoholics and their families—some 11,000 individuals (including 1200 treatment-seeking alcoholics). They were able to identify several biological patterns.

Their research confirmed earlier studies with twins that showed that at least 50% of the risk for alcohol dependence stems from inherited genetic factors[129] and that sons of alcoholic fathers are approximately four times more likely to develop alcoholism compared to the sons of non-alcoholics.[130]

Other research has provided evidence that the children of alcoholics are at a 7-fold risk of developing alcoholism.[131] And research has shown that this is the case even when children have been adopted by non-alcoholic parents very early in life.

In his book, *The 13th Step—Addiction in the Age of Brain Science*—respected addiction researcher Markus Heilig writes:

"Heritability of alcoholism seems to be almost identical for men and women…. heritability estimates from the twin studies are if anything likely to be underestimates…the true heritability of alcoholism is likely closer to 70%."[4]

Of families with a strong history of alcoholism, Heilig says, "we can simply advise people at high genetic risk to abstain from a drug that might otherwise kill them, even though others may be able to use the same substance without much harm and with enjoyment."[4]

Genes and Early Drinking

From the very first drink they take, some alcoholics experience alcohol differently than non-alcoholics. It just feels different—and this makes them vulnerable to addiction.

Alcohol for some alcoholics may feel like a much more pleasurable, stronger drug feels to a non-alcoholic. Researchers call this "subjective response" to alcohol.

This finding is related to variations in genes found in greater quantities in alcoholics with a family history of alcoholism.

Animals and humans who carry these particular genetic variations are simply pre-programmed to be more vulnerable to alcohol dependence. They have been shown to:

- Report greater reinforcement from alcohol.[132][133]

- Metabolize alcohol more quickly. (For example, the speed of oxidation is eight times faster for a man who is homozygous for the ADH1B-2 and ADH1C-1 alleles, as compared to a man who is homozygous for the ADH1B-1 and ADH1C-2 alleles.)[134]

- Display increased stimulation to alcohol.[135]

- Consume more alcohol and prefer it more than do others.[135]

- Experience a greater response to alcohol cues in the mesocorticolimbic areas of the brain.[136]

- Experience a stronger striatal dopamine response to alcohol.[137]

- Show greater response sensitivity in the ventral striatum during anticipation and reward.

- Experience significantly more rewarding effects such as strong vigor and positive mood.[138]

These are the people who, before serious debilitating dependence sets in, may seem to come alive on alcohol. They may simply enjoy the experience of drinking on many levels that someone without this genetic preprogramming does not.

Later in the book there is another chapter dedicated to the genetics of alcoholism. But now, let's move onto an important phenomena called neuroplasticity.

Neuroplasticity

So genetics and environment are key variables in the development of alcoholism.

And scientists believe that one or both affect neuroplasticity.

Neuroplasticity is a mouthful of a word. It's a term that describes the amazing ability of the brain to change and adapt.

Examples of neuroplasticity can be seen in many aspects of life. For example, one study showed that the more time London taxi drivers spent on the job, the larger their hippocampus (the part of the brain associated with navigation) grew.[139] That's due to neuroplasticity.

Neuroplasticity allows the brain to rewire itself in response both to the internal and external environment. No other part of the body can do this. It can delete neural connections and strengthen others. It can rebuild neural circuits allowing uninjured parts of the brain to take over from damaged parts.

Neuroplasticity can be fleeting—lasting hours or weeks—or permanent—continuing until the day you die.

And while neuroplasticity helps us survive, it can backfire.

Neuroplasticity works against alcoholics as the brain of the alcoholic responds and adapts to the foreign substance—alcohol—that has entered the brain.

What one scientist calls "repeated pharmacological insult to the brain circuits,"[140] causes pathological changes in the brain. It causes changes that solidify deeply automated habits.

When an alcoholic passes through the stages from initiation of substance use and eventually into dependence on alcohol, irreversible neuroplasticity is occurring.

In some ways, the brain of someone with alcohol dependence is an extremely well-trained machine.

It may have been designed to drink (through subjective response) more than the non-alcoholic brain in the first place. And now through constant intake of alcohol ('training sessions') it has retrained itself–it has neuroadapted to a stasis where the brain is more comfortable when it contains alcohol.

But unfortunately neuroadaptation in alcoholics seems to be very much a one way street with no going back.

Just like the taxi driver's brain changed physically, so does the brain of the alcoholic.[129] But whereas in the taxi driver, these changes may reverse themselves months or years after they no longer needed, in the alcoholic, the changes can be irreversible, helping to sustain the disease.[1]

Many years after detoxification, even after decades of abstinence, due to the neural adaptations in the brains of alcoholics, they remain at risk for relapse, falling back again into excessive and uncontrolled drinking.[117]

Homeostasis

One of the primary jobs of the brain is to maintain balance–or homeostasis.

The thermostat in your home also has the job of maintaining balance. By turning the furnace and air conditioning on and off it constantly recalibrates the temperature, aiming for a predetermined temperature set-point.

If cold air enters the window of your home, the thermostat senses the drop in temperature–the imbalance–and turns on the furnace so that hot air gets pumped into the house.

Drinking alcohol is like letting that cold air in through a window on purpose. Alcohol enters the brain and disturbs the balance of chemicals so that we can feel the relaxing and enjoyable effects of the imbalance.

Just like the thermostat, the brain realizes that it is not in equilibrium—not maintaining its set-point. So it reacts to try to recalibrate, trying to regain its balance point (or 'homeostasis'). Some of the chemicals it uses to do this are GABA, glutamate, and dopamine.

These chemicals, as well as serotonin, norepinephrine, and other neurotransmitters play important roles in the brain related to reward, relief, obsession, and habit learning.

These systems of transmitters, neurotransmitters, and brain matter affect cognition, mood, emotion, and pain.

When we drink, the pleasurable effect we feel is the result of the brain becoming unnaturally overstimulated by dopamine.

Dopamine is part of the reward system in the brain, and is a chemical that allows us to anticipate and feel pleasure.

Increasing dopamine in the brain is like turning up the dance music at a party. The highs of life are experienced via the reward system—getting a compliment, the fun of a roller coaster, laughter with friends are all made possible via dopamine and the reward system.

GABA slows the brain down. It's like the body's natural relaxant which is why it is called an inhibitory neurotransmitter.

GABA is an important 'feel good' chemical in our brain—it is a calming and relaxing chemical whose role is to relieve anxiety, pain, confusion and stress. That relaxed feeling you get when you are having a massage—GABA is probably a big part of that. Balanced levels of GABA are essential for contentment, peace of mind and emotional stability.

High amounts of GABA can create a 'fog', as well as the comforting feeling of contentment or the experience of 'feeling no pain' that we feel when alcohol is in their system. GABA also creates the slowing, sedative effect of alcohol. Speech, movement, and thoughts are all effectively slowed causing slurred speech, slow, clumsy movements, and inhibiting thought processes.

Glutamate speeds up and stimulates reactions. It's the body's natural stimulant, which is why it is called an excitatory neurotransmitter.

Alcohol inhibits glutamate, increases GABA, and increases dopamine. These changes result in slowing down the brain; relaxing it; while letting it feel good.

As these changes occur, the brain recognizes that its equilibrium is off.

The brain identifies that it does not need as much effect from the GABA as it is receiving. It tries to reduce the amount of GABA as well as turning off the receptors that are receiving the GABA.

Over time, as with neuroplasticity, the brains ability to recalibrate backfires on the alcoholic.

The brain starts to identify its balance of brain chemicals as the 'new normal'–the new set-point. Through neuroplasticity it adapts to that new normal–fewer GABA receptors are now being used–even after alcohol leaves the system. *The revised brain is now less capable of calming itself down.*

The same process occurs with glutamate, which was initially inhibited by the alcohol.

In a reaction to the sedative, foggy, slowing impact of the flood of GABA, the brain tries to recalibrate and re-stimulate the brain by increasing glutamate and the number of glutamate receptors. As with GABA, the brain gets used to the increase, and through neuroplasticity, the new set-point is a brain with more glutamate and glutamate receptors. *The revised brain is more stimulated and alert.*

And again, the same process occurs with dopamine. Alcohol increases the dopamine levels to create good feelings. The brain identifies the rush of dopamine and recalibrates to lower the effect of dopamine, downregulating positive reward pathways, reducing dopamine and dopamine receptors. The new set-point or 'new normal' becomes a brain with less dopamine and fewer dopamine receptors. *The revised brain is less receptive to feeling good.*

Unfortunately, once alcohol is no longer in the system, the brain can't immediately readapt and is now left to function with more glutamate, less GABA and less dopamine (the exact opposite of the effect that alcohol was used to create in the first place.)

Now, with a new set-point, it is harder for the brain to feel the same effects of the alcohol as before. And so in future binges, more and more alcohol must be consumed to achieve an effect that was easier to reach in previous binges. This is called the development of tolerance.[141]

Tolerance makes the alcoholic drink more to try to achieve the desired effects. The brain recalibrates further and the vicious cycle goes on and on reinforcing itself with each cycle.

Whether or not the alcoholic's brain was wired differently to begin with, it certainly is now.

With these changes, or 'neuroadaptations' in the brain, the brain of the alcoholic no longer functions like that of the non-alcoholic.

When a non-alcoholic is 'sober' our brains maintain a balance of chemicals that allow us to feel happiness, contentment, not too much anxiety, and emotional stability.

But when an alcoholic is 'sober' it means that they are living with a brain that has been adapted for alcohol.

If there is an exact opposite of 'drunk', it is what the alcoholic now lives with and experiences. (Imagine a continuum that describes feeling, with 'sober' in the middle, 'drunk' on one end, and 'opposite of drunk' on the other end.)

Living with a sensitized glutamate system is like being a passenger in a car where the driver keeps a nervous foot on the accelerator pedal.

The imbalanced glutamate system means the alcoholic is less ability to calm the ragged edges of life. Without alcohol, the brain suddenly is experiencing less calm—more anxiety, less contentment, more of what is called 'negative effect' or 'nervous system hyperactivity.'

The individual may feel restless, irritable and on edge. This is the reason why alcohol is described as a depressant—after alcohol has left the system the brain is impaired in its ability to maintain contentment—it has trouble responding normally to stress and anxiety-provoking events.[142]

Life without alcohol may go on, but the alcoholic's brain has been effectively rewired.

As a sober person, the alcoholic's handicapped brain is now less physically capable of feeling and enjoying the highs of life.

All the things that make us feel good, happy, optimistic, deeply content and excited do not make as much of an impact. The number of GABA receptors needed to achieve a normal level of calm are missing. The brain is literally unable to feel as much enjoyment of life as before the damage occurred.[143]

These descriptions of the permanent recalibration that takes place in the brains of alcoholics is not theoretical. They have been well documented by scientists.

One of the ways that scientists can measure GABA, glutamate and other alcohol-induced neuroadaptation is through the use of Magnetic Resonance Spectroscopy (MRS).

Scientists using an MRS to measure GABA and glutamate concentrations and imbalances have found for example that in some abstinent alcoholics, GABA levels are as much as 30% lower than in non-alcoholics.[144]

MRS testing can also measure other aspects of alcohol-induced neuroadaptation by measuring other chemicals in the brain.

One chemical is called N-acetyl aspartate (NAA). A lower concentration in the brain of NAA indicates damage within the brain and is linked to lower neurocognitive and motor functioning as well as poorer performances on measures of executive skills and working memory.

Lower levels of NAA affect our ability to remember things we have heard (auditory-verbal memory) and pay attention.

MRS testing has shown lower NAA levels in the brains of alcoholics, suggesting damage to neurons, and other components of the brain at the cellular level.[144]

Treatment Targets

By learning all that they have about the first three stages, and how alcoholics differ in their experience of these stages, scientists are able to come up with treatment targets.

These targets for stage 1, 2, and 3 might include now, or in the future:

- Targeting Environmental Causes: Preventative measures against environmental causes such as social programs that attempt to better protect children; and alcohol pricing and marketing policies that make alcohol less accessible.

- Targeting Genetic Vulnerabilities: Preventative measures that identify and counsel individuals at high genetic risk; gene therapy which changes genetic makeup; treatment that interferes with the expression of genes.

- Targeting Neuroplasticity: treatment that helps the brain use its own neuroplasticity to revert back to a normal homeostasis.

STINKING THINKING: PREOCCUPATION

FROM ROUTINE DRINKING TO DEPENDENCE

Once dependence is in place, we see the alcoholic begin to cycle through addiction's sub-phases: Binge–Withdrawal–Preoccupation.

Scientists draw these three sub-phases as a circle, one leading to the next and to the next and then back to the beginning again.

But in reality, there may actually be a great deal of overlap between the Withdrawal and Preoccupation phases since the experiences of each stage can (and often are) experienced at the same time.

We'll start by looking at the Preoccupation (Anticipation & Craving) sub-phase.

This is a sub-phase that characterized by drive and desire–the experience of wanting.

AA doesn't use subphases to describe the science of alcoholism. But they do have a term that describes the Preoccupation stage very well, and this is 'Stinking Thinking'.

What is going on biologically in the brain to generate drive and intense desire for alcohol? This section looks at some of the enemies of sobriety an alcoholic must conquer to avoid relapse.

These include cues and other triggers, craving, conditioned and automated responses.

TRIGGER & RESPONSE

Often there is an experience or event–a trigger–that undermines good intention, is not dealt with effectively and precipitates a relapse.

Triggers can have two components:

1) Craving (emerging from alcohol cues)

2) Stress (emerging from life)

When we are triggered, how we deal with the response to the trigger is critical. To avoid relapse we need to be able to control our response to the trigger and employ a positive coping behavior.

But unfortunately, triggers can be difficult for the alcoholic brain to cope with. That's because:

- Drinking-cues (which may be experienced at an unconscious level) trigger intense desire/craving for alcohol and generate automated, habitual reactions;

- Alcoholic brains are less capable of dealing with stress, and due to the surrounding destruction the illness causes, they may have many more stressful events to overcome;

- Alcoholic brains are weaker than others in elements that make up self-control and the ability to implement coping behaviors.

Or in other words, while we expect alcoholics to do their best to control their behavior and cope in a positive way, damage and neuroadaptation to their brains has set them up particularly well to fail in this regard.

Many of the elements needed to battle dependence (how one reacts to stress; a feeling of mental well-being, the ability to make sound, measured unimpulsive choices) seem to be the exact set of skills that are casualties of the damage incurred in the brain through alcoholism.

If someone were to design the perfect disease—one that controlled your offence and at the same time took away the capability of putting up a good defense—alcoholism might be the result.

Let's look at these elements one at a time.

Trigger 1: Craving via Drinking Cues

Cravings are often triggered by drinking or alcohol cues. A drinking cue is anything that an alcoholic has been conditioned to associate with drinking.

When we are conditioned by something, we react automatically, before even becoming aware that we are reacting. When an alcoholic sees or experiences a drinking-cue, an automatic conditioned response occurs that generates thoughts and craving for alcohol.

Drinking cues can be photos of alcohol, the presence of a drinking buddy, driving past a liquor store, feelings of loneliness or memories of difficult situations which had previously been associated with alcohol intake, or even feelings of happiness and excitement previously associated with alcohol consumption.[118]

Cues and Relapse

The craving that results from drinking-cues is dangerous because, as scientists have shown, the greater the craving experienced by an alcoholic, the more likely the alcoholic is to relapse.[145]

It has also been shown in brain imaging studies that patients who suffer from multiple relapses and who relapse quickly after detoxification experience much stronger cue-induced activations of part of the brain than patients who were able to abstain from alcohol for longer periods of time.[118]

It's not that the longer-abstaining patients were stronger or 'trying harder' to remain abstinent.

What is occurring is that the brains of the patients who relapse quickly respond to alcohol cues much more fiercely.

Cue and Craving Example with Food

Imagine you smell, see or just imagine an image of your favorite food (for example, for you, it may be chocolate, roasted garlic, fresh baked bread, fried bacon, or the scent of vanilla in an apple pie). This is a 'food-cue'.

Immediately you may automatically notice that the craving and desire to eat that food may increase. You might notice now the saliva in your mouth has increased even before you recognized the presence of a craving for one of those delicious foods.

This is because your brain has become hardwired to associate the scent or image of the enjoyable food (the 'food-cue') with the enjoyment experienced when the food is actually consumed. It's a conditioned response.

Even if you are shown pictures and scents of the food, but you know that there is no food available for you to eat, it does not stop your brain from craving the food.

Your brain has been programmed over time by the activation of the dopamine system to have this conditioned response, whether you know you can have the food or not. Your brain is now expecting the food, anticipating it, waiting for that food. You may be a little preoccupied by that craving.

You may even have had the experience of being unable to shake the craving until you finally give in to it, eating the food that you are desiring.

This is because the dopamine and opioid systems don't just make us feel good when we experience a specific thing we enjoy, but perhaps more importantly, they make us really want the thing in the first place until we get it.

Dopamine is tied to 'wanting' and the prediction of reward.[146] The food cue doesn't necessarily make you feel good–it makes you *want the thing* that makes you feel good.

Or more simply: We see/smell it → we want it → we feel discomfort until we get it → when we get it we feel the original good feeling it brings, and we also feel the relief brought about by no longer wanting it.

The same thing happens when an alcoholic is shown an alcohol cue. These cues trigger the dopamine system at a subconscious level, creating the craving for alcohol which was the original source of the enjoyment these cues are associated with.

Relief from this uncomfortable craving experience is not felt until the alcohol is a) consumed and b) achieves the desired feeling.[146]

Addictive drugs (including alcohol) are addictive specifically because they generate an intense craving and experience of discomfort unless the craving is relieved.

The craving experience for that delicious piece of food you may now be imagining might be compared to the annoyance of hearing a tiny mosquito buzzing around in another room.

The craving experience for someone with a drug addiction may be more like walking through life with two hundred mosquitos flying around your head.

It takes a great deal of self-control not to take a swat at them from time to time. And when under stress, raising a hand to take a swat becomes almost an automatic reaction that is impossible to control.

Craving & Dopamine in Alcoholics

Because of the brain's rebalancing process described earlier, the brains of alcoholics have far fewer dopamine receptors than non-alcoholics.[147] And this is the case even many months after protracted detoxification.[146] Alcoholics also have more mu-opiate receptors in the brain's ventral striatum.

These imbalances make the experience of craving alcohol far more intense than the craving a brain with healthy levels of necessary chemicals would experience.

These two long-term imbalances—fewer dopamine receptors, and more mu-opiate receptors—are measurable, and directly correlate with levels of craving.[147118]

In alcoholics, the fewer dopamine receptors, the more the brain lights up with activity when it is shown alcohol-related imagery and given drinking-cues.[147]

This dopamine/alcohol cue connection is also what helps transform a habit into a compulsion (or dependence).

One of the parts of the brain where dopamine increases when alcoholics see alcohol cues is called the dorsal striatum.

The dorsal striatum is involved in hardwiring habits. Because the alcohol-cue effect also involves the dorsal striatum, a habit is created and strengthened. Ultimately the habit becomes a compulsion.[146]

Types of Cravings

We experience different kinds of cravings. And different parts of the brain are responsible for generating the variations of cravings we experience.

The Psychobiological Pathway Model of Craving, developed by Verheul in 1999 breaks craving down into three brain pathways, with different neurotransmitters and receptors involved:

1) Reward Craving–dopamine and opioid systems

2) Relief Craving–GABA and glutamate systems

3) Obsessive Craving–serotonin systems

Reward craving involves the dopamine and opioid systems (the reward systems) in the brain.

A *reward craving* is one where we desire reward, stimulation or enhancement.

For example, when my mouth waters as I look at a juicy steak sizzling on a barbecue, I am experiencing a reward craving. I want that good feeling of eating the steak.

Relief craving involves GABA and glutamate in the brain. When I have a relief craving, I desire the cessation of an experience I feel to be negative. I want the reduction of tension or anxiety.

For example, when I have studied night and day for an important exam and will feel a constant pressure and tenseness until I have completed my exam I am craving relief. If my child has gone missing and I feel wound up, nervous, anxious and a yearning feeling until my child is back with me, I am experiencing relief craving.

Obsessive craving involves the serotonin system. Lack of control, obsession, compulsiveness and disinhibition characterizes obsessive craving. When I know there is a chocolate bar sitting on the shelf near my desk and I just can't draw my mind away from it; I can't stop thinking about it, this is obsessive craving.

The feeling of salivating over a steak or yearning for the return of a child are very different feelings in some ways, and very similar in others.

Both involve a sense of 'wanting' though the motivating components (desire for something good, or the cessation of something bad) are very different.

My examples used a steak and a child.

But for alcoholics, while the motivating component can be different, the object of desire can be the same—alcohol.

Alcohol can be craved for its reward, as well as for its ability to lessen anxiety and tension.

There are some theories, discussed later in this book about Type A and Type B alcoholics and their unique characteristics.

Type A alcoholics are those who have a later onset of the disease whereas Type B alcoholics may experience the disease earlier in life ('early-onset').

It's theorized that Type A alcoholics experience craving more as 'Relief Craving,' whereas, Type B alcoholics intensely experience 'Reward Craving.'[47]

Trigger 2: Stress

An alcohol-cue resulting in craving is just one kind of a trigger, which can precipitate a relapse.

There are other triggers, many of which create stress. Stress is the enemy of the alcoholic.

Our ability to cope is critical.

For example, a person who is able to execute a coping strategy—such as leaving the room, meditating, calling a friend, etc., is less likely to relapse than someone without the ability to execute a coping strategy.[75]

A brain that is strong in other ways may be able to employ a positive coping strategy, and not give in to the trigger.

But alcoholic brains are far more responsive to stress than the non-alcoholic brain. A 2008 functional magnetic resonance imaging study published in Addiction Biology by Dr. Jodi Gilman and Dr. Daniel Hommer illustrated this vividly.

Frightening, negative images intended to illicit anxiety were shown to detoxified alcoholics and non-alcoholics.

The exaggerated stress response could be seen as parts of the brain (the ventral, object-related visual processing stream, the insular cortex and the right parahippocampal gyrus) lit up vividly in alcoholics—far more so than in the non-alcoholics.[148]

So a stressful event to you and I may be proportionally much more stressing to an alcoholic.

This increased sensitivity to stress only worsens with repeated withdrawals.[118]

And of course this heightened stress response makes it even more challenging to cope with the trigger.

So once again—one of the things we expect and sometimes demand of the alcohol—to simply choose a different course when in a stressful situation—is a challenge that the alcoholic brain is much less equipped to handle, than the non-alcoholic brain.

Alcoholism is indeed a cunning disease.

COPING MECHANISMS & SELF CONTROL

Alcohol cues and stressful triggers create a landslide of automated, unconscious processes and responses (craving, obsessive thoughts, and other habitual responses).

This cascade creates a barrage of pressure that tests self-control and the ability to employ positive coping mechanisms.

And unfortunately, weakened self-control is a further casualty of the neuroadaptations which have gone on in the alcoholic's brain.

Damage from the alcoholism affects systems utilizing the signaling molecules dopamine, opioid peptides, gamma-aminobutyric acid, glutamate, and serotonin, as well as systems modulating the brain's stress response.[149]

With systems like these intact, healthy minds can exert self-control by weighing the consequences of our actions, processing and evaluating information before making an impulsive decision, and changing our direction if a conditioned response or desire is taking us down the wrong path.

It is this set of actions and behaviors that are the ingredients of self-control.

But brains damaged so globally are less able to exert self-control.

Scientists break self-control up into three components:

- Delayed discounting

- Reflection-impulsivity

- Intentional action

When people with addictions are measured on these abilities, they score poorly, because the areas of their brains that need to be strong to score well have changed.

'Delayed discounting' is the ability and willingness to put off present gratification in the interest of a bigger long-term reward. People with addictions are more likely to take a smaller reward now than a larger reward later. Their brains don't calculate the value and associated motivation of the later reward in the same way that the brains of non-addicts do.

'Reflection-impulsivity' reflects consideration of information over time. It is greater in individuals who respond to challenges more quickly, with less information processing time needed than those with lower reflection impulsivity. People with addictions typically have high reflection impulsivity.

And 'intentional action' is the ability to consciously stop an automatic behavior once it has been set in motion.

Let's look at this important ability.

Neurons that control automatic responses are activated before we are even aware of the intention. That means that your brain has already sensed a trigger and started to take action on this trigger before you even know it.

If you have ever reached out and caught a glass toppling off a counter, found yourself half way home to a house you no longer live in, or brushed your teeth and don't remember it, then you've experienced this yourself.

Maybe you spent a lot of time in ball sports growing up. I did, and this training conditioned me to catch things automatically.

Recently I was playing darts with a friend and the dart I had just thrown glanced off the dartboard and rebounded into the air toward me. I automatically stepped forward and caught it in my hand—sharp end first.

I know you aren't supposed to catch a dart and as I started to move to catch it I became aware of this. However, by the time my thinking caught up with my automatic reflex, the dart was already in my finger.

Had I been able to stop this automatic behavior before catching the dart, my fronto-median cortex would have lit up.

This is the part of the brain that steps in to stop reflective behavior.

But for people with addictions (and perhaps for me too), the response in their fronto-median cortexes is not as strong as for people without addictions.[58]

Studies have shown that these deficits in alcoholics are caused by impairment of the dopamine system within areas of the brain such as the orbitofrontal cortex, cingulate gyrus, and dorsolateral prefrontal cortex, the ventral tegmental area and the ventral striatum.

The impairment of this system has devastating results in many areas. Deficits in this system have been shown to result in:

- An increase in compulsive behaviors;

- Problems with the attention processing systems (focused on alcohol; not focused on other things);[118]

- Increased inability to divert attention away from conditioned cues;[118]

- The loss of inhibitory control resulting in the initiation of impulsive behavior;

- An inability to stop certain behaviors, especially automatic ones, once they have started;

- The loss of executive function which results in the failure to follow through on intentional actions;[146]

- Temporal discounting–less ability to choose the larger reward that is farther away than the smaller reward that is immediately before them;[1]

- Decreased ability for the brain to respond to 'new reward-indicating stimuli' (such as new social interactions, hobbies or interests)'[118]

- Increased reaction to alcohol cues.[118]

All of these impairments caused by damage to the dopamine system have a substantial impact on the alcoholic.

In fact, scientists have seen that the more slowly the dopamine system recovers, the greater the risk of relapse will be during early abstinence.[147]

Really–the brain is an incredible thing.

In addiction, we see a brain that has redesigned itself to be the perfect addiction machine.

You couldn't design a brain more susceptible to relapse if you tried.

TREATMENT TARGETS

In this stage we have looked at cues, cravings, conditioned responses, automated responses, stress and elements of self-control.

All these mechanisms behind addiction are products of brain function and create targets for scientists.

Many of the medications in this book are effective because they interrupt these elements of addiction, and drugs will continue to be developed that get better and better at this.

For example, medications can:

- Stop cues from generating automatic responses like craving

- Stop the feeling of craving

- Interrupt conditioned and automated responses

- Reduce exaggerated stress responses

- Rebalance dopamine and dopamine receptors

- Decrease compulsive behavior

- Increase strength of executive control over automated responses

- Increase response to other reward stimuli

Some of the medications that seem to target at least the top half of that list (interrupting craving, automated response to alcohol cues, and reducing stress response) include baclofen, acamprosate, and topiramate.

GOING BACK OUT: BINGE/INTOXICATION

As we've learned, well before an alcoholic relapses, they are battling with cues, conditioned response, craving, and triggers. And we've learned that the mechanism they need to exhibit self-control against this barrage of enemies has been weakened.

The Binge (Intoxication) sub-phase occurs when the onslaught proves too much, and the alcoholic's defense mechanisms fail. Loss of control occurs and the drinking begins.

The Binge/Intoxication phase is often called relapse.

Or in AA vernacular, members say he or she "went back out."

In a weak moment, this can happen to any alcoholic.

Relapse isn't a failure. It's a symptom.

Markus Heilig in his book writes:

> *"Relapse does not have to be a disaster… it is an expected element of any chronic disorder such as addiction, much the way it is with hypertension, asthma, or diabetes. It should be approached with calmness, optimism, and a belief that something can be learned from each episode."*

ALCOHOL DEPRIVATION EFFECT: A BIOLOGICAL MECHANISM CONTRIBUTING TO RELAPSE

Relapse is also something we see in animal models of alcoholism. (And not just in animals with bad attitudes.)

The Alcohol Deprivation Effect (ADE) is a phenomenon that is not often heard about in our discussions of alcoholism yet it has been known about for decades by scientists and is an important underlying mechanism of relapse.

It is not a term I have ever heard in an AA room, yet understanding its existence helps us understand the biologically-motivated underpinnings of relapse.

The ADE was first discovered by Drs. Sinclair and Senter in 1968[150] in rat studies and has been recreated and studied by respected scientists dozens of times since.[117]

Sinclair and Senter gave rats access to alcohol for extended periods of time (effectively addicting them) and then suddenly forced them into abstinence, depriving them of alcohol for lengths of time.

They found that when alcohol was once again made available to the rats that they would drink more–2 to 3 times more–than they had done before.

They would drink compulsively and heavily, shifting their drinking behavior to drink more highly concentrated alcohol solutions to rapidly increase blood alcohol concentrations and achieve intoxication. Their behavior mimicked the behavior of alcoholics who abstained for periods of time and then began drinking again.

Scientists following in footsteps of early ADE researchers discovered other patterns within the Alcohol Deprivation Effect.

They found for example in rats that the size of the relapse binge depended upon the duration of the original drinking, and the length of abstinence. The size of the relapse was also strongly dependent upon the rats' genetic background. (The rats used in testing are of a genetic-strain which can become addicted to alcohol–there are other genetic-strains that are less vulnerable to alcoholism, again revealing the genetic culpability of the disease).

The ADE is such a robust phenomenon that it has been described as is almost "mathematically" predictable in its behavior.[117]

Scientists noticed that the longer the rat had been drinking, the more desperate they were to drink once the abstinence phase was reintroduced.

For example, after a short-term alcohol experience, some rats chose a delicious sugary solution instead of a bitter alcohol solution, exhibiting the ability to exert some self-control over their behavior.

But after much longer-term alcohol addiction, rats would choose the bitter alcohol over the sugary solution regardless of its disgusting taste.

Heavily addicted rats would also completely change their regular drinking patterns, abandoning normal sleeping/eating patterns in favor of drinking.

NOT IF BUT WHEN

If one is an alcoholic, in regards to relapse, the question may not be 'will they?', but 'when will they?'

With no further intervention after complete detoxification (even if treated as inpatients until complete remission of physical withdrawal symptoms) research has shown that up to 85% of all patients relapse.[118]

And amazingly, brain imaging studies of abstinent alcoholics can predict with incredible accuracy, who will and will not relapse, based on the levels of two chemicals in the brain.

In a study, at 1 month of abstinence, alcoholics with decreased frontal white matter chemical 'NAA' were 3.4 times more likely to relapse. Alcoholics with decreased frontal gray matter chemical 'Cho' were 4.8 times more likely to relapse.[118]

By adding other factors (the presence of mood disorders and brain processing speed) to the analysis, the model accurately predicted more than 90% of the relapsers and 80% of the abstainers—proving that relapse is far more a matter of biology than of willpower, attitude or meeting attendance.[118]

The scientists also felt that if they could add knowledge of the individuals' genetic makeup (such as whether the person carried key variations in the COMT or OPRM1 genes), that they would be able to even further improve the accuracy of their relapse predictions beyond 90%.[144]

•••

With each relapse, an alcoholic's brain must react again and again to high volumes of toxic alcohol, further damaging and changing its circuitry. Over time, as damage progresses, the original motivators for drinking change.

Before an alcoholic becomes dependent upon alcohol, they may have been motivated by the positive effects of alcohol–the feeling of the rush of dopamine and soothing feeling of alcohol in their system.

However, the longer the addiction progresses, the less attainable these positive feelings become, and over time, the addict tends to drink more to avoid the negative feelings flooding their system, and is less motivated by the rush of the reward system.

TREATMENT TARGETS

The binge phase utilizes treatments that target two areas:

- Lessening the 'payoff'

- Breaking the conditioning

Medications such as naltrexone and nalmefene (and any drug used 'as needed') target this sub-phase, using a phenomena called pharmacological extinction, which was pioneered many years ago by the late Dr. David Sinclair.

Anyone who has successfully used a smoking cessation drug–such as Champix (varenicline) has experienced extinction. (Varenicline also happens to be a medication for alcoholism found on the B-List in this book.)

Smokers who take varenicline while smoking soon discover that it dulls the effect of their drug of choice (nicotine). Alcoholics taking nalmefene and naltrexone have reported that the feeling of alcohol is dulled.

This lessens the enjoyment of alcohol, but it also has a more significant effect, which is to diminish the strength of the brain's conditioning.

In those for whom this approach is effective, drinking simply seems to become less and less attractive, and the brain's connection between drinking and reward weakens.

For those of us who are not alcoholic–imagine that we have an intense craving for chocolate that is triggered each time you pass a chocolate store. If every time we passed the chocolate store we went in and ate horrible tasting chocolate, and did not receive the rush of pleasure we were used to, eventually, the conditioned response to seeing and smelling the chocolate store would weaken and go away. While overly simplistic, this is how medications targeting this phase work too.

DRY DRUNK: WITHDRAWAL

"I'm gonna need someone to hold me down. I'm gonna need someone to care. I'm gonna writhe and shake my body. I'll start pulling out my hair... Son of a bitch. Give me a drink. One more night. This can't be me. Son of a bitch. If I can't get clean I'm gonna drink my life away...

...My heart was aching, hands are shaking. Bugs are crawling all over me."

From 'SOB', Nathaniel Rateliff & The Night Sweats

For friends and family watching an alcoholic caught in the disease, it is when the alcoholic is drinking that the experience of alcoholism may be the worst. Sometimes we have a misconception that if only the alcoholic would stop drinking, everything would be okay. So it's a relief when finally, for whatever reason, the alcoholic is able to stop drinking.

For the alcoholic, it may be just the opposite, as it is when the drinking has ended that the most difficult and painful parts of alcoholism are experienced.

Sobriety can be excruciating.

Initially, there are physical withdrawal symptoms that can be extremely uncomfortable, and sometimes life threatening.

But the 'unseen' psychological symptoms caused by the very real dysregulation of brain chemicals and changes in the brain may be much harder to tolerate, and last much longer than any physical symptom.

PHYSICAL SYMPTOMS

Physical withdrawal symptoms occur when the level of alcohol has dropped drastically in the body and brain and the brain reacts sharply and quickly to try to recalibrate and readjust its chemistry.

Many of us are familiar with the feeling of a hangover. A hangover occurs after drinking has been discontinued and usually lasts for about a day.

Alcoholics experience what is called 'Alcohol Withdrawal Syndrome' (AWS).

AWS lasts longer than a hangover and occurs in people who are caught in the addiction cycle.

It usually begins 8 hours after blood alcohol levels decrease and peaks at 72 hours. These symptoms may last several days or even weeks depending upon severity, and can be life threatening.[141]

The symptoms of AWS can include upset stomach, sweating, shaking, uncomfortable anxiety, paranoia, the feeling of being overwhelmed, body temperature fluctuations, nightmares, agitation, increased pulse, increased respiration rates, cardiac arrhythmia, fatigue, increased blood pressure, hand tremor, and insomnia.

A group of especially severe withdrawal symptoms is called DTs (delirium tremens) and includes visual and sensory disturbances, confusion, hallucinations, and seizure.

When people die from AWS, it is usually from hyperthermia, cardiac arrhythmias, and complications of seizures.[141]

WITHDRAWAL & COLD TURKEY

When someone is on medication for depression or anxiety or another illness related to the brain, doctors advise strongly against immediately discontinuing or stopping the medication without a tapering process.

This is because the sudden absence in the brain and body of a chemical it has adapted to is dangerous.

But when an alcoholic enters a detox facility or is supported in some other way to stop a binge, usually the availability of alcohol is removed completely. This is probably done not for any sound medical reason, but as part of the punishment we inflict on alcoholics for relapse.

Several drugs have been tested for their ability to help moderate the withdrawal process and in fact, it was through this research that the properties of several of the drugs in this book (baclofen among others) were discovered to be helpful in a more long-term way for alcoholics.

PSYCHOLOGICAL SYMPTOMS

After the experience of physical withdrawal has passed, the alcoholic may be left with a psychological condition called Negative Effect.

As discussed earlier, the 'new normal' of the alcoholic brain is completely off balance.

Anyone who has experienced ongoing, chronic anxiety or depression or the inability to find pleasure in life, may understand the discomfort and psychic pain of a chronically depressed brain.

AA recognizes alcoholics who are experiencing the effects of the brain's recalibration. They call them 'dry drunks.'

AA's Big Book describe the 'dry drunk' as "restless, irritable, and discontented." Dry Drunks have also been characterized as "angry, displaying superiority, selfishness, impulsivity and negative judgment."

AA literature describes the dry drunk as a 'horse thief':

> "A person with chemical dependency issues who is abstinent but regressing. This may include little/no 12 step meeting attendance, minimal/no active sponsor relationship and little/no involvement in 12 step fellowships... Anger opposes all 12 Step principles. It overrides reason. It insulates us from God and the spiritual help necessary for our recovery...If you sober up a horse thief, what do you get? A sober horse thief."
>
> —AA Literature

AA attributes the dry drunk personality to a lack of commitment to the program and encourages the dry drunk to participate more fully in AA, increasing frequency of meeting attendance, and participation.

While AA has pinpointed many of the neurological deficits seen in sober alcoholics, attributing these deficits to a lack of commitment to the program, or underlying personality defects is incorrect.

At the very least it's more likely that this behavior is part of the chronic imbalance of negative affect due to neuroadaptation.

And at its worse, it may be that dry drunk behavior is heavily influenced by persistent brain damage that has targeted the neural circuits that control motivational processes, cognitive ability and appropriate emotional responses.[129]

Brain Damage

Magnetic Resonance Imaging (MRIs) and post-mortem studies of alcoholics show a loss of brain tissue in the frontal lobes and thinning of the corpus callosum.

Additional brain damage can be seen in the amygdala and hippocampus and the white matter of the cerebellum.

These are all areas that are essential for emotional functioning. In alcoholics, the impact of this damage has been observed in their perception and evaluation of emotional facial expressions, interpretation of emotional intonations in vocal utterances, and appreciation of the meaning of emotional materials.[151]

The MRIs below show the differences between a non-alcoholic 'Control Man' and an 'Alcoholic Man'.

Even to a layperson, there is a significant difference in its appearance. It appears as if part of the alcoholic's brain is completely missing.

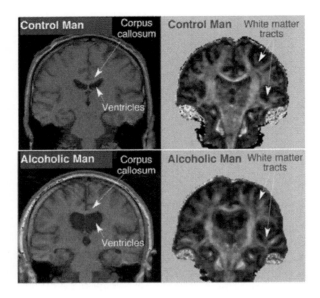

Korsakoff Syndrome

MRIs can be used to compare a non-alcoholic ("Control"), an alcoholic ("Alcoholic"), and an individual with Korsakoff syndrome (Korsakoff).

Korsakoff is caused by brain damage due to a lack of thiamine and is caused by chronic alcoholism. Brain damaged areas (missing areas) can be seen in the MRIs of both the alcoholic and Korsakoff brain.

When the effects of alcoholism become so bad that Korsakoff syndrome or another disease called Wernicke encephalopathy has taken hold, 'dry drunk' symptoms are elevated to a whole new level.

An individual with wet brain (another term for these diseases), may show memory impairment, confusion, problems with gait and coordination, eyelid drooping, a tendency to make up stories and muscle atrophy.

With or without brain damage, the addiction cycle lurches forward.

Eventually, preoccupation, anticipating and craving sets in once again. The stinking thinking of the 'preoccupation/anticipation' phase takes hold, and the vicious circle begins again.

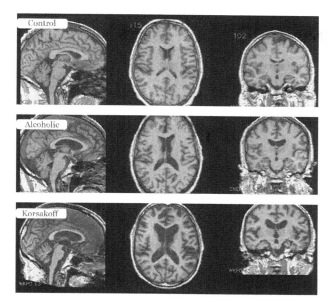

TREATMENT TARGETS

In this sub phase, we looked at the physical and psychological symptoms experienced during withdrawal and later during the experience of negative effect. Medications that target this phase focus on the following:

- Lessening the physical damage and impact of the withdrawal experience;

- Rebalancing depleted nutrients and vitamins that exacerbate physical and psychological symptoms

- Rebalancing brain chemicals that generate negative effect

Medications that can lessen the physical damage and impact of withdrawal, as well as those that can rebalance nutritional deficiencies are not a focus of this book, but are worth investigation for any alcoholic.

Be Cautious of Antidepressants

Sometimes the same medications that attempt to counteract negative effect are often similar drugs that are used to counter other mental illness such as depression and anxiety.

Since depression is so common in alcoholics, there is a major pitfall for treatment seeking alcoholics related to this.

Antidepressants (especially SSRIs) and antipsychotics need to be taken with great caution, and must be very carefully selected.

There are some (not all) medications in this category that have been shown to actually increase drinking in alcoholics (and most doctors are completely unaware of this fact).

For a list of other medications that have been shown to increase drinking, make sure you look at the 'D-List' ('Use Caution') in this book.

09 | GENETIC RISK FACTORS

"Heritability of alcoholism seems to be almost identical for men and women…. heritability estimates from the twin studies are if anything likely to be underestimates…the true heritability of alcoholism is likely closer to 70%."[4]

–Dr. Markus Heilig, The 13th Step – Addiction in the Age of Brain Science

PHARMACOGENETICS

Some of the most interesting work scientists are doing right now (in any field of medicine) is called pharmacogenetics, an area which is sometimes called 'personalized medicine'.

Pharmacogenetics has revealed that the effectiveness of medication is often related to your genes.

It has shown the medications described later in the book are particularly effective (or particularly ineffective) in people with very specific genetic variations.

So if you've tried medication in this book before and it had no effect on you, it's likely your genetic makeup didn't make you a good target for the medication in the first place. A different medication may be more effective.

One of the things that researchers have been plagued with in the study of medications for alcoholism is that occasionally in one study alcoholics will respond to medication effectively–in a way that is statistically significant. And then in another study, testing the same drug, the results just aren't conclusive.

We can see this anecdotally elsewhere too. For example, go on any of the online forums where people with alcoholism are trying different medications.

Person A will report that a medication is immediately effective; Person B reports a blunted feeling when drinking that makes them no longer motivated to take it, and Person C reports having no effect of the medication whatsoever.

What is likely happening is that all three individuals are dependent on alcohol, but they each may have a very different combination of genes that have led them to that dependence.

One could say that they have different kinds of alcoholism.

ALCOHOLISM GENES

Alcoholism isn't binary–it's not a case of a single gene determining whether you will be an alcoholic or not.

Instead, many genes and variations within those genes have been found in higher ratios in alcoholics and their family members, than in non-alcoholics and their family members. Alcoholics have different combinations of these genes and an alcoholic may have many of them, or very few.[129]

Evidence from genome research has provided evidence that some complex diseases are manifested through variations in multiple genes–not just one.[152] This is also the case for other mental illnesses, such as bipolar disorder and schizophrenia.[153]

The first gene that was identified (ALDH1) was found in the 1980s and related to the metabolism of alcohol in the body[123]. Since then, many more have been identified.

Scientists have generated a list of thousands of genes that have some evidence (human or animal) implicating them in alcoholism.[153] Of these, it's possible that a hundred or more are of particular importance in their contribution to alcoholism.[123][125]

The genes which have been identified are known to influence a broad range of brain and body systems. Some of the genes that have been identified work on the brain's GABA system, some work on taste receptors, some work on the way alcohol is metabolized.

Others work on the glutamine, serotonin, and dopamine systems. They work in the systems that impact craving, resiliency, responses to stress, and in systems controlling a range of behaviors and reactions.

I think of the impact of the genes that are related to alcoholism like the 6-inch tall citizens of Lilliput that surrounded Gulliver on his travels.

A handful of little Lilliputians could not take the giant Gulliver down, but hundreds of unique little people, each working on his or her own square inch of his body, were able to pull the enormous man down to the ground.

204 · MEDICATIONS FOR ALCOHOLISM

In alcoholism, some genes may only have a very minor influence on one's feelings, reactions and actions, but the strength of possibly hundreds of altered genes, working from different directions, on many different brain and thought processes, all pushing toward alcoholic tendencies and behaviors, can have a very powerful Gulliver-sized effect.

Because of the contribution of heredity to alcoholism, genetic research is critical for alcohol medication development.

And not just genetic research—but genetic research that includes a large enough population of test subjects to find statistically significant results where the effect of multiple gene and complex variations is at play.

Scientists are just starting to gain access to these kinds of populations.

For example, recently, a GWAS—a Genome-wide association study—was able to explore a pool of individuals large enough to reveal further insight into the genetics behind alcoholism.

In the largest GWAS study of alcohol dependence to date (with 16,087 subjects), the size of the study enabled the researchers to finally, for the first time, identify a gene that increases the risk of alcoholism in the African American population.[154]

GENES AND DEVELOPING DEPENDENCE

Genes can influence behaviors which make young adults more vulnerable to developing dependence during the early phases of alcoholism.

Here are a few research findings:

- The ADH gene in adolescents is associated with early drinking and subsequent alcoholism.

- GABA receptor gene variations are associated with alcohol dependence.[123] And the gene known as GABRA2 is related to increased drunkenness during the transition between adolescence and adulthood.[155]

- Young carriers of CHRM2 variations are likely to have early symptoms of depression; and adolescent carriers of GABRA2 variations more frequently display sensation-seeking behaviors[155] and increased rule breaking behavior such as trouble with the police, fighting, and expulsion from school.[123]

- Variations within the cluster of genes which include CHRNA5—CHRNA3-CHRNB3 not only increase the risk of dependence on multiple substances but also influence the initial responses to alcohol in adolescents.[125]

- Teenagers who carry a certain variant of the OPRM1 gene experience more alcohol-related problems and are more likely to be dependent on alcohol.

- Nearly 52% of youth with alcohol dependence carry at least one copy of the OPRM1 gene variation (the G allele) compared to 16.3% of young people who carry it and do not have alcoholism.

- The OPRM1 gene can manifest itself in the addiction development process is through the way that it enhances the sensations related to drinking for those that carry the variation. Carriers may feel more pleasure and greater intoxication from drinking than those without it.[156]

- Variations in the CRHR1 gene (related to stress response) have been shown to predict many alcoholism-related outcomes including adolescent binge drinking and greater alcohol drinking when exposed to stress.[157]

Alcoholics who drink to calm anxiety and excessive stress may be medicating feelings associated with CRHR1 gene variations.

One researcher hypothesizes that the may be "drinking to feel normal—they may drink to tame a hyperactive CRF stress system in the brain…In the absence of alcohol, the alcoholic feels ill because his or her body cannot easily reverse these artificial levels."[158]

PHENOTYPES: UNIQUE TRAITS

A phenotype is an clue that an individual may have an illness, even before that illness has appeared.

For example, there is a genetic illness called Waardenburg syndrome which causes people to sometimes have unusually widely set eyes. This characteristic is a phenotype for the syndrome.

This phenotype doesn't *cause* the problems the syndrome is known for (such as hearing loss and intestinal disorders).

And widely-set eyes don't *always* indicate that the syndrome is present.

However, the genetic variations that cause this physical feature are present statistically more often in those who have the syndrome than in those that don't. So unusually widely set eyes is a risk factor and a phenotype for Waardenburg syndrome.

Because alcoholism is highly hereditary and involves so many genes, there are many phenotypical clues that can give away someone's potential of developing alcohol dependence long before it develops.

None of the phenotypes for alcoholism are perfect—they don't predict future dependence accurately—but they can make us aware of vulnerability in ourselves or in others.

Genes don't just give us obvious traits like eye color—they also determine a thousand little (and big) details about us.

Even many personality traits and behavioral patterns that are often seen in people who develop alcoholism are actually genetically-influenced attributes.

Some of these attributes emerge very early and contribute to the early descent into alcoholism.

For example, traits sometimes seen in alcoholics even prior to dependence (which may be rooted in genetic variations) include: moodiness and emotional issues, propensity for compulsive behavior, impulsivity, risk-taking, sensation seeking, nonconformity, a sense of social alienation, heightened stress, abnormal decision-making behavior, harm avoidance, reward dependence, and weaker coping skills.[144]

And there actually is a connection between eye-color and alcoholism.

What could eye color and alcoholism possibly have to do with one another? Eye color clearly isn't something that influences personality or even early adolescent behavior that may lead to drinking.

But scientists in 2015 learned that genes which control eye color have relationships with genes that control other characteristics. They even found that genetic variations associated with alcoholism were more likely to be present in people who carried genetic coding for light blue eyes.[159]

The following is a list of other phenotypes, traits and behavioural patterns that are often seen in alcoholics and which have their grounding in DNA variations.

Smoking

If you have ever attended an AA meeting, you may have noticed the heavy reliance on cigarette smoking that members seem to have, which is disproportional to smoking in the general public.[155]

In fact, studies have shown that approximately 80% of alcohol-dependent individuals in North America are regular smokers.[144]

This is not coincidental, as two genes (DRD2 and CHRNA5) that have been identified to influence the risk of becoming alcohol dependent are also strongly linked to habitual smoking.

Recent research also found it likely that smoking facilitates the transition to alcohol dependence and increases compulsive alcohol drinking.[160]

Sweet Preference, Novelty Seeking

Another behavior seen in many alcoholics is the (sometimes compulsive) consumption of sugar at certain points in their abstinence. Many alcoholics struggle with eating large amounts of food with high sugar content when they are not drinking.

This is a genetic trait that many individuals at risk for alcoholism are born with. Scientists have found that "sweet and alcohol preference are genetically linked, at some concentrations to almost 80%."[1]

There is also research that showed that this genetic marker can correlate to effectiveness of naltrexone. Higher sweet preference was significantly related to successful treatment outcomes in a 2011 study.[161]

The linkage between sweet preference and alcoholism has been shown in several studies.

In one, it was shown that 61% of individuals with a strong family history of alcoholism preferred the strongest sucrose solution presented to them, compared with 19% of individuals with no family history of alcoholism.[162][163]

Researchers have concluded that individuals with what is called the 'sweet-liking phenotype'–people who choose increasing concentrations of sucrose in studies–is a characteristic which is "significantly and positively associated with the genetic risk of alcohol use disorder.[164]

Several studies have shown that the preference for stronger sweet taste is "more prevalent in children of alcoholic families than in children from non-alcoholic families, regardless of the child's drinking status."[164]

Another variation related to taste was also found to be a significant risk factor in alcoholism–one related to a receptor that is involved in decreased sensitivity to bitter tasting compounds.[123]

There is a third dimension to the sweet/alcohol phenotype–and that is the presence of certain behavioral characteristics. Human studies have reported an association between family history of alcoholism, sweet-liking and impulsive and novelty seeking behaviour.

One study found that individuals who had both traits (novelty seeking and sweet liking) had the greatest risk of future problems with alcoholic behavior.[165]

Recent Magnetic Resonance Imaging (MRIs) studies have also shown that that the brains of individuals with very high alcohol intake respond significantly differently to sweet tastes than the brains of those with much lower average alcohol intake levels.

The greater the response in the left orbitofrontal region of the brain to sweet tastes, the higher the subjects' reported daily drink average was.[166]

Inhibition

Some researchers feel that the results of the Reduced P300 Amplitude' test are the closest thing to a perfect phenotype for early onset alcoholism as we are likely to find.

In the P300 test, subjects are shown a stimulus, like a bright flash of light, and then scientists measure the spike in electrical signal strength in the brain that occurs between 300 and 500 milliseconds after the flash.

In alcoholics (even abstinent ones), the electrical signal strength is distinctly muted (at a lower voltage) compared to its strength in the brains of non-alcoholics.

Scientists have been able to see this difference even in the at-risk children of alcoholic parents[144]–indicating that this difference is not caused by drinking, but is a genetic trait that is a risk factor for becoming an alcoholic later in life.

The lower P300 voltages seen in young boys at high risk of developing alcoholism (due to heredity), before exposure to alcohol, is striking.

It has been replicated in many studies (over 17), with and without alcohol administration, in both older and younger subjects at risk, as well as in female and male offspring.[131]

Other studies which have shown differences in measurements of brainwave frequency amongst alcoholics and their offspring have also emerged. But scientists believe that the P300 test may be one of the most robust tests to identify individuals at risk for alcoholism.

How does this weakened brain response manifest?

People who are weak in this area are more prone to acting on impulses originating in lower brain regions.[123]

When we feel an impulse the ventral striatum becomes hyperactive, and it is the job of the prefrontal cortex to put the brakes on, minimizing impulsive behaviour.

But in the alcoholic brain, there is a marked imbalance in the ventral striatum/prefrontal cortex dynamic that can cause weakened powers of inhibition.

It's common for early-onset alcoholics not only to distinctly remember the very first drink they ever had, but recall that it was the first time in their lives they ever felt 'normal' or 'in balance.'

Some scientists hypothesize that alcoholics drink as a way to regulate their brains to achieve the psychological state which is associated with different brain wave activity.[130]

Low Response, Depression or Max Drinks

'COGA,' stands for 'Collaborative Studies on Genetics of Alcoholism, and is an important research initiative funded by the NIAAA. COGA research has helped to identify additional characteristics which appear in people who are likely to become alcoholics (before the development of any dependence).

Some of the phenotypes identified by COGA include:

- 'Low Response': This is a powerful predictor of the development of alcohol dependence, and is genetically influenced. If you have low response, then you must consume larger amounts than others before feeling the effects of alcohol.[123][167] This is the case even before dependence sets in during later stages.

- 'Alcoholism or Depression': Major Depressive disorder shares some genetic factors with alcoholism. Both alcoholism and depression occur commonly in families of alcoholics.[167]

- 'Maximum Number of Drinks': Researchers have identified that individuals with one genetic variation were significantly more likely to have consumed large quantities of alcohol within a single 24-hour period (at a time before becoming alcoholic).

  Sixty-five percent of men and 53% of women who reported having at one time consumed 9 or more drinks in a 24-hour period and who had this variation were eventually diagnosed with alcohol dependence.[167]

ARE YOU AT RISK OF ADDICTION?

If you have a strong family history of alcoholism, you are at higher risk of developing alcohol addiction through drinking unless you take preventative measures.

Unfortunately, there is not yet a commercially available DNA test that can identify variations you have that make you at risk for dependence.

So, understanding of your heredity and phenotypical characteristics related to genetic variations are the best way to identify potential risk.

The following is a list of characteristics that may be rooted in hereditary factors that are often seen in alcoholics and in people with a strong family history of alcoholism.

Parents should take strong note of these attributes in their children.

And if you see yourself in more than a few of the following descriptions it may be time to put the brakes on further drinking if you still can:

- You have a parent or sibling who often over-drinks or some other history of alcoholism in your biological family.

- You enjoy ice-cream, candies, sugary pop or other sweet-tasting sugary foods. Sometimes your consumption is binge-like.

- You consider yourself a thrill seeker. You strongly desire and seek thrilling, exciting experiences that bring rewarding physical sensations and the feeling of a 'high'.

- You drink differently from others–needing more alcohol than others seem to need to get the same effect.

- You often overdrink, especially in comparison with others your age.

- You started overdrinking early in life–before the age of 24.

- You drink regularly to minimize anxiety or discomfort.

- You remember your first drink very well–it seemed to stabilize you in some way, or made you feel normal for the first time.

- You feel more emotionally balanced when you drink.

- Without alcohol, you don't feel like you fit in and you feel different from others.

- You are often moody, depressed or stressed, struggling with emotional balance.

- You can be highly impulsive and uninhibited at times.

- You have ADHD.[4]

- You are a smoker.

- You often think about drinking.

- You have an eating disorder or experience other mental health issues related to compulsivity, anti-social or risky behavior.

You seem to be unable to stop yourself from pursuing certain actions once you have started, even when you know better.

3

PART 3: YOUR MEDICATION JOURNEY

10 | HOW THE MEDICATIONS WORK

"Given that many neurotransmitter systems are affected...numerous druggable targets have been identified; consequently, a "cocktail" of different compounds will further improve the treatment situation."[168]

–Dr. Rainer Spanagel, Director of the Institute of Psychopharmacology, University of Heidelberg

How Medications for Alcoholism Work

Between environmental contributors, genes and brain neuroadaptation, alcoholism generates a lot of feelings and behaviors that contribute to the development and reinforcement of alcohol dependence.

For example, alcoholism can manifest characteristics that influence alcoholics to:

- be more impulsive

- be less able to halt impulsive, automatic actions

- seek thrills

- experience a strong enjoyment of alcohol

- be highly reactive to alcohol cues

- become drunk more quickly than others

- feel less affected by drinking (dependence)

- experience chronic anxiety, depression or other mental illness

- develop deep conditioned responses more quickly

- react more strongly to stressors

- experience obsessive thoughts and cravings

- feel uninterested in anything but drinking

- have difficulty valuing negative consequences

Some people experience all of these. Some experience few. Everyone is different.

If you were freed from just one of these feelings and behaviors—for example—'chronic anxiety', or if you were only able to remove 'obsessive thoughts and cravings', maybe it would allow you to stop the addiction cycle.

Or, perhaps if every one of these feelings and behaviors remained, but were just lessened by 10%, you would be able to regain control.

Researchers recognize the importance of minimizing these feelings and behaviors, and so in developing medications for alcoholism, researchers look at these feelings and behaviors and try to identify the parts of the brain that are generating them.

All of the characteristics described above are produced inside the brain, and there are many different systems in the brain, such as the dopamine system, and systems that the dopamine system involves, such as glutamate, GABA, corticotropin-releasing factor, 4-HT and opioid that are involved in generating them.

Knowing that these systems are involved in alcoholism, researchers try to identify drug compounds (existing or new ones) that target these systems.

And by targeting and interfering with these systems, researchers hope to interfere with the thoughts and feelings that contribute to alcoholism.

For example, let's look at one target—the opioid system.

We know that the opioid system (part of the reward system which is related to feel-good endorphins), is involved in the reinforcing effects of alcohol.

We also know that there are variations in at least four genes that are related to the opioid system that are found in alcoholic populations.

For example, OPRM1 is a gene that is related to at least three opioid receptors in humans. So something is occurring in the opioid system of alcoholics to contribute to their alcoholism, that may not occur in non-alcoholics.

Therefore, for scientists looking for a way to interrupt the addiction process—the behaviors and feelings associated with alcoholism, the opioid system becomes a natural 'target'.

Naltrexone is a drug that is known to interfere with the opioid system.

It binds to opioid receptors, blocking them so that the rewarding feeling of alcohol may be muted. Over time, it can also help reverse the altered balance in the brain (caused through homeostasis described earlier), undoing alcohol conditioning.

By undoing conditioning, fewer cravings for alcohol may be experienced.

So, by targeting the opioid system with the medication naltrexone, at least three of the feelings and behaviors associated with alcoholism can be weakened or eradicated:

- experience a strong enjoyment of alcohol

- develop deep conditioned responses more quickly

- experience obsessive thoughts and cravings

Whether for depression, Alzheimer's, or alcoholism, targeting brain systems is an imprecise science.

It's generally known which systems a drug is interfering with, but not what the outcome of the interference will be.

And when the outcome is good (for example, by reducing craving), researchers don't necessarily even understand why the drug is working.

That's why, for many of the medicines in this book the 'mechanism of action', or in other words, how the drug actually works, is nothing more than an extremely well-educated guess.

You'll notice that naltrexone may be helpful with three feelings and behaviors associated with alcoholism and the reward system.

But how about all of the other feelings and characteristics?

Others may be more a result of issues in other brain systems, and so these other brain systems become another 'target' for researchers, and drugs that are designed to interfere with these targets can be applied.

While the numerous targets make alcoholism very complex, it also means lots of opportunity.

As scientists wrote in one journal article in 2013, "there is no other field in psychiatric research that has, in recent years, yielded so many novel, druggable targets and innovative treatment strategies than for alcohol addiction."[168]

CAUSES OF ADDICTION VERSUS DAMAGE CAUSED BY ADDICTION

As you are thinking about the behaviors and feelings that contribute to your alcoholism, it may be helpful to think about how you felt when alcoholism was first developing, and how you feel now. These can be valuable clues to help you understand what you need to tackle.

For example, did you drink routinely and heavily because you were trying to manage stress or anxiety? Or did you do so because drinking was so enjoyable?

And now that you are drinking more than you want to, what is it that you feel before you relapse? Severe cravings? Anxiety? Or perhaps you don't sense cravings, but seem to automatically just head for the bottle.

The more you understand how your own brain and body is being motivated and affected, the better chance you will have of choosing medications that might help you.

For example, whereas the rewards of thrill and sensation seeking may have driven you to addiction in the first place, it might be a state of anxiety, stress, and depression caused by the addiction that now contributes to each consecutive relapse.

One is related to causal factors, and the other is related to the chronic damage caused by the disease. For these two separate dimensions, different treatments may be appropriate.[1]

Multi-prong strategies may be very necessary, involving various types of treatments and combinations of treatments (pharmaceutical and other), which target multiple goals.[146]

Some of these treatment and medication goals which include a variety of different areas and systems of the brain, and might target both the causes and the chronic effects of alcoholism might include a "cocktail of compounds"[168] involved in:

- decreasing the reward value of the drug

- increasing the reward value of non-drug reinforcers

- weakening conditioned drug behaviors and motivators

- decreasing obsession and craving

- strengthening frontal inhibitory and executive control

- reducing reactivity to stressors

SHORT CIRCUITING ADDICTION

Every now and then a major discovery is made that throws other discoveries before it into question (or solves their mysteries), as well as paving the way for new insights and treatments.

In 2007 such a discovery was made: Scientists studying stroke patients realized that an injury to the insula could instantly and permanently break a smoking habit.[169]

The Director of the National Institute on Drug Abuse (Dr. George Koob) said of the discovery, "This is the first time we've shown anything like this, that damage to a specific brain area could remove the problem of addiction entirely...It's absolutely mind-boggling."[169]

Scientists knew that the insula was a structure in the brain that was involved in addiction, but they had no idea just how important it was.

It is still a mysterious and complex part of the brain, nicknamed by one researcher as the 'hidden island of addiction' and related to highly evolved processes.

It is thought to "integrate introceptive states into conscious feelings and into decision-making processes that involve uncertain risk and reward." It seems to be related to the experience of craving and intuition.[170]

Researchers found that patients with damage to the insula underwent a complete disruption of smoking addiction which was:

"...characterized by the ability to quit smoking easily, immediately, without relapse and without a persistence of the urge to smoke.

In one case, this disruption of addiction after insula damage was so profound as to lead one patient to proclaim that his 'body forgot the urge to smoke.'"[170]

In other words, damage to the insula eradicated the addiction to smoking. No behavioral therapy, soul searching, fighting of urges and cravings was necessary–through damage to the insula, smoking addiction was simply wiped out.

How is this related to alcoholism?

I'm not recommending you go out and try to injure your insula.

While being an important discovery on many other levels, what the discovery shows is that alcohol addiction researchers are on the right track when it comes to targeting the brain's biology.

It provides validity to the notion that irrespective of the environment you grew up in or the psychological baggage you carry, if changes to a specific section of the brain in an addicted smoker can extinguish addiction, then it can be achieved (maybe through a different mechanism, or a different area), in alcoholics too.

Dr. Koob is correct when he says that this is the first time we've seen anything like this–in that this experiment showed such a profound and complete reversal of addiction in nearly every insula injury.

However, this phenomena has also been seen in alcoholics taking specific medications too.

For example, in the treatment he developed and tested on himself using baclofen, Dr. Olivier Amiesen describes a 'switch'–a point at which addiction is 'turned off' in treatment.

When Amiesen (and many others since) experienced this switch point, their experience was one in which the intense craving for alcohol one day simply disappeared.

Other individuals, such as many for whom naltrexone has been successful, have experienced the same effect–that eventually at a point in their treatment, they simply no longer feel the extreme obsession and drive to drink and inability to stop, any more.

11 | THREE TREATMENT STEPS

"So with no other disease do we expect people to wait until they're a danger to themselves or others to self-diagnose and seek treatment.

Every other disease — you got a broken leg, you got diabetes, you got some sort of sickness, we understand that we got to get you help.

And we also understand when it comes to other diseases that if we don't give you help, and let you suffer by yourself, then other people could get sick.

Well, this is an illness. And we got to treat it, as such. We have to change our mindset."[30]

—*US President Barack Obama*

STEP 1: GETTING PREPARED

If you didn't read the legal statements early in this book, please go back and read it now. It contains important information that you should not read further without.

GOALS & GOAL TRACKING

ABSTINENCE OR REDUCTION

> *"If an addict has made major advances, taken steps in positive directions that few would argue with, then it is absurd to suggest that this person is not recovering. A switch from 10 bottles or 10 bags a week to 2 bottles or 2 bags a week is a huge improvement and obviously should qualify as 'recovery'."*[11]

What would you like your treatment goal to be?

Your goal will impact which medications you choose to take and even how you decide to take them.

Let's step back and talk first about the goals now available for treatment.

•••

There is a significant shift in perspective occurring in our thinking around what a treatment goal can and should be for someone with alcoholism.

If you have been in treatment or a 12-step program, you may believe that the only possible goal is abstinence. And perhaps that still is the best goal for you. (Or maybe it never was a realistic goal for you, and never will be).

Abstinence is the very black and white goal that AA has laid out for alcoholics.

And for people in the program, even status and tenure are measured on the basis of that goal—one day at a time.

Anniversaries of sobriety–1 day, 1 month, 1 year–and more are hard won and celebrated. Fall off the wagon and you start again at day 1. Sobriety or nothing–there is no middle ground–'cutting down' counts for nada.

Unfortunately, abstinence simply doesn't work as a treatment option for many people with this disease. If you are one of them, then another goal maybe more realistic for you.

Abstinence from alcohol works about as well for many as abstinence from sex works as a form of birth control–a nice idea but not very practical. And as with AA's philosophy of abstinence, it's an idea from an earlier time.

HARM REDUCTION

For people who are not interested in a solution that involves abstinence, there are other options. These options are categorized under the term 'harm reduction', or simply 'reduction'. Many organizations and support groups espouse this approach that can be found by simply searching for 'alcohol harm reduction' online. One example can be found at hamsnetwork.org, ("Where better is better!")

Harm reduction strategies are aimed at reducing the negative consequences associated with alcohol dependence.

This is an important approach to the treatment of a progressive disease that is often fatal.

ABSTINENCE GOALS: A BARRIER TO TREATMENT?

One of the reasons that people do not pursue treatment is because in the past treatment has *always* meant abstinence.

Heavy drinkers (often with the greatest risk of harm from alcoholism) often desperately want the option of moderating their drinking if they can, instead of trying to give it up altogether.[56]

The black and white 'abstinence or nothing' approach is a major barrier to helping alcoholics. In one study 50% of those who knew they needed it did not seek treatment because they were not ready to give up alcohol.[171]

This is worth repeating—half of the people who knew they needed help did not get it because they were not prepared to stop drinking. They were not ready for any treatment that had abstinence as a goal.

These are the people who desperately need treatment options that help them to decrease their consumption.

Another reason people don't pursue treatment is because of the perception that treatment means involvement in a program.

The following are additional reasons why people who knew they needed help did not seek it (numbers rounded).[171] Notice how each one is related to an element of program participation:

- No transportation/inconvenient—7%
- No program having type of treatment—8%
- No openings in a program—1%
- Did not know where to go for treatment—7%
- Might cause community to have negative opinion—6%
- Might have negative effect on job—7%
- Did not have time—3%
- Did not want others to find out—2%

In total, 43% of individuals who knew they needed help for their alcohol dependence did not get it because of issues around program participation.[171]

Again—worth repeating—43 percent of the people who knew they needed help did not get it because of issues likely related to participating in a program.

These are the people who—even if they *are* willing to accept abstinence as a goal—will not receive any treatment for their illness if it is program-based.

But as with those who aren't willing to give up drinking, for these program-averse people, medication (confidential, non-time consuming, non-participatory), is an option that they might be open to.

For those individuals, if only one medication is tried, and that medication was effective for only one in three individuals (the 'number needed to treat' for baclofen), that would mean that one in three people could see improvement in a disease that they would otherwise not be getting treatment for—one which could otherwise be progressively killing them.

The president of pharmaceutical company Lundbeck (Ulf Wiinberg) reiterates this perspective. Lundbeck has launched the 'as needed' medication Selincro in Europe that is targeted toward individuals seeking a reduction in consumption.

He says, "If we can get addicts to reduce their consumption from 50-100 drinks a week to 20-25, then we will have come a long way. In this way, these people could regain control of their own lives. This would be a viable solution for certain groups of users."[172]

IS 'REDUCTION' A NAÏVE GOAL?

Is treatment that only aims for a reduction in consumption naïve?

For some people, it may be just the opposite. As researchers point out–it is not *drinking* that causes so many health problems for alcoholics–it's *heavy drinking* that leads to the burden of disease and cost associated with alcoholism.[173]

Therefore, if heavy drinking can be reduced to moderate drinking, many lives could be saved. For example, research shows that:

- For an alcoholic drinking 8 glasses of alcohol per day, if he reduces his intake by just 2 glasses per day, his one-year mortality risk is nearly cut in half.[174]

- In heavy drinkers (those who drink 100g or more per day), cutting consumption in half reduces the chance of death by 800%.[173]

Given these statistics, it's hard to understand why there was not a focus on using medication to help alcoholics reduce consumption, years ago. Why *wouldn't* we look for ways to reduce consumption if we could?

Clearly, reduction is not a naïve approach—especially given that the alternative for many is not abstinence–but simply continued drinking at high levels.

Reduction can also be an intermediate step in the right direction for those who eventually choose abstinence as a goal.

There are many anecdotal stories from people who have taken medications and been able to reduce their drinking, and who, once they were able to cut down, decided that abstinence was possible and preferable for them.

ABSTINENCE CAN BE DANGEROUS

The idea that abstinence (from alcohol as well as medical assistance) is the only definition of true recovery is not only old but, more importantly, it's outdated–and dangerous.

In a study of 1800 treated drinkers done in 2007 that looked at the aftermath of treatment which focused on abstinence versus moderation, they found that individuals that chose abstinence experienced negative consequences (due to drinking, or relapsing), at the same rate as individuals whose goal had been to moderate drinking.[56]

Other research on the Abstinence Violation Effect has shown that when an alcoholic believes a lapse is a shameful and devastating personal failure (as the abstinence philosophy implies), they are much more likely to continue to a full-blown binge, instead of stopping and regrouping.[75]

SHIFTING PHILOSOPHY

Thankfully, the 'all-or-nothing medication-free abstinence' approach is slowly starting to come under fire in the US, but North America is lagging behind Europe in this way of thinking.

Recent research shows that in Europe at least, "many clinicians and patients consider reduction of alcohol consumption as a valuable treatment option to reduce the consequences of harmful alcohol use or, at least, as an intermediate goal towards abstinence, and research evidence supports this."[175]

And the European Medicines Agency (equivalent to the US FDA) has guidelines that recognize both treatment goals: abstinence and reduction in alcohol consumption.

Practitioners and patients are starting to recognize reduction as a viable goal. And even the tone of articles and government reports indicate a subtle undercurrent that a "philosophy of abstinence" may not, and should not, be for everyone.

What This Means For You

Once you have thought about and determined what your goal is, this will help you (and your medical advisor) to choose which medications to try.

As you read the information about each drug in the next section, you'll see information on each one regarding the goals the medication might assist you with.

For example, if your goal is abstinence, you will want to avoid any medication (or more accurately—any *methods* of taking that medication) on an 'as needed' basis. Alcohol consumption is a key component of the science behind 'as needed' methods. (You can take 'as needed' medications and abstain too, but you'll be following a different method. As this is confusing, see the naltrexone section for a detailed explanation).

Perhaps you can seek medications that help with your trigger points instead–such as those that have been seen to address strong cravings, anxiety, or alcohol cue reactivity.

If your goal is a reduction in drinking, most of the medications are an option for you.

Nalmefene is an example of a drug that is taken 'as needed'–meaning it is taken an hour before drinking–to help reduce drinking.

Therefore, abstinence isn't its (initial) goal.

Naltrexone and topiramate are two other medications known for their ability to help reduce drinking.

TRACKING

"What gets measured gets managed."
–Peter Drucker

Tracking important measures helps us manage many illnesses.

For example, if you have type 1 diabetes, doctors recommend that you check your blood sugar four to eight times per day. Blood pressure is another metric commonly measured to manage disease.

Not everyone is good at tracking—it takes a certain amount of discipline to do so—and courage to look at the numbers when they may not be as good as we would like.

But, as with other diseases, if you have alcohol dependence and track the amount you drink, it may help you manage this disease too.

Tracking will help you see whether what you are doing is helping, or if another strategy should be considered.

If you bring your data to your doctor, it will also help your doctor see that you are committed to change. It may help them get on board with you on your journey—something that will be extremely valuable to you if you are going to go down the path of experimenting to see if one or more medications can help you.

Two metrics are commonly measured by people who are tracking their consumption:

- Number of drinks per day

- Number of drink-free days

Also, if you find that these are factors in your drinking, and really want to diligently track your progress or triggers, you could also track (on a scale of 1 to 10) any of the following:

- The amount of craving you are experiencing

- The amount of stress you are experiencing

- The amount of anxiety you are experiencing

People track using different tools.

For example:

- A notebook you carry with you (a 'drinking diary')

- A simple notepad app on a cell phone

- By taking a photo with your phone of each drink you start, and counting later

- A cell phone app that is specifically used for measuring drinking

There are quite a few cell phone apps now available–some of which are free, and some of which cost a few dollars.

Using an app can help take away the problem of determining whether drinks are equivalent or not.

For example, if I drink four glasses of wine today, and four bottles of beer tomorrow, did I drink the same amount each day? Yes, I drank the same number of drinks, but certainly not the same amount of alcohol.

Some apps can help you compare apples to apples by allowing you to categorize drinks as you enter them, and then letting the app determine actual alcohol consumption.

A quick search online for cell phone apps found:

- AlcoDroid Alcohol Tracker

- SoberApp Alcohol Calculator

- My Daily Journal

- Drinking Buddy

- DrinkControl

If it sounds like a lot of work–well maybe it is–but have you ever redecorated a room and wished you had taken a 'before' picture before you started?

Tracking your drinking is like that. If you are able to reduce your consumption, there is a great deal of reward gained when you can see the numbers go down. It may take weeks or months for that to happen, but when it does, you'll be glad that you tracked.

In some of the online forums mentioned later, people anonymously post their drinking diary data (sometimes in their signature, so it appears after every posting), and update them daily or once a week.

Here's an example of how this looks.

The first number represents the number of drinks per week, and the second represents the number of 'Alcohol Free' ('AF') days the individual experienced:

Week 1–25–1 AF

Week 2–41–0 AF

Week 3–40–0 AF

Week 4–52–0 AF

Week 5–37–0 AF

Week 6–37–0 AF

Week 7–37–1 AF

Week 8–24–3 AF

Seeing other people's diaries is motivating–you can see that for some people medication works very quickly, while for others, it take a long time to work (if it ever works). It helps to know other people are in the same boat, and you aren't alone.

And if you decide to track and post your drinking diary in a forum too, you may be surprised at the encouragement you receive from others in your journey.

YOUR MEDICAL TREATMENT OPTIONS

WHAT TO EXPECT FROM YOUR DOCTOR

What should you expect from your doctor?

Nothing. You should be prepared to be underwhelmed, unfortunately.

When you start to talk to your doctor about pharmaceutical treatment for your alcoholism, you may suddenly feel like you are Alice in Wonderland.

This is because you might find yourself in a situation where you will be asking him or her for:

- Medical Treatment for a medical condition

- FDA-approved medication that has been used safely for decades

- Medication in large enough doses to treat your condition

- Treatment protocols for dosing that are backed by published research by respected scientists.

Not much to ask for really.

And yet, you may find that he or she:

- Has never heard of either the medications or treatments you are referencing and won't take your request seriously;

- Suggests that you go to a 12-step religion-based program like AA (with no medical/scientific evidence backing it);

- Might haltingly be convinced to prescribe you with the medication you are seeking, but in much lower doses than the effective (proven) dosages.

Welcome to Wonderland.

When it comes to medical, pharmacological treatment of alcohol addiction, you and I are pioneers and most (but not all) doctors are still back in 1939 with Bill Wilson. So be prepared.

Imagine if you went in with diabetes and asked for proper treatment and he/she responded in the same way—told you go find your higher power and dismissed your request for treatment? It might be lawsuit time.

We are just in a very different place in the treatment of alcoholism. Know it, be prepared for it, and don't take no for an answer—don't be another tragedy in the making.

If your doctor positively responds to all your requests on the first try, then you are seeing one of a small handful of very rare, very enlightened doctors in the world. Congratulations. You are incredibly lucky! With their support and cooperation, you have a strong chance of actually making life with this disease much more manageable. (But it probably won't be that way–not today anyway).

If and when you are lucky enough to obtain some of the medications written about in this book you will be on a new path. Not just new to you–new to the world.

This pathway can be very challenging–managing side effects, wondering whether anything is working, experimenting with correct dosages and combinations. Again–unless you are incredibly lucky–your doctor won't be much help to you in these areas.

But please–don't confuse your doctor's lack of knowledge as meaning that these medical options are not excellent, effective, life-changing medical treatments...your doctor just doesn't have experience with them, education about them, or colleagues who have more expertise than themselves in this area.

There are many resources mentioned in this book where you can learn much more about treatments and what to expect than your family physician will ever be able to offer you. Use those resources.

Manage your own recovery and research, and you will soon know much more about the treatment of alcoholism than your doctor will.

And you can (and probably will) be the first of your doctor's patients to go through this process, which means you'll be helping to train your doctor and make treatment easier for every other patient that comes after you. You can help save the lives of people you'll never meet in this way.

If your doctor won't work with you to find a solution using medications in this book, then what are your options?

You have a few.

Each of these approaches is discussed a little later. You might not like all of them. I'm not telling you to do any of them–all I want for you is to know your options and manage your health with your own best interests in mind.

Try to Manage Your Doctor

Do your best to attempt to nurture a partnership with your doctor.

He/she might just hold the keys to your illness in their hand. See this as a business partnership if you can and help guide your doctor to the knowledge that can help them help you. For example:

- Print out relevant parts of this book, the research, and something similar to the letter below. You may want to drop it all off in advance.

- Book time with your doctor for a talk.

- Dress and act as professionally as possible. If you have the means, try to wear what you would wear to a business meeting. Appearance makes a difference. It shouldn't. It does.

- Book time when you will be at your most lucid and sober.

- Bring a friend who can help advocate for you.

- Search online for "how to advocate with your doctor" for tips and ideas.

- There are ways to speak with your doctor that will help guide them in the direction you wish to go. Learn about these and practice them. For example, "I found this on the internet" might not be a good start, but "a doctor at the addiction treatment center recommended I look into this," may keep them listening to you for longer.

- Be relentless. It's your life and your health—not theirs.

Start with a First Line Drug

If your doctor has little experience with treating alcoholism with medication, then this may be a critical piece of advice for you: start out with a first line drug.

A first line drug (I'll explain exactly what this is soon) will be far more within your doctor's comfort zone than other drugs.

Acamprosate and naltrexone are both great starting points because they are the only two drugs on the A-List that are FDA-approved for the treatment of alcoholism in most places in the world.

Nalmefene is a good place to start if you are in Europe because it was recently launched there for alcoholism treatment and there is substantial pharmaceutical marketing creating a push for it with doctors right now. (It's not available in North America though). Lundbeck has placed some excellent resources online for physicians that can get them up to speed on the medication.

Baclofen is a good starting point for people in France because it was recently approved there to be prescribed specifically for the treatment of alcoholism. Doctors have more familiarity with baclofen in France for alcoholism treatment than they do in North America or other parts of Europe.

By starting with any of these, you won't be asking your doctor to prescribe you a medication for alcoholism that was approved for another medical condition (an 'off-label' medication).

All four are quite effective in some individuals, and there is a great deal of research evidence you can bring to your doctor to back up these choices.

Most doctors who have heard of or prescribed any medication for alcoholism will start with disulfiram.

If you are just starting out, read up carefully on this medication (it's on the B-List), as there are some good reasons (that your doctor may not know about) *not* to start with this one.

Acamprosate, naltrexone and disulfiram are all often considered to be 'first line' medications.

A 'first line' treatment is usually the first 'go-to' medication that a doctor might prescribe for a medical condition. (Though, in the treatment of alcoholism, very few people are ever prescribed any pharmaceutical treatment, so this term is something of a misnomer here).

Whether a medication is first or second line is subjective. This designation reflects both the effectiveness of the medication, but perhaps more so it simply reflects the length of time that doctors have prescribed the drug, thus building a level of confidence in its safety.

A medication can be highly effective and not be considered a first or second line treatment–particularly if the medical community has not been prescribing it for any length of time.

Despite the potential effectiveness of other medications, when asking your doctor for a prescription, it may be easier to get the doctor to prescribe you a medication that you can show him is a first line medication.

Even if the first line medication does not work for you, it's possible that by starting with these medications you can start a partnership with your doctor on your journey, and maybe they will feel more confident about prescribing you another medication that is a second or third line treatment.

Look for another Doctor

If you simply can't convince your doctor to work with you on this, then you may need to look for another doctor.

Here are a few things to keep in mind:

- Research doctors online–see if you can learn anything about their flexibility and accommodation in working with their patients in other areas.

  Online reviews can tell you a lot about a doctor's approach in general. For example, I've never asked my doctor for medication for alcoholism, but I know that when I have researched medications for other issues, if I bring her information about it, she will consider it for me and work with me. She is neither arrogant, nor dismissive.

  These are the traits to look for in online reviews, and if you have several options to choose from, doctors who are unwilling to consider a well-versed patient's input are doctors you may wish to avoid.

- Some forums (links are later in the book) provide lists of doctors that are known to treat alcoholism with medication. You could also post a question on a forum asking for recommendations in your area. Or you could choose to travel a little farther to a doctor who has been identified as knowledgeable in this area.

It may be well worth your time to travel a few hours in order to see a doctor with experience in this area and who is willing to work with you.

- If you find a new doctor (especially a new one that may not have experience with alcohol medication, but who you think may exhibit traits you are looking for), you may wish to build a relationship with the new doctor first with a few visits for some other minor issue.

Be profession, reliable, credible and build a rapport with them. Sadly alcoholism is still stigmatized. It's unfair, but a doctor may be more likely to see you as a credible human being if you don't initially present yourself as having an addiction problem.

WHAT TO BRING TO YOUR DOCTOR

Part 4 of this book was written to help you learn the most important information about each medication, but also so that you will have research and medical information to bring to your doctor when you discuss the drugs with him or her.

The information about each drug has been written in the order in which it would be most useful to a doctor to read.

Each of the drug sections provides the following:

- A paragraph or two introducing some of the key facts about the medication;

- A Q&A section that answers many of the most important things you and your doctor need to know about each medication as possible;

- A list of significant research and the main findings of each piece of research in order of most recent to oldest.

- A little more background information about the drug that may be of interest to some.

- Thoughts and comments from alcoholics who have experience taking the medication.

You may wish to photocopy and bring the entire section on the medication or medications you are interested in. Please feel free to do so.

You may also want to look up and print out the most recent research that is referenced in sections that cover each medication. All of the resources listed there would be appropriate and even quite useful to give to a doctor and are linked to from the book website.

Bring a professional-looking package with you and be prepared to drop it off a week or two in advance of the appointment or leave it behind for the doctor to review.

The following is a letter you may wish to include. You could include a photocopy of it, with a handwritten note from yourself.

Your note could say something like, "Looking forward to our appointment at 3 on Thursday the 7th. I'm hoping that we can discuss my options with one of these medications. Perhaps something of interest here." Or something to that effect.

LETTER TO YOUR DOCTOR

Dear Doctor,

The patient carrying this letter to you would like your help in the treatment of their alcohol dependence.

While it may not be widely known, there are several prescription medications that can help reduce craving, increase the time to relapse and reduce drinking quantity.

These drugs include: naltrexone, acamprosate (both approved by FDA, Health Canada and European Medicines Agency for the treatment of alcohol dependence); as well as baclofen, topiramate, nalmefene, gabapentin, ondansetron, sertraline, prazosin/doxazosin, varenicline and zonisamide (all widely approved off-label; baclofen approved on-label for alcohol dependence in France and nalmefene approved on-label for alcohol dependence in Europe).

Your patient has an interest in one or more of these medications and has brought additional information to you that it's hoped will be of assistance to you in determining whether or not the medication is appropriate for your patient.

In the interest of evidence-based medicine, and so you can determine the best approach, the information brought by your patient includes a list of significant research findings for the medication(s) of interest, general information about the medication, as well as a list of relevant research reports.

You can access the research reports (or their abstracts) at the website associated with this book which contains links to each journal article mentioned. Or simply search for them on Google Scholar (scholar.google.com).

Thank-you for your support and for the incredibly important role you play.

And thank-you in advance for taking time from your busy schedule to carefully read and review the information provided.

Sincerely,

Your Patient

THREE OTHER OPTIONS

Some people have found that no matter how they approach their doctor, they cannot succeed in obtaining medical treatment from within their own healthcare system for their dependence on alcohol.

Individuals who have come up to a brick wall have found some other options. These include:

1) Seeking medical treatment outside their own country;

2) Seeking treatment for a different illness that is treated with the same medications; and/or

3) Purchasing medication themselves without a prescription via an online pharmacy.

NOBODY in this century, living in any first world country, should need to resort to any of these options. People (particularly the same doctors that won't prescribe you the medications in this book) will call them dangerous. I think some of them are dangerous. I don't think that anyone should feel that in order to save their own lives they must resort to any of these options.

But as we've discussed earlier, there is a treatment gap that 20.7 million alcoholics in the United States are falling into.[3]

Authorities say, "there simply is no other disease where appropriate medical treatment is not provided by the health care system."[3]

And the Director of the Harvard Medical School herself says, "there is no other comparable example in medicine where you have evidence-based treatments that are not available.[3]

So that sterile waiting room at your doctor's office may look like it's from this century; your doctor's education may be the best training there is; there may be a cutting edge computer sitting on the office desk.

But in some cases, you may as well be sitting in Doc Baker's Walnut Grove office from Little House on the Prairie for all the help you'll receive.

What's more dangerous—taking matters into your own hands for a disease that can destroy your life and kill you? Or sitting in a 'treatment gap' in your doctor's office waiting for help that never comes?

Leave the Country

One approach that some individuals take is to cross the border to the 'border-town' clinics and pharmacies that exist for that purpose in some countries.

If, for example, you live in Canada, and wish to obtain naltrexone by monthly injection (not yet approved in Canada), then one approach is to travel across the border to the United States once a month to obtain the injection there. (One bonus of this option is that because it's an injection you won't be bringing medication back into the country).

Disulfiram is no longer approved by the government in Canada so those looking for it may need to go to a compounding pharmacy (a pharmacy that will literally make the medication for you). But an alternative may be to obtain it in the United States instead.

If you are outside, but close to France, it may be somewhere you could visit to obtain medical supervision for baclofen.

Nalmefene is currently only available in parts of Europe and is another medication that might be more easily obtained from cross-border visits to parts of Europe.

'Medical tourism' is a big industry—many people plan trips to other parts of the world to obtain medical treatment and prescriptions there.

Of course, if you go outside your country, buyer beware. Be careful and cautious. The same principles you'd apply to every other area of your health apply here to.

Don't be that person who gets cheap Botox injections in Tijuana and then wonders why her face is on fire.

Don't break the law.

Do your research, no matter where you go.

And make sure you know the rules for bringing medications back across the border before you take the trip. It may be wise to look at shipping medication over the border to yourself instead of trying to carry them back (but again—make sure the approach you take is legal).

You can contact the customs office for the country you will be exiting and re-entering, to find out specific rules for what you can and cannot bring across the border.

Seek Treatment for a Different Illness

I'm not advocating this—I'm just reporting here on what others have done.

Many medications in this book are FDA approved for other purposes, and doctors are more comfortable prescribing them for those other purposes.

For example, topiramate is often prescribed for migraines and varenicline is widely known as a smoking cessation treatment.

Sometimes, for some people, if faced with not receiving any kind of treatment or medical supervision at all (and all other avenues are exhausted), this is the only option they are left with.

Treat Yourself

Some individuals have successfully found overseas pharmacies which will provide them with a prescription and will ship medication to them, thus completely bypassing their physician.

I estimate that a significant percentage of people (perhaps 20-50%) writing about their experiences with these medications within forums obtain the medication they are using from online pharmacies.

Some online pharmacies require a prescription from a doctor to be provided to them before they will ship the order.

Others will allow you to pay a little extra for an assessment by a pharmacy-employed doctor who will then provide a prescription for the medication.

One reputable online pharmacy that I have ordered from provides an online assessment, so that the individual placing the order never interacts with or speaks to a physician before the prescription is made.

There are many scams on the internet, and many people that will gladly take your money or steal your identity and give you nothing in return. Some of these scams involve online pharmacies.

Please be very cautious if you take this approach. Order only a very small amount if you are trying a place for the first time. Get a more savvy friend to help you if you can. And attempt to get a recommendation from someone you have developed trust with on an online forum about reputable places to order online medications.

However, if you consider yourself quite internet-savvy and have run out of other viable options, many of the medications in this book can be purchased successfully and cost-effectively from online pharmacies.

I have personally purchased liquid baclofen, baclofen tablets, topiramate and naltrexone at a lower cost, with fewer hassles, than I would have been able to buy it in my country, and had it shipped to a delivery address with few problems.

I did notice that one of the packages was held up at customs, and that in some cases the medication took much longer to arrive than a typical online purchase would. So if you go this route may sure you err strongly on the side of caution if you need to order repeat medications so that you do not run out. Allow yourself at least a month, if not longer for a shipment.

It is much easier to purchase from online pharmacies if you live in the United States than from Canada, so if you have an address or friends with an address in the United States, this may be an easier alternative for Canadians. (Most, but not all online pharmacies do not ship to Canada).

If you run into problems with side effects, go to your doctor immediately and be honest about taking any medications you think may be causing them. These are serious medications that can have some rare, but real side-effects that can harm you.

If you choose this route, be an educated consumer–read everything you can about the medication you are considering taking and be aware of all drug interactions, black label warnings, and side effects before you begin. Be smart and do your research.

DRUGS AND THERAPY

The term 'Medication Assisted Treatment' subtly implies that there is something else besides medication being implemented in treatment.

This subtle suggestion is probably more about positioning (with psychiatrists, counselors, treatment providers and 12-steppers) than anything grounded in science.

Nearly everyone can benefit from 'Assistance', in the form of therapy or counselling. And certainly patients need a great deal more support than they are getting from their medical providers today.

However, from a purely evidence-based perspective, of the hundreds of research reports I read, there was not a single one that showed there was a *conclusive* and *significant* difference in outcome if the medication was paired with intensive therapy or counselling of any kind.

Some, such as Cognitive Behavioral Therapy (CBT) have been shown to be complimentary, but therapy is by no means a critical success factor in Medication Assisted Treatment.

I think as you read the research you'll notice too, that it's the 'Medication', with less emphasis on the 'Assisted' part of Medication Assisted Treatment that is the critical component here.

DEALING WITH NAYSAYERS & THE CRUTCH

BE READY TO BE TOLD NOT TO BOTHER

We live in a culture with a very skewed perspective on the disease of alcoholism.

We looked at this extensively in part 1, but if you skipped over that to this section then all you need to know is that you may run up against a lot of people in positions of authority (at treatment centres, in the medical system, social workers, nurses, doctors, treatment professionals, etc.), that are under the influence of this skewed perspective and will not be supportive of your efforts to be treated medically.

If you start to go down the path of considering or trying medications, be ready for what you will hear from others.

People don't know about these drugs and the AA effect has really biased society away from anything that is not 12-step based.

Talk to enough people, and you *will* be told:

- Medication doesn't work

- Medication is a crutch

- Medication is not 'pure sobriety'

- Don't bother

- Medications aren't effective and don't work

- All these medications are addictive

All of these things are entirely untrue.

Please don't listen to them. The people that will tell you certainly haven't read the research and have themselves been immersed in mistruths, maybe for decades.

Tell them to come back and talk to you when they've read this book–the whole book.

When asked about medications, here are the kinds of things that people in 'the industry' will say, as quoted from a Newsweek article from 2008 (but you can find this type of sentiment everywhere):

"We need four or five more years to see how [Vivitrol] does," says staff psychiatrist Garrett O'Connor at the Betty Ford Center, in Rancho Mirage, Calif. "And we need to be very cautious, because a failed treatment will set a person back."[58]

The Ford Center and the Hazelden Foundation, in Minnesota, use drugs sparingly, and mostly just in the first days or weeks of recovery, the "detox" phase.

"Hazelden will never turn its back on pharmaceutical solutions, but a pill all by itself is not the cure," says William Moyers, Hazelden's vice president of external affairs. "We're afraid that people are seeking a medical route that says treatment is the end, not the beginning."[58]

These kinds of cautious, unfounded responses spread misinformation. They are insidious. They sound like they know what they are talking about, and these people hold senior positions in respected organizations. Why wouldn't you believe them?

But what they say is nonsense. It's fearmongering by 12-step advocates designed to scare anyone considering medications away.

Let's break this down...

Statement:

"We need four or five more years to see how [Vivitrol] does."

Response:

Naltrexone (which is the medication in Vivitrol) has now been researched for over 23 years (since 1992), and the extended release version (Vivitrol), has been studied in humans for over 10 years, since 2005.

And as early as 2002, one report showed that up to 2001 there had already been 14 trials assessing the effectiveness of naltrexone compared with placebo for treating alcoholism, enrolling 2127 subjects, in five countries. It stated, "there is strong evidence that naltrexone significantly reduces alcohol relapses to heavy drinking, the frequency and quantity of alcohol consumption in those who do drink, and alcohol craving."[46]

Highly respected researchers have said:

- "Meta-analyses of available trials, even when the negative study is included in the analysis, unequivocally support NTX [naltrexone injection] efficacy."[1]

- "There is abundant evidence supporting the use of naltrexone for the treatment of alcohol dependence (Level A)."[176]

The first quote comes from Markus Heilig, one of top 10 researchers of AUD worldwide; former NIAAA Clinical Director; active medical practitioner; author of more than 200 peer-reviewed journal articles, including papers in Science, PNAS, Lancet, Archives of General Psychiatry. His research work has 8000+ citations. Egli and Soyka's credentials are just as impressive.

Statement:

"And we need to be very cautious, because a failed treatment will set a person back."

Response:

This is fear-mongering with no basis in reality. It implies that medication is likely to fail, with severely negative consequences. But the other available treatments fail consistently–over 90% of the time in fact. So if people are being 'set back' by treatment failure, it is happening every day, with every other treatment anyways. And alcoholism is a chronic, medical condition, of which relapse is a symptom. So there will be setbacks for some people with every treatment.

Why does medication deserve more caution? Does anyone say you should be 'very cautious' about going to AA?

Well, actually some do–and justifiably so–Google the phrases 'thirteenth step AA' or 'predators in AA' if you'd like more information on the problems vulnerable newcomers and women have experienced in 12-step programs.

Statement:

"Hazelden will never turn its back on pharmaceutical solutions, but…"

Response:

This is like when a person says, "I don't mean to offend, but.", and then insults you.

One recovering lawyer quoted in an article on addiction commented on this kind of response from places like Hazelden saying:

"It's a paradox that some of addicts' biggest advocates have been the most resistant to new treatments...But a lot of them come to the field after recovering from their own addictions, and they can be very stubborn about what works and what doesn't."[58]

More pointedly, she adds, "some people feel recovery from addiction should not be easy or convenient."[58]

So... be ready for the inevitable naysayers you will meet.

And keep in mind—they just don't know any better.

WHEN IS A MEDICATION 'A CRUTCH'?

"The ideal, of course, is to be physically and emotionally healthy without medications. Just turns out that hasn't been the case for me.
I kinda see the medications as a crutch. But when you're disabled—either temporarily or permanently—you need a crutch.
And oh, how I can run when I have my crutch!!!"
—Recovering Alcoholic

People who have been involved in 12-step programs often struggle with the idea of incorporating other treatment approaches—instead of or in addition to AA—into their lifestyles. From time to time I have heard people who are influenced by AA guiltily describing taking medications for alcohol dependence as a 'crutch.'

Sadly, while this belief is outdated and irrational, it's still widely taught and believed in 12-step groups.

When the 12-step based Hazelton treatment center started including medication as a treatment for addiction they had enormous resistance from program members.

Medical Director Marvin Seppala describes the way pressure is sometimes applied to members who choose to take medications:

> "We have had resistance within the 12-step communities. No 12-step groups have resisted specifically what we are talking about or even spoke against it in any public forum.
>
> In keeping with their traditions that hasn't happened.
>
> Individuals, however, certainly have come forward and said things like, "You're ruining AA" and "We don't want your patients on medicine in our meetings."
>
> They refuse to sponsor people on those medications. It's been troublesome from that perspective … we've actually developed an approach called Stigma Management for our patients. If they're placed on medication and they're attending 12-step meetings, we help them find meetings that are amendable to these medications…
>
> Some people at some meetings won't let people talk about this. They'll really give them a hard time and tell them to get off the medications even though a doctor at one of our facilities has prescribed them."[73]

In Gabrielle Glaser's excellent article, 'The Irrationality of AA', she writes:

> "It's not that AA started out as irrational, but when you stand still and do not evolve, while the world evolves and changes around you and you don't question yourself, you can become irrational in comparison."

The crutch concept started out rationally.

There was not a single effective medication for any mental illness in the 1930s when AA was started.

Back then, the lobotomy was still considered cutting edge and treatment for mental illness was more like torture.

The very first medication for alcoholism was opium. And later, the Keeley Cure helped civil war surgeon Leslie Keeley grow rich by selling a 'scientific' treatment–containing 28% alcohol.

The Keeley Institute treated alcoholics with the 'cure' up until 1939, incidentally the same year the big book of AA was first published.

Other medicinal 'cures' followed–many of them useless, harmful, addictive or all of the above.

So in 1939, and for decades after that, when mental illness was untreatable and alcoholism medication was ineffective at best and addictive at worst, it made a lot of sense to dissuade AA members from relying on any substance or treatment other than AA.

In addition, alcoholism is such an insidious disease–hijacking ones' own thought processes and decision-making–that susceptibility to other addictive substances is something alcoholics must be vigilant about.

In the early thirties, forties and fifties, when there were no good medication options for any kind of mental illness, let alone alcoholism, drawing a line in the sand and saying 'medication is a crutch' was simply a way to help alcoholics steer clear of pitfalls.

There's an analogy that I believe fits AA in many aspects of its existence. It's a story about a lady who used to cut the top inch off of every turkey she cooked before it went in the oven. When asked why, she said she didn't know why it was done, but it was the way her mother had taught her.

One day, she asked her mother why she used this approach, and her mother responded, "my oven was always too small to fit the bird in it–so I cut a piece off the top to get it in."

It's easy to understand AA's original intention and approach, but once again, like many of AA's notions, the idea that medications are unequivocally unacceptable is now doing more harm than good.

If you are someone who is strongly influenced by 12-step principles, and the 'medication is a crutch' issue is problematic for you, then it's time for you to stop cutting the top off the turkey.

And maybe it's time to look at AA as the crutch instead.

There is a place for AA in the future—alcoholics still need a great deal of support—something AA provides well.

But anyone dissuading an alcoholic from taking medication in this century—anyone who thinks they know better than the thousands of gifted medical researchers and addiction specialists whose research is cited in this book—should consider that they may be helping to sign that alcoholic's death certificate.

Avoid MOM

Medication Option Myopia—MOM for short—is a common downfall that you need to avoid in this process. This book—which presents not just one, but many medication solutions—is attempting to counter this pitfall.

There is a curious phenomenon that affects how we make choices and how we recommend options to others. I'm calling it 'option myopia' for lack of a better term.

When I read Claudia Christian's book about her experiences with alcoholism and finding naltrexone and then watched her documentary, 'One Little Pill,' I became convinced that her direction was the 'right' direction. I disregarded information about other medication I came across.

Later, when I read Dr. Ameisen's book about his experiences and how baclofen (and only baclofen) worked for him, I could see that he was very focused on helping others to access baclofen—and only baclofen. In fact, in some of his writing, I'm sad to say that he criticized those prescribing any medication other than baclofen.

I think it works like this... we think that 'what saved me' is most likely to save you too. And the bigger the impact that solution had on our own lives, the more 'stuck' we are on the idea that it is the ONLY way for anyone else.

And, if you are on the receiving end of advice from someone who is truly passionate and honest about their experience, the more likely we may be to feel that 'what saved them' will 'save me too.'

Option Myopia applies to doctors too (and maybe this is one reason why they aren't prescribing these medications).

But you can see it everywhere—it may be why you want your son to be a lawyer just like you; or why my friend wants me to buy the same kind of car she drives; or why your daughter wants you to be vegan and gluten-free just like her. It's one of the reasons that AA members are also so adamant about AA.

While Option Myopia comes from a good place, it can be very dangerous. You may find it affects you in these ways:

- You will be less likely to get support from others who are emotionally invested in their own recovery solutions.

- You may become quite emotionally invested in one solution; and if that solution doesn't work for you, may be devastated by the outcome and hesitant to try anything else.

I am here (admittedly with my own biases and myopia) to suggest that you do not pin your hope on one medication: avoid MOM and be completely option neutral.

Come on this journey with the long-term view—that if the first medication doesn't work, there are at least 10 more to try.

And maybe you'll have to try ten before you hit on what works for you. Think of this as a marathon, not a sprint. Do not become emotionally invested in one medication or solution. Be like the scientists—test it, and if it doesn't work, learn and move on.

Recognize it's okay if you don't get support from people who are option myopic themselves—this is inevitable; ignore them.

Remember it is a very few lucky ones who hit on the right medication first—Ameisen, for example, tried AA, short-term rehab, long-term rehab, psychological counseling, disulfiram, naltrexone, acamprosate and topiramate with very little effect before finding that high-dose baclofen worked for him.

And in the end, it was a combination of three solutions that helped Ameisen the most. What brought Ameisen serenity was to apply what he had learned in AA and psychological counseling to a new life with baclofen.

What if you try numerous medications and nothing works?

Then take a break for a few years. And then, one day try again: things are now changing more quickly in this space than they have for decades—so if the current solutions don't work for you, take a break but don't give up.

By the way, don't get option myopic about the broader idea of medication for alcohol treatment either.

Perhaps mindfulness and meditation or some other approach will work for you more effectively. That's perfectly okay.

Maybe ultimately you'll discover that taking magic mushrooms and praying to God while you hang upside down from your heels every night is just the thing that helps you find your way.

That's wonderful—more power to you!

[But do us all a favor and don't create a cult that professes this will work for everyone if they just work hard enough at it. Thank-you.]

Remember: be solution neutral, not option-myopic.

WHEN TO START

Why *would* you wait?

Is medication the last resort for someone who has tried every other way to reduce or quit drinking?

Hell no. The earlier, the better.

There is no evidence that medication should be the treatment of last resort, and in fact, given that alcoholism is a disease that becomes progressively more severe and the alcoholic loses more and more control as its progress continues, it is logical that medication should be one of the first solutions examined.

Doctors do not wait to prescribe effective medications to people who are diagnosed with other serious illnesses (including mental illnesses) until every other possible means of 'natural' or 'spiritual' alternative is extinguished.

Many individuals who are first diagnosed with mental illness not only are often prescribed medication in the very same appointment, but are told that if they *don't* take the medication that other treatment will not be made available to them.

So, particularly given the fact that many of them are very safe, commonly used medications for other illnesses, why should doctors wait to treat alcohol dependence with medication?

It's well documented that progressive alcoholism causes physiological and brain damage ('neuroadaptations') to sufferers. There is no reason to let this damage progress.

Waiting not only weakens one's ability over time to gain control over dependence, but the risk of illness and death increases significantly with every year—so it makes sense that alcohol dependence is treated—right from its identification—in a much more aggressive way perhaps even than other mental illnesses.

The medication may have more of a fighting chance in someone with a weaker addiction, and whose body and mind are still in some ways healthy (versus many years down the road when other medications and illnesses could further hamper recovery), and who still have social supports, such as friends and family and employment, in place.

BRING YOUR GRAIN OF SALT

One of the themes of this book is educating yourself.

But as you are reading through research, or hearing the comments of others about personal or scientific findings (whether it's online or in a doctor's office) I recommend taking their conclusions with a grain of salt.

With so little knowledge and clear information available about treatments for alcoholism, mistruths are rife.

In one forum I remember reading a posting about one medication that said, "scientists thought that XYZ was true, but that was completely disproven in a recent study."

You can't draw a conclusion from a single study—unlike the poster stated, a single study cannot completely prove or disprove anything.

Conclusions can only be drawn with some degree of accuracy after multiple well-run studies have been conducted properly by different scientists, that reproduce the finding of the first study. So I caution you never to base your conclusions on one study or one comment.

Even in scientific research, it seems that sometimes there is an agenda behind certain conclusions. (And that is just one reason why a high-quality body of research–not just one or two studies–is important to take into consideration).

For example, one of the things that have surprised me as I read through all of the research I have is how easy it is to 'prove' that something doesn't work if you really want to.

Some of the research I have read almost seems like it is setting a medication up for failure on purpose. (In these cases I wonder what political or financial gain is behind the design of the test.)

For example, one piece of research that caught my eye is an article called, "Comparison of baclofen vs. naltrexone treatment during abstinence on the reinstatement of alcohol self-administration in baboons"[177] which was published in the *Journal of Drug and Alcohol Dependence* in 2015.

The first part of all research reports contain an abstract, which is a summary of the experiment, its results, and conclusions. The stark results of this piece of research were stated at the end of the abstract: "Conclusions: These data do not support the use of baclofen during early abstinence to reduce relapse to heavy drinking."

It's so easy to scan this research and conclude simply that 'baclofen doesn't work,' from this conclusion.

However, the way that baclofen was administered to baboons in this experiment is completely different to the way researchers have found baclofen must be administered to humans in order to be effective.

Specifically, baboons were given small doses of baclofen beginning on day 1 of a 5-day forced abstinence period and it was found that they drank just as much on day 6 as baboons taking another alcohol dependence drug–naltrexone (which is known to decrease drinking).

However, baclofen has been shown to work best under completely different circumstances.

It's recommended to slowly taper up dosage over the course of weeks or months, maintain a very high maximum dose (a much higher maximum amount than the grams per kg tested with the baboons), for a month or more until a switch point where reduced craving and desire for alcohol is achieved, and then slowly taper down to a maintenance level. An entirely different scenario than those poor drunken baboons experienced.

The conclusion for the baboon test should perhaps instead have been: "When administered in a way that has never been shown to work, and we didn't really think would work, baclofen does not work."

STEP 2: DESIGN YOUR PATHWAY

WHICH DRUG WORKS BEST?

After facing a barren landscape of non-medical treatment options for alcoholism for years, you may now find yourself overwhelmed by the plethora of pharmaceuticals that actually are realistic options for you.

So, the question is, which one do you start with?

If I (or anyone) could tell you which drug will work best for you, they would be sitting on their own private island drinking beer out of a golden stein right now.

I promise you that the best that science has to offer is at most a pretty uneducated guess about which medications you should try first, and second and third…

If someone is 'certain' about anything related to these drugs (certain they will work, or certain they won't work, or certain about the 'best' one), then I can tell you with 100% confidence that person is not someone whose advice you should hold in high regard.

That is because the *only* certainty in this field right now, today, is that nobody can tell you that.

We just do not know enough about alcoholism and how each drug works to predict which drug will work for which person. At this time, it is impossible to rule out a drug (due to lack of predicted effectiveness) in anybody.

The only way to know for sure if a medication will help you is to try it.

And that is why, when deciding which drugs to try first, I recommend you think about your plan as a 'Medication Pathway.'

And by this I mean, instead of selecting *the drug*, create a list of drugs. As yourself–based on what I know about myself and these medications–which might be the first drug I try, and then the second drug I try, and then the third one, and then the fourth, and so on.

Don't choose a drug–choose a pathway.

•••

Do you remember the game 'Mastermind'?

It's a code breaking game. The code maker hides a set of four colored pegs at the end of a plastic board. The codebreaker tries different combinations of pegs, one set of four at a time. After each attempt, the code maker gives hints about the accuracy of the guess. The code breaker gets 12 different tries to get it right, solving the code through trial and error.

Choosing a medication for alcoholism is a lot like a game of Mastermind.

That's not very helpful when it comes to narrowing down where to begin, though.

So here is how you will go about determining which medications you need to try.

CREATE A LONG LIST

To start with, keep reading.

- This book covers the characteristics that give hints as to which medications may or may not work. So as you read, write down your personal characteristics–whether you think you are a Type A or B alcoholic or a combination; if you have other health concerns; if you smoke or not; if your alcoholism is what you use to treat another illness like anxiety or depression; write down your goals.

- Then read through the list of medications. As you read, take a few notes about the ones you think might be helpful for you based on your own personal characteristics.

Those notes (and any other information you gather elsewhere) will help you create a 'long list' of drugs.

The A-List and B-Lists contain 15 medications in total. You may be able to cross a few off your list, or lower their priority just through what you learn about yourself and the medications.

Research has given us 'directional clues' about medication.

For example, research has shown that some medications work better for Type B than Type A alcoholism, and other medications seem to work better for those motivated to drink by reward (versus motivated by anxiety). (Type and drinking motivation are discussed in more detail later).

These directional clues can help you choose where to start or what to try next.

But keep in mind that for every little clue we have that suggests a drug *may not* work for someone, there are examples where that drug worked very well for that person.

And for every clue we have that a particular drug *will* and *should* work for someone, there are examples of people it has been completely ineffective in.

And as frustrating and as hit-or-miss as this may be, the fact that you can't rule too many drugs out because there's little proof it *won't* work is, at least, a hopeful thing. (It means it's very difficult to run out of options).

This hit-or-miss approach is the one recommended by scientists.

Raye Z. Litten, Ph.D. Associate Director Division of Treatment and Recovery Research National Institute on Alcohol Abuse and Alcoholism (NIAAA) says, "what we hope to do is to actually have a menu of treatments that clinicians could choose from. If one drug doesn't work or they can't tolerate it," patients would "try another one and so forth, and hopefully they'll find one that is effective."[3]

If that process leaves you confused, know that any one of the medications on the A-List has a wealth of data supporting its effectiveness, so starting with one or two drugs on that list may be as good a start as any.

You could simply do this—start with the first medication on the A-List and begin with that one, and work your way down.

NARROW TO A SHORT LIST

Next, your long list can be made into a shorter list due to other factors.

These factors are less to do with effectiveness and more to do with aspects like availability, commitment and safety than effectiveness.

For example, when choosing a medication to start with, ask yourself these questions:

Availability:

- Is it available in my country?

- Will my doctor prescribe it?

- Can I afford it?

Commitment:

- Are the potential side effects tolerable? Am I willing to take the medication even if they make me feel sick, spacey or tired?

- If availability will be a barrier, am I willing to pursue other ways of obtaining it?

Safety:

- Will it interact with other medications I take?

- Can I take it despite existing health concerns?

LEARN FROM YOUR EXPERIENCES

Once you begin to try a medication, pay very close attention to your behaviors, thoughts and actions. Identify any variations you can. These will be clues in your journey.

For example—let's say you feel a strong effect from naltrexone. Maybe the first few times you try it, instead of drinking that whole bottle of wine, you just walk away from it.

Later you drink on it but you don't feel what you are looking for from the alcohol.

A few days later, you avoid taking the pill before you drink and you give up on naltrexone.

Great! That's not a failure.

You've learned four valuable things:

1) Your brain responds to naltrexone.

2) Naltrexone removes some pleasure from your drinking.

3) Your alcoholism may be tied to the reward system in the brain (the part that includes dopamine and the opioid system which makes drinking feel good).

4) You have trouble with 'as needed' medication.

What can you do with that information?

You can:

• Try another naltrexone method (such as monthly injection).

• Try another medication that works differently but targets the reward system—such as topiramate.

• You can add another medication on that helps you with that impulsiveness that leads you to jump straight to the drink without the pill. Like acamprosate or even disulfiram.

• You can try some combination of the above options.

Learning these things and applying them to the process is exactly what will move you down that game board toward success.

And as you eliminate medications by trying them, use what you have learned to revise that pathway. One day you may land upon the perfect combination for you.

Mastermind!

WHAT TYPE ARE YOU?

One of the most important clues you can use to determine which medications to take is the type of alcoholic you are. Read on to learn more about determining whether you are Type A, or Type B.

But first, imagine this scenario:

There may be 10 people in a room, all who drink excessively, none of whom have the ability to control their alcohol intake, and whose drinking is damaging to themselves and to those around them.

All ten might be considered to have 'textbook alcoholism'. All ten would receive the same diagnosis.[131]

But do all ten have the same disease?

Probably not.

They each may have very different sets of genes and environmental variables that put them at risk. And these very different genes may contribute to very different imbalances in their brains and bodies that all ultimately result in alcohol addiction.

Understanding this is the key to understanding why one medication for alcoholism will work extremely well in one alcoholic, and have no effect whatsoever in another.

There is more and more evidence that there are at least two types of alcoholism: Type A and Type B.[178] As research progresses, other types will be identified.

Type A and Type B are probably made up of two separate (but sometimes intersecting) pools of very different genetic variations. But because we don't have conclusive genetic testing for alcoholism, the way that we determine Alcoholism type is based on two factors driven by those genetic variations.

Those two factors are:

1) When your heavy drinking began.

2) Whether you have a family history of alcoholism or not.

As research progresses, types (and their corresponding medical treatments) will probably be at least partially (if not completely) delineated based on findings related to your DNA.

Genetic variations hold the key to whether a medication will work for you or not. And correspondingly, we have been able to see that some gene variations seem to occur more frequently in Type A alcoholics, and other variations appear more frequently in Type B's.

So it may be very useful for you to try to classify yourself–if possible–as one of the two types. You may find that you are the very definition of one of the types, or you may find that you have overlapping characteristics shared by both.

Here is how both are described:

Type B alcoholism ('Early Onset Alcoholism') is described as[178]:

- the most distinct form

- thought to be present in 65% of alcohol-dependent people[179]

- due to its higher severity, this subtype is seen more frequently in treatment or medical facilities

- characterized by an early age of onset (before the age of 25)

- tendency toward high impulsivity

- strong family history of alcoholism

- motivated early on by strong enjoyment of drinking

Type A alcoholism ('Late Onset Alcoholism') is described as[178]:

- everyone else

- thought to be present 35% of alcohol-dependent subjects[179]

- anxious personality traits may be a characteristic feature

If you are struggling to determine which type you may be, researcher Bankole Johnson suggests that the best way to determine whether you are a type A or B alcoholic is to ask a single question: "…at what age did drinking become a problem for you?"[178]

If it became a problem early–before the age of 25, then you may be Type B; if it was later–after the age of 25, then you may be a Type A.

If you find it hard to remember which type is which, this trick might help: The word 'late' has a distinctive 'A' sound in it. Remember the word 'lAte' associated with type A alcoholism and you won't get confused.

And the phrase 'the early bird gets the worm' can help too, since 'bird' starts with a 'B', and Type Bs start early.

RELATIONSHIP BETWEEN TYPES & MEDS

It is thought that in Type B alcoholics, early alcohol consumption is driven by a strong biological need for positive reinforcement of the brain's reward system.

In other words, Type B alcoholics may crave from an early age the feelings and experiences that alcohol brings.

In contrast, Type A alcoholics' consumption may be driven by an entirely different process–for example, an imbalance in the stress hormone system which generates feelings that the individual seeks to numb and lessen with alcohol.

In short, it's hypothesized that in general, Type A's are driven by pleasure (and alcoholism may be more reinforced by malfunctions in the reward centres of the brain), and Type B's are driven to numb pain (and perhaps related more to stress systems).

It's this thinking that reveals why medicines work for different types. Pleasure/reward and pain/stress are generated and controlled by very different brain systems. And different medications are used to target these different brain systems.

Earlier in the book I mentioned how knowing the type of alcoholism you may have can help you narrow down the medications to try.

As you read through descriptions of medications and research highlights in the next part of the book you'll come across examples where research into specific medications showed different results for Type A alcoholics than Type B alcoholics.

Ondansetron is an example of one of the medications where this has been found to be the case. Researcher Dr. Bankole Johnson showed that ondansetron reduced drinking in Type B alcoholics, but was ineffective in Type A patients.

Johnson hypothesized that this is because ondansetron impacts receptors in the brain that interfere with the positive reinforcement the brain provides when alcohol is present. In other words–it interferes with the pleasure that Type B's seek. And over time it may weaken the brain's conditioning, decreasing craving and drive for alcohol.

Bankole was also able to connect the success of ondansetron specifically to a group of Type B alcoholics with specific genetic variations. He found that alcoholics carrying a combination of the same five gene variations were able to reduce their drinking when taking ondansetron.

One of the combinations within these 5 gene variations were held by individuals who responded in such a positive way to ondansetron that he termed this group 'super-responders'.[180]

And notably, for alcoholics in the study *without* these genetic markers, being treated with ondansetron actually worsened their alcohol consumption.

Johnson suggests that a DNA test that looks for these five genetic markers will one day predict the outcome of treatment by ondansetron in alcoholics.

He is not the only researcher who thinks DNA testing will help alcoholics find the best treatment. The Director of the National Institute on Alcohol Abuse and Alcoholism (NIAAA), Dr. George Koob says, "Our hope is that down the line, we might be able to do a simple blood test that tells if you will be a naltrexone person, an acamprosate person, a ghrelin person.[181]

Better yet, perhaps eventually, we'll use this testing to prevent alcoholism in the first place.

As researcher Dr. Marc A Schuckit says, "it's theoretically possible to take kids before they first drink, find out whether they have any gene variations, and say to them, 'If you choose to be a drinker, then be careful.'"[3]

Unfortunately, this kind of DNA testing is not yet available to the general public. But with private DNA testing services like 23andme.com popping up online, it's only a matter of time. (At this time, 23andme.com does not provide this type of testing, they are simply given as an example of the type of company that eventually might).

Johnson's work is not the only work that is connecting the dots between alcoholism, genes, and medications.

At least six of the medications discussed in this book respond to alcoholism in individuals with specific genetic variants.

For example, topiramate has been shown to work more effectively on carriers of a variation of the GRIK1 gene.

Naltrexone's efficacy seems tied to variations of OPRM1 and DRD4; sertraline shows promise in carriers of variations of 5HTTLPR[182]; and people with a variation of the gene GATA4 have shown improvement with acamprosate.[47]

For doxazosin, scientists that saw that alcoholics with a strong family history saw a drinking reduction, but for those with little family history of alcoholism, increased drinking was seen.[183]

OFF-LABEL MEDICATIONS

"My doctor won't prescribe it to me because it is off label, and he says he could lose his license."

Understanding what 'off-label' means and what its implications are, is critical to being able to advocate for yourself with your doctor.

This is because the statement above, written by someone in an online forum who was seeking a prescription for topiramate for the treatment of their alcoholism—represents a common, but false misconception.

The term 'FDA-Approved', means a medication has been approved by the United States Food and Drug Administration.

If you are in Canada, the equivalent term is that a drug has been 'Approved by Health Canada'.

In Europe, the drug has been 'Approved by the European Medicines Agency (EMA)'.

All three of these organizations are responsible for evaluating and regulating medicinal products within their regions.

A drug company interested in selling a prescription drug must test it in various ways. First are lab and animal experiments and next are human tests to see if the drug is safe and effective in humans.

After testing, the drug company sends the FDA an application with the test results and a proposed label. The label indicates the illnesses it has been shown effective for, possible risks, and the approved dosage.

For example, many years ago, a drug called Quinine was FDA-Approved as an anti-malaria medication. This means it went through testing and was shown safe and effective specifically for this purpose. So, when prescribed in the FDA-approved manner, it is prescribed only as protection against malaria—as per the label instruction.

Quinine is now far more likely to be prescribed by doctors for people who suffer from nighttime leg cramps than as protection against malaria.

When it is prescribed for that purpose, it is prescribed 'off-label.'

If it were prescribed for anti-malaria purposes, but at *double* the FDA-approved dosage, it would also be called an 'off-label' prescription.

Drug companies often learn about other uses for their medications before submitting the FDA application but choose not to seek regulatory approval for the other use.

The entire process of testing and application development is very expensive, so whether the drug company decides to submit another application for the other use or not is based solely on a cost-benefit analysis.

The effectiveness of a medication, and its on- or off-label status are much less related than you might assume.

It is important to know that a medication is not 'off-label' because it is not proven or effective. ('Off-label' and effectiveness are completely unrelated).

A drug can be extremely safe and effective and be better than on-label treatments yet be off-label *simply* because it has not been in a drug company's best financial interests to apply for approval for the specific purpose of treatment of alcohol use disorders. Drug development and approval is motivated solely by shareholder value—not altruism.

The three drugs that have had on-label approval for alcoholism in North America are the same three mentioned earlier as being 'first line': acamprosate, naltrexone, and disulfiram.

It is illegal for pharmaceutical companies to market drugs for their known off-label purposes.

So, for example, even though Quinine can be legally prescribed by doctors as a medication that helps nighttime leg cramps, drug companies are not allowed to promote or market or even speak to doctors about Quinine's use for leg cramps.

Quinine could have a thousand research studies supporting its incredible leg cramp capability but without going through an approval process and gaining FDA-approval, the drug company that owns it can never–will never–say a word to a doctor about it.

Whether or not to prescribe medication for an on-label or off-label purpose is solely the decision of the doctor. It is an entirely legal and very common practice.

Prescribing off-label can be very beneficial to patients (for example–those suffering nighttime leg cramps), but doctors can be averse to doing so because it also has its risks.

Doctors don't want to open themselves up to the risk that patients under their care will be harmed by a drug that has not been tested for the purpose for which the drug is being prescribed.[184]

For example, Quinine was never tested for the purpose for which it is used most.

In 2011, Health Canada issued an advisory that it had received 71 reports of serious adverse reactions to Quinine, 67 of which were for prescriptions for leg cramps, not malaria.

But despite doctor's fears, off-label prescribing happens every day, is completely within the doctor's legal rights to do, and is necessary to patient care.

The American Medical Association says that the deciding factor in off-label prescribing is up to the doctor and based on "the best interest of the patient."[22]

The FDA only regulates drug approval–not drug prescribing. According to one expert, doctors are:

> *"Free to prescribe a drug for any reason they think is medically appropriate and off-label use is so common that virtually every drug is used off-label in some circumstances."*[185]

Off-label prescribing is extremely common. Over 23 percent (more than one in five) of all prescriptions and over 60 percent in cancer care are off-label.[22]

In Canada, nearly 80% of prescriptions for rare diseases are off-label.[186]

And in fact, regarding doctor's prescribing habits, and the ethics around them, so few medicines are approved for rare diseases that doctors would be acting unethically if they only prescribed on-label medications for rare illnesses.

Alcoholism is the same in this regard–with so few approved medications for its treatment–it could be argued that any doctor refusing to prescribe off-label medication for its treatment is also acting unethically.

There is one other thing that is important to know about off-label prescribing and it relates to drug coverage.

Medications that are prescribed for off-label treatments can fall into a loophole in many insurance coverage plans. Some plans may restrict reimbursement to medications prescribed for on-label purposes only.

Of course, this can create burdensome cost implications for anyone seeking treatment for alcohol use disorders and can (and probably will) severely limit the medications you may be able to get coverage for.

So knowing in advance whether your coverage plan will cover an off-label use of medication you are requesting from your doctor can impact the way you may choose to go about selecting and obtaining medication.

But the bottom line is that if a doctor is telling you that they can lose their license for prescribing one of the drugs in this book to you (particularly if it is one of the ones in the heavily-researched A-List), then it may be time to try to educate the old one, or look for a new one.

ARE THESE DRUGS ADDICTIVE?

Of all of the medications found in this book, there are only two which raise any kind of concerns in regard to addictive qualities.

The first is Sodium Oxybate, which is found very last on the B-List.

I wasn't sure whether to include it on the B-List or not because of its addictive nature, and that is why it is very last on the list.

Finally, I included it because, despite its addictive qualities: (a) there is a great deal of research showing its exceptional effectiveness; (b) a new formulation is being developed which will include deterrents to its use in addictive behavior; and (c) it has been used for many years successfully as a treatment in Italy for alcoholism.

I think that, should the new formulation (with addiction-deterrents) be successful, then Sodium Oxybate could one day find itself on the A-List.

The second is gabapentin, which is found on the A-List.

This drug is not addictive by itself. It is also a common medication prescribed in high volumes by many physicians around the world.

However, it has been found to be used as a booster (a drug that makes another drug more potent) for other addictive behavior in a very small number of cases.

If your addiction is limited to alcohol, and you do not abuse any other substance, then you need not have any concerns about gabapentin in regard to addiction.

COMBINING MEDICATIONS

Adjunctive therapy is the term used to describe adding a second medication or other treatment to make a first one more effective.

For example, adjunctive therapy might include adding acamprosate to your naltrexone regime, or it could mean adding cognitive behavioral therapy to your naltrexone regime.

For the treatment of alcoholism, adjunctive therapy—with a second or even a third medication—has a higher probability of working for you than treatment with only one medication. (Though because so many alcoholics have trouble even getting the first prescription for even one medication, it's only a lucky few who are able to access this kind of multi-drug treatment).

There is good reason for this approach and it is one that holds greater promise as more research is done.[178]

First, more than one neurotransmitter system in the brain is affected by alcoholism and different medications target different systems, which target different feelings and behaviors found in alcoholism.

So one medication can be working on one system while another medication is working on another.

Second, multiple medications can target other psychiatric conditions that often come hand-in-hand with alcoholism—from depression to anxiety to bipolar or schizophrenia.

Third, a lower dose of each of two drugs can minimize the side effects experienced with a higher dose of a single drug; and this, in turn, can improve adherence to the treatment.

Fourth, by combining medications, synergistic effects can be found—the drugs can build on each other resulting in a better end-result for the patient compared to improvements of each drug individually.

And finally, choosing a medication is very hit or miss—a medication often will work for only one out of five to ten individuals (similar to anti-depressants), so it increases your odds of finding a solution sooner if you are able to try more than one at a time, especially when the ones you are trying are acting on different systems in the brain.

A recent study by respected NIAAA researcher Dr. Lorenzo Leggio looked at seventeen different clinical studies (eleven of which were high quality, randomized, double-blind and placebo controlled) that investigated combinations of medications in alcoholism.

It found that ten of the eleven high-quality studies showed the combination of drugs to be superior to placebo and that three out of eleven showed an overall advantage of the combination.[187]

While several of the drugs in this book have been combined in some research and shown promising results, there is still little research on the combining of medications to treat alcoholism. (There is a shortage of funding for research and development in alcohol addiction as it is, and so research that looks at multiple medications at once is lacking).

However, for individuals who are pursuing their own treatment, looking at medication combinations could be very promising.

So as you read through the rest of the book, if you plan to pursue medication options, ask yourself whether combinations may be worth looking into.

You may wish to consider a multi-medication strategy.

Multi-Medication Strategy Example

A multi-medication strategy could be used to break down the elements of alcoholism you struggle with and target them separately.

For example, you may want to look at one drug as a way to weaken your cravings and decrease responsiveness to stress or alcohol cues; while another medication could be selected based on your experience when drinking on it (lessening the pleasure of drinking or increasing your ability to stop after fewer drinks).

So for example, if you are trying to remain abstinent perhaps a combination of acamprosate and naltrexone could be considered.

The acamprosate may help you manage cravings which could lead to relapse; and the naltrexone may lessen the reward of drinking so that you drink less if you do lapse.

And if you do relapse, while this book does not cover medications that help with alcohol withdrawal, several medications can make withdrawal- and getting back on your feet again afterward less physically and mentally defeating.

For example, two in this book: baclofen and gabapentin, have been shown to help with withdrawal severity.

So a plan which attacks your alcoholism with a three-pronged approach might work for you: One to deter you from relapse for as long as possible; one to minimize the extent of the lapse itself; and a third to help you recover from the lapse as quickly as possible, to regain your equilibrium and health quickly.

While this may not be a 'cure' for your alcoholism, the severity and impact on your life could be greatly minimized by an approach such as this.

I'm not suggesting that you start dosing yourself with massive quantities of every kind of pill you can obtain.

The point I'm trying to make here is to be strategic.

If you can stand back and with your doctor's help assess the areas where you need the greatest support, then it's possible you could put a combination of medications in place that allow you to manage your alcoholism. Other chronic diseases are managed in the same way—with multiple medications that target different elements of the disease, allowing life to be livable.

Instead of having it continue to destroy you, it's possible that you might be able to use medications and other tools available to minimize alcoholism's impact on your life and health.

When considering combinations always look at the available research on combinations (see the Q&A section for each medication for combinations that have been researched together), and always check for drug interactions.

This can be done at online medication checkers, with your doctor or your pharmacist.

OTHER CONSIDERATIONS

There are many considerations you may wish to take into account when determining which medication to try (or to try next).

AVAILABILITY

What you can Obtain—At the Correct Dosage

Your doctor may not wish to prescribe medication to you at the doses that have been shown to be effective by research.

For example, research has shown that baclofen at very high doses (even as high as 300mg per day or more) may be required for effectiveness for some individuals. Sadly, many doctors are only comfortable prescribing up to 30mg of Baclofen per day for alcoholism.

If this is the most you are able to have prescribed to you, then it might be better to try another option instead.

Or, some individuals have reported that they will accept the prescription from their doctor anyways and then looked for other avenues where the dosage amount can be topped up—such as purchasing from an online pharmacy. In this way, some people are still able to have a doctor medically overlook their treatment, though they are actually dosing themselves at higher amounts. (As mentioned earlier–I don't recommend this–taking greater doses of medication without your doctor's knowledge can be extremely dangerous. However I also recognize the extreme treatment gap many patients face.)

If you have already tried one or more of the medications in this book and found them ineffective, it may be worthwhile for you to revisit just *how* they were prescribed to you. It's possible, (especially if you tried baclofen), that you were not prescribed an effective dose.

Don't rely solely on a single doctor's knowledge about dosage or what will or will not work. Learn as much as you can from research and online from others so that *you* can determine the approach you want to take– and then work hard to get that plan implemented *with* your doctor.

What's approved in Your Country or One you can Visit

Not all medications are available in all countries. Earlier I wrote about ways that some people have gotten around this–for example, by going to another country or ordering online.

If ordering online or leaving the country for treatment are not steps you wish to take then you may need to cross some medications off of your long list.

For anyone in Canada, naltrexone injection will need to be crossed off the list.

And unless you are in a country like Italy, where GHB has more acceptance and traction, GHB will probably be one to cross off too.

And because a version of GHB is illicit, don't even consider trying to buy it online or take it over a border.

If you'd like to try nalmefene, you may only be able to get it in Europe at the moment, so naltrexone may be a close alternative to try.

Cost and Health Plan Coverage

There are a few ways that may make medication less expensive for you. Here are a few:

- Lower costs by asking for generic drugs where they are available or by buying outside your area or over the internet if you can find a good quality source. Medications have very different price tags in different countries and in states and provinces within those countries.

- Look for ways to apply discounts (for example on the Vivitrol website—naltrexone injection—there is an opportunity to apply for an immediate $500 discount on the cost of the injection).

- Ask your doctor for free samples of prescribed drugs to help cover costs. (In Europe, samples for nalmefene, which is being marketed by Lundbeck to doctors there may be available to physicians who ask).

- Investigate insurance options which might cover certain medications. In Canada for example, there is an extensive list of medications not typically automatically covered, but for which you can apply to the government for coverage. You may need to dig a little to find out these types of options no matter where you live.

- Consider not just the per-pill cost of medication, but the cost of the medication at full dose for an extended period of time to be effective. (But if this seems exorbitant, don't forget to consider the cost to you and your family of your drinking and alcoholism over time too—as it may be far more 'expensive').

- Because of healthcare reforms and the 2008 mental health parity law, plans that did not cover you a few years ago may cover you now. The law that was put in place was intended to end discrimination in health insurance coverage seen in coverage of mental illness. Coverage providers may not be aware that alcohol dependence is a mental illness and should be covered by insurance just as treatment for any other mental illness would be.

SAFETY

Currently Drinking or Abstinent

Most of the medications on the A- and B-Lists (while not necessarily recommended) can be initiated and taken safely during detox and even while drinking.

The only significant exception to this is disulfiram—which is designed to cause major physical discomfort if it is in your system at the same time as alcohol. Never drink with disulfiram in your system.

There are two medications—naltrexone and nalmefene—that doctors are now being encouraged to prescribe in an 'as needed' manner. This means that they would be taken an hour before drinking. So if you are abstinent and wish to stay that way, the 'as needed' approach would not be for you.

However, research has also shown that for some people both of those medications can be taken (and may be helpful) even if you are abstinent and wish to remain so.

Side Effects

You may experience intolerable side effects with the same medication that others experience no side effects for. If you do experience side effects, under the care of a physician, here are a few things you can do:

- Slowly taper down your dose until you reach a dose that is more tolerable, and then very slowly and gradually increase the dosage until you get to the desired dose again. Sometimes your body needs more time to adjust.

- If you must stay at a lower dose, consider adding a second medication to your approach.

- Look at additional online information for the drug to see whether others experienced the side effects and found a way to minimize or tolerate them (or if they diminished over time).

- Remember—you and your support system are in the driver's seat here—take an active role in investigating and minimizing side effects. Always pay attention to what you are experiencing and then investigate their seriousness.

- These are serious medications that can have some rare, but real side-effects that can harm you. Go to your doctor if you have concerns.

- Be an educated consumer—read everything you can about the medication you are considering taking and be aware of all drug interactions, black label warnings, and side effects before you begin. Be smart and do your research.

- Sometimes there are simple over-the-counter products that can help with side-effects. For example, stomach problems and head-aches can be treated effectively separately. Sleeping pills can be prescribed that will help with insomnia. For loss of appetite, meal-replacement drinks can be helpful temporarily. Anti-nausea medication like gravol, or stronger medication can help with nausea. Problem-solve and try to research and find solutions for the side-effects before choosing to discontinue medication because of the effects.

- As long as you have checked with your doctor and side-effects are not health-threatening in any way, why not hold on for another week?

Existing Health Concerns and Drug Interactions

Alcoholism is confusing and stubborn enough without trying to treat it in tandem with another illness.

However, the fact is that concurrent mental and physical illnesses are extremely common experiences for those with alcoholism. In some cases they probably share some of the same genes.

If you have a concurrent illness, please be particularly careful to check drug interactions, dose up slowly and with caution, observe yourself carefully and ask your support system to give you feedback if they notice unusual emotional or physical changes in you. If you have a concurrent illness, it's even more important that you only take medication under a doctor's care.

Another health concern to be very careful with is liver damage. Alcoholism can seriously strain and damage your liver, so existing liver damage may narrow down your choices of medication too.

Some of the drugs in the book have been found to be quite safe for people with liver conditions, but work with your doctor closely on this. A government database related to drug-induced liver injury can be a helpful resource in this regard and is found at:

livertox.nih.gov

For some individuals, it may be most important to treat a concurrent illness first before trying a medication in this book.

If you are managing multiple illnesses, it's even more important that you find a doctor that can work closely and flexibly with you. If your current doctor is inflexible, then that may be the first issue you need to remedy.

Run any other pharmaceuticals or non-prescribed medications (for example opioids) through an online drug interaction checker to ensure that one medication will not interact with another you are taking.

Or ask a pharmacist to assess the interaction between one drug and another.

Drug interactions can be life threatening—make sure your approach is a safe one.

Safety & Trade-offs

Nobody *wants* to take medication for anything.

And safety concerns are very valid. The medications in this book can harm you if taken the wrong way.

However, if safety is a major barrier for you, consider the alternatives.

Compare the risks of taking these medications with the risk of continuing on the path you are on.

For some people, the path they are on will kill them—sooner rather than later. And for these people, the question I might put to them is: 'what do you really have to lose by trying?'

Maybe it is helpful to put this in a different perspective.

If you were told that radiation and chemotherapy were required to put your cancer in remission, there would be very few people who would opt not to undergo the treatment.

Yet radiation and chemotherapy expose people to both harmful short-term side-effects and enormous, long-term medical risks.

The side-effects and long-term health risks of current alcohol treatment drugs are mild or practically non-existent, in comparison. And these are medications that are fighting a disease that is just as serious as cancer.

If you have severe alcoholism, what choice do you really have?

For me, it's a no-brainer. If I were an alcoholic, I wouldn't hesitate. And if my parent or my child were alcoholic I would encourage them in this direction in a heartbeat. But that's just me.

COMMITMENT

You may be able to walk into their doctor's office with the right materials and approach, and convince them to prescribe either of the two first-line medications, naltrexone or acamprosate.

And if you are lucky, these drugs will be the right ones for you and you can begin to regain control of your life again.

However for others, this process will take a much larger degree of commitment. You will run into some barriers.

You'll need to jump through hoops finding a doctor that will work with you to access medications that are not first line.

They may be expensive; you may have to go to another country to obtain them; after working hard to obtain the medication, it may not be effective for you; you'll try medications where the side effects are uncomfortable.

This process may not be easy. I can practically guarantee you that it will not be easy.

But the only *true* barrier is your commitment to the process.

If you assume now that you will have barriers like these, then when you come to them they will be less difficult to accept. You'll know that all you have to do is keep pushing and looking for alternatives.

You can check every barrier you come to off on the list of 'problems in the system' and then try to work to change them later when you have your life back.

So determine your level of commitment now, and stick to it.

Compliance

'Compliance' sounds like a word used by accountants or interrogators. Or even worse, accountant interrogators.

But in medicine, compliance means you are following the directions that the doctor gave you regarding a prescription.

Some alcoholics are able to take medication, without their brains talking them out of it. Others have more difficulty.

Determining the option that will work best for you requires a certain level of honesty and self-assessment.

There are several medications known to present a challenge to some individuals in the area of compliance. These include disulfiram and naltrexone (and also perhaps nalmefene).

The effect of drinking alcohol while disulfiram is in your system is not one that anyone wishes to experience, not to mention being very dangerous to your health.

So if you simply cannot stay away from drinking, disulfiram may not be a good choice for you as you'll have trouble with compliance on this medication.

Naltrexone (via the Sinclair Method) and nalmefene are taken as needed–this means that you must have the ability to choose to take these drugs an hour before drinking, each and every time you drink. If that is not something you can commit to, then they may not be a good choice.

Baclofen requires several doses at varying times during the day–this not only requires commitment but also a certain level of sobriety to be able to carry through with the correct dosing.

For people where compliance is a serious problem, naltrexone by monthly injection may be a good option because commitment and follow-through only have to happen 12 times a year.

282 · MEDICATIONS FOR ALCOHOLISM

You may not realize you have trouble with compliance until you begin taking a medication, and then don't follow through on it.

That's okay. Learn from it, and move on to an alternative approach.

STEP 3: THE BIGGER PLAN

SPOKES ON A WHEEL

You medication plan is part of a bigger plan. (And I'm not talking about 'that' bigger plan).

This book focusses on medication. But just like any illness, you need to consider and take into account the balance of your entire lifestyle.

Think of your bigger plan like a wheel—with you in the center surrounded by spokes.

Each spoke represents an important part of your health. For example:

- Getting enough sleep

- Eating a healthy diet

- Connecting with others

- Continuing to gather knowledge

- Dealing with other medical issues

- Gathering support from positive sources

- Medication and treatment plan

- Physical activity

- Minimizing stress

- Dealing with financial issues

- Maintaining mental health

The stronger each of those spokes are, the greater likelihood that you will be okay if one of those spokes breaks. You'll still be held up by the others.

For example-if you are getting enough sleep, eating well, connecting with others, building your knowledge and addressing all other medical conditions, then if you come across major obstacles in your medication and treatment plan, those obstacles won't affect you as much.

However, if you are overtired, undernourished, lonely, uninformed, and sick, and then run into obstacles, you are going to have a much weaker ability to tackle them.

Assess how you are doing in all of those areas. And shore up ones that are weak if you can. There are books and websites that cover every one of those spokes and can help you strengthen them.

REACH OUT

FRIENDS AND FAMILY

When you are an alcoholic, relationships with friends and family can be fraught with difficulty. It's called a 'family disease' for good reason.

But they are a critical part of your success.

Remember that the three best predictors of success in recovery are:

- Social support from family and friends

- Social standing–the things that give you esteem and dignity–like your job and your home

- Cognitive functioning–how well your brain continues to function

And data has shown that one-year recovery rates for alcoholics are 60 to 80% if you have both intact family and intact job. With only one of those it drops to 30 to 40% after one year. If you were missing both, it drops in half again to 15 to 20%.[73]

When you don't have support from important people in your life, this can help lead to setbacks. Interpersonal problems (relationship problems) are a large factor in relapse with data showing that negative emotional states and interpersonal problems serve as triggers for more than one-half of all relapses.[75]

All of this points to the importance of working on rebuilding or strengthening connections with the people that are important to you. (Or if it's too late for that, building new relationships with new supports).

As with other spokes on the wheel, there is a lot of available information on building and strengthening relationships available in books and online.

From the perspective of your medication journey, however, one of the most important things to keep in mind is that your family and friends can get the 'option myopia' problem we discussed earlier too.

They can be very focused and set on a particular solution for you, and unsupportive of all other solutions.

They can pin their hopes and dreams on you and on a particular solution working. And when you relapse they can feel despair and hopelessness, and this can lead to anger.

Remember, they are a product of this society—one which looks at alcoholism as a personality disorder—just as much as anyone may be.

Your family may need gentle help to open their eyes to other available solutions. And if they are on board with the solution you choose to pursue (whatever that may be), then it will be easier for you to gain their support and encouragement.

One major pitfall to watch out for is this: If you have tried to be abstinent, and then choose to try an 'as needed' approach that encourages drinking to be successful, then it is critical that you try to help your friends and family understand the approach first.

Otherwise you may find yourself with little support.

If picking up a bottle again will signal the end of your marriage and career, then an 'as needed' medication may not be the one to start with.

If you have decided to pursue medication then one thing which may help is to introduce them to the same materials that you have looked at. I hope that this book might be one of those materials. The top resources I would recommend showing them include:

- Book—The End of My Addiction by Dr. Olivier Ameisen[22] (Particularly if you decide to take baclofen).

- Documentary—One Little Pill by Adam Schomer and Claudia Christian, which is available to stream online.[188] (Particularly if you decide to take any 'as needed' medication, such as naltrexone or nalmefene).

- Article—The Irrationality of Alcoholics Anonymous, published in The Atlantic (theatlantic.com)[15]

- Forums—mywayout.org/community and thesinclairmethod.net

- Additional resources specific to each medication are found in the FAQ section of this book

SUPPORTS AROUND YOU

No matter what kind of illness you have, the greater the support you have for recovery, the more likely you will be to succeed.

Some individuals have been very successful with disulfiram, perhaps because they have had the assistance of committed partner who watches them take it each and every day. This requires commitment and support.

Tolerating side-effects, tolerating drinking, the cost of medication, trying multiple medications before succeeding, and going through the hassle of a medical and recovery system that has not advanced as quickly as it should have in regards to addiction treatment is not easy for the alcoholic or your support network.

It's hard to watch someone we love struggle. But it's a little easier if they are going down a treatment path that we understand.

Assess the support you have around you in relation to the medication you choose. If you have support, engage those individuals early on in the best way you can.

ONLINE

There is a wealth of information and insight to be found in online forums about these drugs. I really cannot recommend these forums enough as an important part of your journey.

Most people in the medical community will advise that there is a lot of misinformation to be found in online forums, and this is very true.

But they also will provide you with insight and support that you may be able to find nowhere else.

In general (there are exceptions to every rule), here is what I have observed to be helpful and not-so-helpful about online forums:

Good for:

- Other's personal experiences—what worked and what didn't

- Immediate help for questions—for example, "Has anyone else experienced this side effect?"

- Encouragement and support from a group of people on the same path as you—an excellent reminder that you are not alone and that you are part of a community (can be helpful if you lack other supports)

- Clarification or translation of medical/research jargon and theory into actual experience and more easily understood language.

- Troubleshooting when you run into barriers. For example, you can ask, "I can't get this medication from my pharmacist anymore—what should I do?'

- A place to help others and feel good about yourself

- Interaction and insights between alcoholics and family/friends of alcoholics (we need help to gain perspective on each other's' worlds and experiences)

I have learned to take with a grain of salt (or ignore altogether):

- Insights into very scientific specifics about why or how the medications work or the inner-workings of alcoholism within one's brain.

- Information about areas that are extremely complicated or require in-depth scientific knowledge.

- Some people may be very opinionated about and focused on their solution (option myopia) and less open-minded about other solutions.

- People on forums suffer from the same stereotypes and stigma as people everywhere—even alcoholics spread stigma.

Negativity—there are sick people everywhere and 'hurt people can hurt people'.

12 | FOR CAREGIVERS

Courage to change the things I can,
and the wisdom to know the difference.

Rethinking Enabling

I think one of the saddest things about many illnesses–but particularly brain illnesses–is that it is sometimes difficult to ask for help–and then when we do, sometimes it feels like a door is shut in our face over and over again.

The hurdles and hoops people with alcoholism have to jump through to reach help sometimes is tragic.

How do you get to the clinic an hour away, on time for the appointment, when you have no money, no vehicle, can't stay sober, can't sleep, are dealing with marital problems, bankruptcy, legal issues?

How do you coherently and convincingly advocate for yourself that you'd like a referral or a prescription or housing assistance, or access to a fax machine or computer to send the referral to the next place, while your doctor (who has either become hardened to you due to your lies and drunken behavior; or doesn't know you from Adam) looks at you suspiciously and dismissively and asks you to go home and please shower.

Obtaining the medications in this book, and the right help is NOT an easy thing.

There are enormous barriers–how do you even find out about them unless you have strong cognitive ability and an appetite for seeking and reading medical research?

What if you don't have access to the internet? No health card? No credit card? No money?

Even if you convince your Doctor to prescribe you one, will they prescribe the next one when that one doesn't work?

The one that could work for you may not even be available in your country. They might not be available at your pharmacy. They might not be available to you in your country through online ordering. They might be exorbitantly priced.

What a headache.

Imagine if we made cancer sufferers go through so much to obtain treatment?

It amazes me that anyone ever gets help.

As caregivers (friends or family of an alcoholic), I know that some of the 'principles' taught to those of us who have addicts in our lives are:

- Don't be an 'enabler'

- They have to want to get (and then go and get) help themselves

- Don't cause a crisis, but don't stand in the way of one either

- They have to hit rock bottom–don't cushion their fall

These principles imply a very 'hands off' approach.

But when it comes to getting and accessing help (and maybe having to get and access many different solutions before one of them does help), I think addicts need all the help, support and enabling behavior they can possibly get.

THE FAMILY DISEASE

If you are the friend or family member of an alcoholic, then you have most likely been affected by the family disease of alcoholism.

An enormous burden is placed on friends and family members of those who suffer from alcoholism.

Obtaining and taking medication (and finding the right medication) can be a straightforward process.

But more often it's not.

You don't have to lead this process of getting your alcoholic on medication, but it's important to know that your involvement–your support, love, time, help and encouragement–may be the difference between life or death for your alcoholic.

Information is power. I encourage you to read this book and do your own research.

And get the right support. You will *not* get support for a medical approach from the vast majority of 12-step program family groups or treatment centers. As the Alanon adage goes—don't go to the hardware store for milk. And don't go to a 12-step program for support for a medical approach.

Look instead to online support groups where family and friends of other alcoholics that are taking medication help each other. There you'll get the right encouragement and support.

RELAPSE HAPPENS

Relapse is a part of the disease of alcoholism. If your loved one never relapses, they probably were never an alcoholic to begin with.

As family and friends, how do we deal with this?

Here is the truth: Your alcoholic's relapse is not a personal affront to you. It has nothing to do with you. It is not a reflection on whether they love you enough or not. Get over that.

If your alcoholic is dependent enough on alcohol, they may have little to no control left over relapse. Alcoholism is a disease where circuits in the brain necessary for free will are eroded.

React the way you would react if anyone you loved relapsed with any other another disease. It's not personal.

This book recommends treating the medical route as a pathway—you could treat it that way too. When your alcoholic relapses, help them learn from it, and move forward.

DON'T BE THE BAD GUY

If you stand back and look at your relationship with the alcoholic and others involved in the drama of alcoholism, what do you see?

Do you see people playing the victim? The rescuer? The bad guy?

If so, you may be caught in an unhealthy triangular family dynamic called the Karpman Drama Triangle. You can learn more about this model simply searching for it online.

There are three roles in the triangle: victim, rescuer and persecutor.

You may be desperately and actively seeking any means of help for your loved one, completely abandoning your own health and livelihood, as well as that of all others in the your family. You may be focussed on picking up all pieces and solving all problems. *If so, you are acting as a Rescuer.*

You may feel the alcoholic and anyone that enables them is to blame for much suffering in your life, and you are completely and utterly powerless to change anything. Woe is me. They are a monster and I'm so hard done by. *You may be acting as a Victim.*

Your old sympathies may have turned to anger and resentment that is eating away at you and causing you to lash out. You might be lashing out angrily not only at the alcoholic, but at every person who seems to be enabling that alcoholic. *If so, you are acting as the Persecutor.*

We don't always stay in the same role—we can shift between them in a changing dynamic. And each role has a drawback and a payoff. Yes—a payoff.

The reason I'm writing about these dynamics in this book is simply because they are part of the disease; and one which can greatly harm family and loved ones.

It was very sad to me to see that in some of the families of alcoholics I met, the rage and resentment of the non-alcoholic members at the alcoholic member was what ultimately split the family apart.

While often alcoholics are ostracized from a family for their destructive behavior, I met many non-alcoholic family members who were the ones ostracized from their families. Their angry behavior was deemed far more destructive by the other members of the family than even the alcoholic's behavior.

All of us get caught up in these roles from time to time. The first step is simply to identify that it is occurring. If you see yourself stuck in this triangle, it's time for you to get help too.

BEING PART OF POSITIVE CHANGE

Let's educate ourselves and others around us. Let's start talking about treatment options like medication—even in 12-step programs.

When we see something wrong—let's complain to the heads of the groups where it is going wrong. Let's stop spreading stigma. This is a medical illness. We know it. Let's treat it that way.

We have the tools now.

I's hard to be taken seriously when you are the friend or family member standing next to someone who smells like vomit.

It's hard to ask for better treatment for an alcoholic who is in the back of a cruiser, or who is being treated like a child who can't be trusted with a cell phone or a cigarette in a detox unit.

When their doctors don't provide actual medical treatment to them, and hospital staff forgets them, it's difficult to speak up.

But do it anyways.

The things that need to be changed aren't going to change overnight.

But if we all do a little bit to chip away at the problems, to make our voices heard then change will come. It is already coming.

PART 4: MEDICATIONS FOR ALCOHOLISM

13 | DRUG BY DRUG DETAIL

"There is no other field in psychiatric research that has, in recent years, yielded so many novel, druggable targets and innovative treatment strategies than for alcohol addiction."[168]

—Dr. Rainer Spanagel, Director of the Institute of Psychopharmacology, University of Heidelberg

THE DRUG LISTS

Here we are—the most important part of this book. This section is all about the drugs.

When you visit your doctor, photocopy the sections on the medications you would like to discuss with your doctor and give him or her a copy—you have my explicit permission to do so (in fact—I hope you do so! They need all the help they can get.)

You can also visit the book website (APrescriptionforAlcoholics.com), find links to some of the recommended research for each medication and print the research for your doctor too.

Drug Groupings

I've divided up the medications covered in this book into several groups. These groupings are somewhat arbitrary because there is no clear way to really rank or rate medications.

Sometimes medications are referred to by the medical community as 'first line', 'second line', etc., depending upon whether a medication is a 'go to' medication for a condition, or a secondary medication to try if the first one fails or is not appropriate.

I have avoided using these terms since they can be misleading.

While I might try to start with one or more of the medications on the A-List myself, there are so many factors to take into consideration (discussed in the previous chapter), that you may find that something on the B-List or even on the Futures List which might just be a very good fit for you.

The groupings I've created include:

1) The A-List: Most Important Medications for Today

2) The B-List: Medications Worth Consideration Today

3) The D-List: Eleven Drugs that May Increase Drinking

4) The Futures List: Sixty+ Drugs to Watch

Please note–don't confuse alcoholism 'Types' with the naming of these lists. They are not related at all.

Both Type A and Type B alcoholics may find medications that work for them on either the A-List or B-List.

About Web Links

There are links in each section to important (and reputable) reference sites.

Some of the links are long, full of characters that can wrap onto the next line. So to avoid problems with links I've used a link shortener.

For example, one of the first links is to information about acamprosate side effects at the US National Library of Medicine website. The link is shown like this:

http://bit.ly/acamprosatesides

But when you type that link into your web browser it will actually take you straight to the MedlinePlus page on the National Library website at this address:

https://www.nlm.nih.gov/medlineplus/druginfo/meds/a604028.html

And note that you don't actually need to type the 'http://' part into your web browser.

In the example above, simply typing the following would work:

bit.ly/acamprosatesides

Using Google Translate

A few of the links provided are in languages other than English. A useful tool for these links is Google Translate.

When you come across a link such as 'baclofene.org' which is a French-language site, simply go to Google Translate and type the website address, baclofene.org, into the box on the left. Then select 'English' above the box on the right, and click 'Translate'.

Google will re-generate the entire site in machine-translated English. Google Translate can be found here:

translate.google.com

THE A-LIST: MOST IMPORTANT MEDICATIONS FOR TODAY

The 'Most Important' medications are those which either have a lot of research and leading researchers backing them; are FDA-approved either for other medical conditions or for the treatment of alcohol dependence; and/or have a lot of promise for some other reason or a combination of reasons for their use against alcohol dependence.

My focus in putting together this list is the evidence of efficacy (effectiveness).

This does not necessarily mean that they will be the easiest to attain.

These are generally the medications most commonly tried by those who are investigating and taking medications for treatment of alcoholism for the first time, and they may also have significant anecdotal support for their effectiveness.

These medications include:

- Acamprosate

- Baclofen (High Dose)

- Topiramate

- Naltrexone (Daily Dosage, As Needed or by Injection)

- Nalmefene

- Gabapentin & Pregabalin

THE B-LIST: MEDICATIONS WORTH CONSIDERATION TODAY

The medications I have classified as 'Worth Consideration Today' have less supporting evidence (possibly due to a lack of research, not necessarily due to lack of potential), or may not seem to be quite as effective or appropriate for as many individuals.

Most of them still have a fair amount of top-level research or pharmaceutical support based on trial evidence.

With further research and greater understanding of how they work, any of these might join the A-List (or drop further down the list).

All of the medications on this list are FDA-Approved, but only one is FDA-Approved for the treatment of alcoholism.

These medications include:

- Ondansetron

- Varenicline

- Disulfiram

- Prazosin & Doxazosin

- Zonisamide

- Olanzapine

- Sertraline

- Sodium Oxybate (SO) (See caveats around this one in the section specifically focusing on SO)

THE D-LIST: USE CAUTION

The F-List contains medications that, in at least one study (in either lab animals or humans), have been shown to *increase* drinking.

These medications include:

- Sertraline

- Doxazosin

- Ondansetron

- Atomoxetine

- Fluoxetine & Venlafaxine

- Flupenthixol Decanoate, Amisulpride, Tiapride

- Lisuride

- Ritanserin

- Tiagabine

THE FUTURES-LIST: SIXTY+ MEDICATIONS TO WATCH

Medications I have classified as 'To Watch' have either recently been researched for alcohol dependence with promising results or findings or have some other indication (such as filing of patents) that indicate they may be worth watching.

These medications could ultimately be proven ineffective or in some way dangerous, or with more research and discovery they could eventually top the A-list.

It's worth noting that at the time that Amiesen started experimenting with baclofen for example (which I've classified as a 'Significant Medication'), it would have also fallen into the 'Medications to Watch' category due to the very limited, but somewhat promising research on it.

14 | A-LIST DRUGS – MOST IMPORTANT MEDICATIONS TODAY

These are the medications that I consider the most important today:

1) Acamprosate*

2) Baclofen (High Dose)*

3) Topiramate*

4) Naltrexone (Daily Dosage, As Needed or by Injection)*

5) Nalmefene

6) Gabapentin & Pregabalin

The importance of these medications is confirmed in the 2012 report *'Addiction Medicine: Closing the Gap Between Science & Practice'*.[3]

This may be the only prominent report published and geared toward medical professionals that not only highlights acamprosate, naltrexone and disulfiram, but also topiramate, baclofen and ondansetron as imporant treatments for alcoholism.

(As nalmefene's oral format is not yet approved by US-regulators for any purpose it made sense that it was not included on their list).[3]

ACAMPROSATE

INTRODUCTION TO ACAMPROSATE

Acamprosate is one of the three medications that is approved throughout the world (by the FDA, or EMA or Health Canada) as an *on-label* medication for the treatment of Alcohol Dependence (the other two are naltrexone and disulfiram). (There are many other FDA medications that are effective in the treatment of alcoholism which may be prescribed *off-label*).

It is possible that acamprosate reduces the Alcohol Deprivation Effect (ADE) which causes relapse drinking.[38]

And because it works with an entirely different mechanism of action than naltrexone, the combination of the two may be effective for some dependent drinkers.

As has been shown in other medications (topiramate, naltrexone, ondansetron, sertraline and disulfiram), acamprosate is more effective in the treatment of individuals with specific genetic markers.

For example, in the case of acamprosate, it was shown in 2011 by Kiefer et al., that those with the genetic variant GATA4 (rs1327367) are less likely to relapse when treated with acamprosate than those without the variant.

In 2014, VM Karapyak et al. found that the genetic variants minor GRIN2B rs2058878 A allele and rs2300272 SNPs were both associated with longer abstinence during the first three months of acamprosate treatment.[189]

Acamprosate is one of the most well-researched substances in regards to its effectiveness. A recent paper pointed out that there are more than 450 published original investigations and clinical trials and 1.5 million treated patients which together has resulted in an impressive body of knowledge around acamprosate as an effective treatment for alcohol dependence.[38]

THE BACK-STORY

In his 2014 piece 'Acamprosate: An Alcoholism Treatment that may not be What We Thought', (published in Neuropsychopharmacology), Markus Heilig writes, "Occasionally, a paper comes along that fundamentally challenges what we thought we knew about a drug mechanism."[190]

Heilig was referring to a study published in 2013 by Spanagel et al., that turned scientists' understanding of the FDA approved alcoholism medication acamprosate, on its head.[38]

What the paper found was that the way many thought acamprosate worked in the brain to stop alcohol cravings is not the way it may work at all. It concluded that calcium–not acetylhomotaurinate as thought–is the active ingredient in acamprosate and that it is due to the high plasma calcium levels left over from acamprosate treatment that led to improvement in time to relapse and cumulative abstinence results.

This discovery was something of an inconvenient truth for researchers. It cast doubts upon the widely held association between the interaction of acamprosate and the glutamate neurotransmission system; it led to the conclusion that large doses of calcium might largely duplicate the effects of this drug; and finally, perhaps most significant of all–it meant that one of the very few FDA-approved drugs that is actually *on-label* for the treatment of alcoholism may not, in fact, be a drug at all.

Ultimately, though, it is yet another reminder that in the sphere of alcoholism treatment, what we think we know must always be re-questioned.

Where the Spanagel study questioned acamprosate's mechanism, it did not cast any doubt on the accuracy of the research that showed acamprosate's effectiveness in study after study.

This is an important distinction.

Whether acamprosate is simply a calcium pill or not, there is not another substance on the planet that has been more researched, or with more studies supporting its safety and effectiveness against alcohol than acamprosate.

Given the fact that it is FDA-approved for the treatment of alcohol dependence, has an extremely safe profile and has been proven to be effective, it is hard to understand why a medical practitioner would NOT prescribe acamprosate to an otherwise healthy individual struggling with alcoholism.

It may not work for everyone, and alone it may only have a modest effect, but as a first line treatment option acamprosate is an excellent first step.

ACAMPROSATE MEDICATION FAQ

MEDICATION OVERVIEW

What is the medication called?

Acamprosate

What are common brand names and generic names for this medication?

Acamprosate oral, Campral, Campral Oral, acamprosate calcium, N-acetyl homotaurine, calcium acetylhomotaurinate, Regtect, calcium bis acetyl homotaurine, Aotal

What 'type' of medication is this?

Synthetic amino acid analog

What is it usually prescribed for?

Alcohol Dependence

How is it described?

- Acamprosate is N-acetyl homotaurine, a synthetic amino acid analog similar to gamma-aminobutyric acid (GABA) and taurine.

- Acamprosate is a drug used for treating alcohol dependence. Originally it was thought to stabilize the chemical balance in the brain that would otherwise be disrupted by alcoholism by blocking glutaminergic N-methyl-D-aspartate receptors while gamma-aminobutyric acid type A receptors are activated.

- More recently there has been questions about its true mechanism of action.

- Acamprosate was the third medication to receive approval for the treatment of alcohol dependence in the US. This drug is widely used in Europe to reduce alcohol cravings in problem drinkers who have quit.

AVAILABILITY & FDA APPROVAL STATUS

A prescription for alcoholism is usually:
On-Label

Is it FDA approved in the USA? When?
Yes—FDA Approved in 2004

Is it HC approved in Canada? When?
Yes—Health Canada approved in 2007

Is it EMA approved in Europe? When?
Yes – EMA Approved in 1989

How is it available?
By prescription in USA, Canada and parts of Europe

STRENGTH AND CREDIBILITY OF RESEARCH FOR ITS USE IN ALCOHOLISM

How many years has this medication been researched specifically for the treatment of alcoholism?
30+ Years (Since at least 1985)

What is the strength of the supporting research?

- "Clinical efficacy of acamprosate is robustly documented in meta-analyses of available studies...the latter of these was a meta-analysis of 17 studies which included 4087 individuals."[1]

- "Acamprosate is available in 29 countries outside the United States, including most of Europe, China, Singapore, and Australia, as well as Central and South American countries. It has been prescribed to more than 1.5 million persons with alcohol abuse or dependence in those countries with no apparent pattern of serious side effects. European data indicate that the drug has no potential for abuse or rebound effect after discontinuation. European data have also indicated that the drug effectively reduces craving for alcohol and can help maintain abstinence in dependent patients."[42]

What credentials does the researcher making the statements above have?

- Markus Heilig is one of top 10 scientists of AUD worldwide; former NIAAA Clinical Director; active medical practitioner; author of more than 200 peer-reviewed journal articles, including papers in Science, PNAS, Lancet, Archives of General Psychiatry. Research work has 8000+ citations.

- Michael Soyka is an extensively published and credentialed researcher and Medical Director, Switzerland.

RESEARCH FINDINGS ABOUT EFFECTIVENESS IN TREATMENT FOR ALCOHOLISM

How many patients need to be treated to see one true medication responder? (Known as the 'Number Needed to Treat–NNT)

The number needed to treat is estimated between 7 and 12.[134] This means that one in seven to twelve people will respond well to treatment with this medication.

How effective is this medication for the treatment of alcoholism?

- Acamprosate was found to be superior to placebo in maintaining abstinence in a 2015 study in patients with alcohol dependence. The 2015 report cited that "these findings concur with 11 randomized, blinded, placebo-controlled clinical trials conducted in Europe."[39]

- Mason's 2012 analysis included 1317 women and 4794 men from 22 studies within 18 countries and found that acamprosate had "significant beneficial effect across 4 efficacy endpoints–percentage of abstinent days, percentage of no heavy drinking days, rate of complete abstinence and rate of no heavy drinking. Acamprosate had a high rate of treatment completion and medication compliance.[40]

- Soyka provides the example of a meta-analysis of data from 11 European clinical trials that included over 3000 patients and showing that "acamprosate nearly doubled the likelihood of preventing relapse to drinking and increased the likelihood that patients would remain in treatment by nearly one-third."[41]

In research, how did this medication compare to other medications for the treatment of alcoholism?

- The NNT (Number Needed to Treat) for acamprosate has been found to be at its low end 7, similar to that for naltrexone, though Markus Heilig points out that "it is important to bear in mind that different outcome variables seem to be differentially affected by the 2 drugs, making a direct comparison of the effect size difficult."[1]

- Yahn found that the most recent meta-analysis comparing acamprosate to naltrexone found that "acamprosate is more effective than naltrexone in maintaining abstinence, while naltrexone reduces heavy drinking and craving to a greater extent than acamprosate."

- Importantly Yahn also stated that the difference in effectiveness of acamprosate versus naltrexone is gene-specific—"depending on patient geno¬type, acamprosate and naltrexone have been shown to outperform one another."[191]

TREATMENT CANDIDATES FOR THIS MEDICATION

Note: this section highlights study findings that have identified some characteristics that may increase odds of effectiveness. This does not mean it won't help individuals without these characteristics.

What treatment goals might this medication help achieve?

Abstinence, no heavy drinking, reduction of desire and craving for alcohol.

What are some typical feelings and motivators of people this medication tends to help?

Research has not yet provided a great deal of insight on this answer. It may be useful for people with strong craving leading to relapse.

Has this medication been shown to be more successful in early-onset or late-onset alcoholics?

Research has not yet provided insight on this answer.

Is this medication typically more effective in people with a strong family history of alcoholism?

Research has not yet provided insight on this answer.

Are there specific genetic markers that have been found to be relevant in treatment with this medication?

- Yes–it was shown in 2011 by Kiefer et al., that those with the genetic variant GATA4 (rs1327367) are less likely to relapse when treated with acamprosate than those without the variant.

- In 2014, VM Karapyak et al found that the genetic variants minor GRIN2B rs2058878 A allele and rs2300272 SNPs were both associated with longer abstinence during the first three months of acamprosate treatment.[189]

Do Alcoholics Have Difficulty Taking this Medication as Prescribed? (i.e. Are there "Compliance" Issues?)

Research has not pointed to any issues with compliance though side-effects may sometimes lead to discontinuation.

Are there other characteristics (gender, taste sensitivity, alcoholism type, co-morbid disorders, smoker status) that may be related to success with this medication?

- Those with a higher severity of alcoholism (i.e. Those requiring detoxification before treatment) may experience more significant results than those who do not.

- In regards to gender, Mason found that acamprosate was equally effective in men and women in a 2012 study that looked at over 6000 individual records.[40]

DIRECTIONS FOR USE & HOW IT WORKS

At what dose and for how long does research suggest the medication should be taken?

- Two 333 mg delayed-release tablets by mouth three times per day (6 pills per day in total), with or without food (a lower dose may be effective with some patients and must be used with those with impaired renal function).

- Pills are swallowed whole, not crushed or broken.

Has this medication been tested with other medications for the treatment of alcoholism and found to be complimentary?

Yes–several studies have shown that the combination of naltrexone and acamprosate can be both safe and effective. Each works on different neurobiological pathways: "Naltrexone has been shown to reduce the positive reinforcing properties of alcohol, and acamprosate reduces the negative reinforcing properties," (such as craving).[187]

What is known about how this medication actually works in alcoholics? What is the 'Mechanism of Action'?

According to researchers: "The primary beneficial mechanism of action remains unclear; however, acamprosate is believed to normalize the balance between excitatory and inhibitory pathways that become adapted to chronic alcohol use and alleviate psychological and physiological discomfort that follows withdrawal. These effects may be due to some combination of antagonizing NMDA glutamate receptors, modulating type 5 metabotropic glutamate receptors, or reducing glutamate accumulation during repeated episodes of alcohol withdrawal."[192]

SAFETY CONCERNS

Is this medication addictive? Does it have abuse potential?

Acamprosate is non-addictive.

How safe is this medication?

- Regarding safety, Mason found, "neither acamprosate nor gabapentin are appreciably metabolized in the liver, and both have been shown to be safe in patients taking concomitant medications and in those with hepatic impairment. This is an important distinction relative to disulfiram and naltrexone, which each have a black box warning for hepatotoxicity."[193]

- Venturella stated acamprosate "does not cause addiction, abuse or withdrawal of its suspension and does not interfere with other medications that patients often alcoholics must take."[194]

Can this medication be taken while drinking?

While it is not recommended to take this medication while drinking, it can be taken while the alcohol-dependent individual is still drinking though side-effects if taken while alcohol is in one's system may be enhanced.

What are the expected side effects of this medication?

Research indicates that expected side effects include stomach upset and diarrhea.

What are other fairly common side effects?

Research has showed fairly common side effects to include diarrhea, gas, upset stomach, loss of appetite, dry mouth, dizziness.

Where can I find a complete list of all side effects, precautions, and instructions in case of emergency or overdose?

You can find this on the US National Library of Medicine website. Search google for 'acamprosate and National Library of Medicine' or visit:

http://bit.ly/acamprosatesides

What does the National Institute of Health (NIH) say about liver impact and where can I find further information on liver impact of this medication?

- Acamprosate has not been linked to serum enzyme elevations during therapy and has not been linked to cases of clinically apparent liver injury.

- Also visit this page at the livertox.nlm.nih.gov website :

http://bit.ly/acamprosatelivertox

What known drug interactions should I watch for and where can I find more information on drug interactions?

- There are no known drug or alcohol interactions with acamprosate.

- Also visit the drug interaction checker at drugs.com:

    http://bit.ly/acamprosateinteract

Where can I find alerts and Black Box Warnings? (Black Box Warnings are cautions affixed to medications by the government)

- Visit this page on nlm.nih.gov:

    http://bit.ly/acamprosatesides

Were there any known black box warnings at the time this book was written?

No—but you may still wish to visit the link above for up-to-date information.

OTHER USEFUL INFORMATION

Note: Links to all recommended information sources can be found on the book's website at www.APrescriptionforAlcoholics.com

Recent Research:

- 2013: Meta-analysis of naltrexone and acamprosate for treating alcohol use disorders: When are these medications most helpful?[195]

- 2013: Safety and efficacy of acamprosate for the treatment of alcohol dependence.[191]

- 2012: Acamprosate for treatment of alcohol dependence: Mechanisms, efficacy, and clinical utility[196]

CONNECTING WITH OTHERS

Online Forum(s):

- The 'MyWayOut' community started out focused on topiramate but is now a good place to read about and connect with others regarding a variety of medications for the treatment of alcoholism.

- Visit MyWayOut at:

    http://bit.ly/mywayoutforum

- A link to Google search results for a search inside the MyWayOut forum for this specific medication:

  http://bit.ly/mywayacamprosate

Reviews from others on Drugs.com:

- For 'acamprosate':

  http://bit.ly/drugsacamprosate

- For brand name:

  http://bit.ly/drugscampr

Reviews from others on WebMD:

- For 'acamprosate':

  http://bit.ly/webmdacamprosate

- For brand name:

  http://bit.ly/webmdcampr

Generic Wikipedia Link:

  http://bit.ly/wikiacamprosate

DrugBank.ca Link (Detailed Drug Data Including Pricing):

  http://bit.ly/drugbankacamprosate

SIGNIFICANT ACAMPROSATE RESEARCH &

FINDINGS

2015–Donoghue–Addiction
The Efficacy of Acamprosate and Naltrexone in the Treatment of Alcohol Dependence, Europe versus the Rest of the World: A Meta-Analysis

---

- The study found that "Both acamprosate and naltrexone appear to reduce the risk of individuals returning to drinking alcohol in those who are alcohol-dependent."[197]

2015–Higuchi, Journal of Clinical Psychiatry
Efficacy of Acamprosate for the Treatment of Alcohol Dependence Long After Recovery from Withdrawal Syndrome

---

- A study within 34 Japanese Medical institutions found that the acamprosate-treated group demonstrated significantly superior efficacy over the placebo group in the primary endpoint: the proportion maintaining complete abstinence.

- Results were: abstinence in the acamprosate group was 47% (77/163 subjects), compared with 36% (59/164 subjects) in the placebo group. The difference in complete abstinence rates between the two groups was 11%.

- The study concluded, "Acamprosate is superior to placebo in maintaining abstinence in Japanese patients with alcohol dependence. These findings concur with 11 randomized, blinded, placebo-controlled clinical trials conducted in Europe."[39]

2015–Mason–The Journal of Clinical Psychiatry
Acamprosate, Alcoholism, and Abstinence

- Mason stated, "A recent sex-specific, individual patient data meta-analysis found acamprosate to have a significant effect compared with placebo in improving rates of abstinence and no heavy drinking in both women and men with alcohol dependence."

- Regarding safety, Mason found, "neither acamprosate nor gabapentin are appreciably metabolized in the liver, and both have been shown to be safe in patients taking concomitant medications and in those with hepatic impairment. This is an important distinction relative to disulfiram and naltrexone, which each have a black box warning for hepatotoxicity."

- Another finding showed that acamprosate was more effective with high severity of illness (i.e. those who initially required detoxification), and where the individual was already abstinent at the initiation of treatment.[193] [note–this finding seems to conflict with Kalk's 2012 work that indicated acamprosate should be started during or as soon as possible after detoxification.]

2014–Karpyak–Translational Psychiatry
Genetic markers associated with abstinence length in alcohol-dependent subjects treated with acamprosate

- In relation to genetic findings, "GRIN2B rs2058878 and rs2300272 SNPs are associated with abstinence length during the first 3 months of acamprosate treatment."[189]

2014–Rosack–Psychiatric News
Once-Promising Alcoholism Drug Runs into FDA Roadblock

- "Acamprosate is available in 29 countries outside the United States, including most of Europe, China, Singapore, and Australia, as well as Central and South American countries. It has been prescribed to more than 1.5 million persons with alcohol abuse or dependence in those countries with no apparent pattern of serious side effects. European data indicate that the drug has no potential for abuse or rebound effect after discontinuation. European data have also indicated that the drug effectively reduces craving for alcohol and can help maintain abstinence in dependent patients."[42]

2014–Venturella–Journal of Biological Research Italy
The Control of Abstinence in the Treatment of Alcohol Dependence: The Use of Acamprosate in Relapse Prevention

---

- Regarding safety, Venturella found, "it does not cause addiction, abuse or withdrawal of its suspension and does not interfere with other medications that patients often alcoholics must take."

- Venturella found that craving becomes absent after 3-4 months of therapy in approximately 89% of patients that were observed. Venturella states, "the strong point seems to be the ability for the user to experience a new sense of normalcy and to remove the desire for significant periods of alcohol."[194]

2013–Spanagel–Neuropsychopharmacology
Acamprosate Produces Its Anti-Relapse Effects via Calcium

- Spanagel stated in groundbreaking research: "we conclude that calcium is the active moiety of acamprosate...we found that patients with high plasma calcium levels due to acamprosate treatment showed better primary efficacy parameters such as time to relapse and cumulative abstinence...the effects of acamprosate described in more than 450 published original investigations and clinical trials and 1.5 million treated patients can possibly be attributed to calcium."[38]

- Spanagel also noted that in the early 1950s clinical studies proposed intensive calcium therapy (called calmonose) for the treatment of alcoholism.[198] He pointed out that "Although this therapy disappeared from the treatment landscape for unknown reasons, in light of our new findings, calcium supplements could be easily re-introduced into treatment programs."[38]

2013–Yahn–Substance Abuse: Research and Treatment
Safety and Efficacy of Acamprosate for the Treatment of Alcohol Dependence

---

- In an extensive review, Yahn found that due to acamprosate's extremely poor bioavailability in humans (11% on an empty stomach), large doses are required to achieve therapeutic effects. Regarding safety, Yahn stated, "since its availability in Europe starting in 1989, pharmacovigilance data from over 1.5 million patients has revealed no serious health risks from acamprosate use. In addition, acamprosate does not possess an abuse potential."[191]

- Regarding results, Yahn reported that in a meta-analysis of 17 randomized, placebo-controlled, double-blind trials there was a "statistically significant benefit of acamprosate over placebo in the primary outcome measure of continuous abstinence at 6 months."

- In another meta-analysis of 22 randomized and controlled clinical trials "acamprosate was associated with significant improvements in the rate of abstinence as well as in days of cumulative abstinence."[191]

- Regarding effectiveness compared to other medications Yahn found that the most recent meta-analysis comparing acamprosate to naltrexone found that "acamprosate is more effective than naltrexone in maintaining abstinence, while naltrexone reduces heavy drinking and craving to a greater extent than acamprosate."

- Importantly Yahn also stated that the difference in effectiveness of acamprosate versus naltrexone is gene-specific—"depending on patient genotype, acamprosate and naltrexone have been shown to outperform one another."[191]

2012–Kalk–British Journal of Clinical Pharmacology
The Clinical Pharmacology of Acamprosate

- Kalk found evidence from several studies that acamprosate should be started "during detoxification" or "as soon as possible after detoxification" to achieve the greatest effect.

- Regarding treatment duration, Kalk referred to documentation that indicated that "acamprosate be given for 1 year as data has shown improvement in drinking outcomes over time."

- Kalk also found that the number needed to treat to result in one more patient becoming abstinent was between 9 and 11.

- She also stated support for "Littleton's hypothesis that acamprosate targets negative reinforcement craving produced by withdrawal."[34]

2012–Mason–Alcoholism: Clinical and Experimental Research
Acamprosate for Alcohol Dependence: A Sex-Specific Meta-Analysis Based on Individual Patient Data

---

- Mason's 2012 analysis included 1317 women and 4794 men from 22 studies within 18 countries and found that acamprosate had "significant beneficial effect" across 4 measures of success—percentage of abstinent days, percentage of no heavy drinking days, rate of complete abstinence and rate of no heavy drinking.

- Acamprosate had a high rate of treatment completion and medication compliance.

- Mason concluded that "acamprosate has a significant effect compared with placebo in improving rates of abstinence and no heavy drinking in both women and men with alcohol dependence."[40]

2012–Miller–The International Journal of Psychiatry in Medicine
Medical Treatment of Alcohol Dependence: A Systematic Review

- Miller's extensive review found that "a total of 85 studies, representing 18,937 subjects, met our criteria for inclusion…Acamprosate shows modest efficacy with recently abstinent patients…."[199]

2012–Witkiewitz–Therapeutics and Clinical Risk Management
Acamprosate for Treatment of Alcohol Dependence: Mechanisms, Efficacy, and Clinical Utility

---

- Witkiewitz stated that Acamprosate demonstrated its efficacy in more than 25 placebo-controlled, double-blind trials of individuals with alcohol dependence and "has generally been found to be more efficacious than placebo in significantly reducing the risk of returning to any drinking and increasing the cumulative duration of abstinence."[196]

2010–Mason–CNS & neurological disorders drug targets
Acamprosate: A Prototypic Neuromodulator in the Treatment of Alcohol
Dependence

- Mason stated, "Acamprosate's excellent safety profile along with several pharmacokinetic and pharmacodynamic characteristics make it well suited for treating a broad population of alcohol-dependent patients."[200]

2010–Rösner–Cochrane Review
Acamprosate for Alcohol Dependence

- Rosner looked at 24 trials with 6915 participants and found that compared to placebo, acamprosate was shown to significantly reduce the risk of any drinking and significantly increase cumulative abstinence duration. Rosner found that acamprosate was an effective and safe treatment in alcohol-dependent individuals to support "continuous abstinence."

- Rosner stated that when added to psychosocial treatment strategies, "acamprosate reduced the risk of returning to any drinking after detoxification compared with treatment with a placebo (number need to treat (NNT) for one person to benefit was nine). The cumulative abstinence time was also clearly increased."[201]

2009–Ooteman–Addiction Biology
Predicting the Effect of Naltrexone and Acamprosate in Alcohol-Dependent
Patients Using Genetic Indicators

- Ooteman stated regarding treatment genetics and the impact of treatment with acamprosate and/or naltrexone, he states that "the benefit of each treatment is dependent upon (a combination of) polymorphisms in four out of the seven candidate genes tested in this study."[202]

2008–Rosner–Journal of Psychopharmacology (Oxford, England)
Acamprosate Supports Abstinence, Naltrexone Prevents Excessive Drinking:
Evidence from a Meta-Analysis with Unreported Outcomes

- In a comparison of naltrexone and acamprosate, the researchers concluded: "acamprosate was shown only to support abstinence; it did not influence alcohol consumption after the first drink. When the efficacy profiles of the two drugs were compared, acamprosate was found to be more effective in preventing a lapse, whereas naltrexone was better in preventing a lapse from becoming a relapse. The superiority of either one drug or over the other one cannot be determined as a general rule, it rather depends on the therapeutic target."[203]

2008–The world journal of biological psychiatry
World Federation of Societies of Biological Psychiatry (WFSBP) Guidelines for Biological Treatment of Substance Use and Related Disorders, Part I: Alcoholism

---

- Regarding the wealth of research data on acamprosate, Soyka stated that acamprosate "significantly reduced relapse rates in alcohol-dependent patients in a number of placebo-controlled, double-blind trials (Level A)."[41]

- He noted that the medication has been studied in more than 5,000 alcohol-dependent individuals in 19 double-blind, placebo-controlled clinical trials conducted in 14 different countries; he also states that analyses provide "clear evidence of the efficacy of acamprosate for the maintenance of abstinence."

- He provides the example of a meta-analysis of data from 11 European clinical trials that included over 3000 patients and showing that "acamprosate nearly doubled the likelihood of preventing relapse to drinking and increased the likelihood that patients would remain in treatment by nearly one-third."[41]

- Soyka says that "perhaps the most robust effect of acamprosate was seen in a German multi-centre study, where the abstinence rate after 1 year was 41%, compared to 22% in the placebo group, an effect that persisted during a 1-year period following the discontinuation of study medication.[41]

2007–Ooteman–European Neuropsychopharmacy
The Effect of Naltrexone and Acamprosate on Cue-Induced Craving, Autonomic Nervous System and Neuroendocrine Reactions to Alcohol-Related Cues in Alcoholics

- "The findings provide some evidence for differential effects of naltrexone and acamprosate: naltrexone may exert its effect, at least partly, by the reduction of cue-induced craving, whereas acamprosate may exert its effect, at least partly, by the reduction of autonomic nervous system reactions to alcohol-related cues."[204]

2006–Jung–Yonsei Medical Journal
Pharmacotherapy for Alcohol Dependence: Anticraving Medications for Relapse Prevention

- "Acamprosate normalizes the dysregulation of N-methyl-D-aspartate (NMDA)-mediated glutamatergic excitation that occurs in alcohol withdrawal and early abstinence."[205]

2005–Verheul–Psychopharmacology
Predictors of Acamprosate Efficacy: Results from a Pooled Analysis of Seven European Trials Including 1485 Alcohol-Dependent Patients

- In a large sample size, Verheul found that none of the following variables could predict a successful (or unsuccessful) outcome of taking acamprosate: high physiological dependence at baseline, negative family history of alcoholism, late age-of-onset, serious anxiety symptomatology at baseline, severe craving at baseline, and female gender.

- He concluded that "acamprosate can be considered as a potentially effective pharmacotherapy for all patients with alcohol dependence. The effect size of acamprosate alone is, however, moderate. Some evidence indicates that the combination of acamprosate with naltrexone or disulfiram leads to substantially better outcomes."[206]

2004–Kim–Psychiatry and Clinical Neurosciences
Effect of the Combination of Naltrexone and Acamprosate on Alcohol Intake in Mice

---

- "When combined with naltrexone, acamprosate reduced alcohol consumption across both doses of naltrexone."

- This effect was sensitive to both dose and number of days of exposure to the naltrexone/acamprosate combination."[207]

2003–Heyser–Neuropsychopharmacology
Effects of Naltrexone Alone and in Combination with Acamprosate on the Alcohol Deprivation Effect in Rats.

- Heyser found that acamprosate blocked the alcohol deprivation effect (ADE). In tests combining naltrexone and acamprosate he concluded that the drugs' mechanisms were different and complimentary, stating that "these results support the hypothesis that naltrexone and acamprosate are effective in modulating aspects of alcohol-seeking behavior, and under certain situations may be more effective in combination."[208]

2003–Weinstein–Addiction Biology
A Pilot Study on the Effects of Treatment with Acamprosate on Craving for Alcohol in Alcohol-Dependent Patients

---

- Weinstein found that duration of treatment is a major factor in the outcome, stating patients "scored lower on craving questionnaires during week 6 compared with week 2. Our results suggest that acamprosate may play a role in reduction of craving for alcohol after 6 weeks of treatment."[209]

1999–Garbutt–JAMA
Pharmacological Treatment of Alcohol Dependence

- In an extensive review of previous trials (41 studies and 11 follow-up or subgroup studies) where the quality of research findings was graded with an A, B, or C, Garbutt found: "Acamprosate (grade A, from large-scale studies in Europe) reduces drinking frequency, although its effects on enhancing abstinence or reducing time to first drink are less clear."[210]

> **1996–Spanagel–European journal of pharmacology**
> Acamprosate (grade A, from large-scale studies in Europe) reduces drinking frequency, although its effects on enhancing abstinence or reducing time to first drink are less clear

- Spanagel stated, "Acamprosate (calcium-acetyl homotaurinate) is a new compound in the treatment of alcoholism," and that "when acamprosate (50-200 mg/kg i.p.) was administered twice daily, alcohol-drinking following an alcohol-deprivation phase was decreased dose-dependently. Given at the highest dose alcohol intake even dropped significantly below baseline drinking. Together, these results show that acamprosate effectively diminishes the alcohol-deprivation effect."[211]

> **1990–Lhuintre–Alcohol and Alcoholism (Oxford, Oxfordshire)**
> Acamprosate Appears to Decrease Alcohol Intake in Weaned Alcoholics

- Five hundred and sixty-nine alcoholics were included in a double-blind placebo-controlled randomized multicenter study of the effects of Acamprosate on alcoholic relapse after withdrawal.

- After 3 months of treatment patients given acamprosate had a significantly lower plasma gamma-glutamyl transpeptidase (GGT) level (an indicator of recent alcohol ingestion).

- The major side-effect of was diarrhea, present in 13% of patients given acamprosate.[212]

> **1985–Lhuintre–Lancet**
> Ability of Calcium Bis Acetyl Homotaurine, a GABA Agonist, to Prevent Relapse in Weaned Alcoholics

- In an early study, Lhuintre found: "The results suggest that acamprosate may be useful in helping severe alcoholics who have been weaned off alcohol not to relapse."[213]

PERSONAL EXPERIENCES WITH ACAMPROSATE

Short Forms Used Below:

- AF–Alcohol-Free (A day when no alcohol is consumed)
- GI–Gastrointestinal Upset

•••

I have heard a lot of people rave about Acamprosate. I took it for three days and didn't last because my issues are more emotional than physical cravings. I did notice that I "forgot" to want a drink on the second evening–it was weird.

•••

I've been taking Acamprosate for a month now. I was a daily drinker of 2 bottles of wine. I found the Acamprosate to be very good. I lasted AF for 21 days then binged. It is possible to override the Acamprosate if you really want to drink. The first days of taking Acamprosate were great and I didn't really think about drinking at all. Maybe it was complacency that got to me. I still have a long way to go to figure out my button pushers! However, I am no longer drinking during the week and this is an achievement. I still intend to be AF totally as it is clear I can't moderate. The side effects from Acamprosate are not too bad just the "wind" and a mild GI upset to start with. Absolutely no effects on the sex drive! I would say give it a go it is helping me–Anything is worth a try!

•••

Acamprosate is very helpful. Don't know why I stopped taking it but am back on it now. I notice not a single side effect, except I can overcome the desire to drink. And if I do drink, it is less and not nearly as enjoyable as before. It is like I drink out of habit but not because I really want to. I think it lessens the buzz so there is really no point. Sex drive not affected. I really do think it is a wonder and would encourage any and everyone to try it. It is not totally magic- but I know of nothing better.

•••

I've been on Acamprosate for nearly a week–had one day of running to the bathroom–several days of gasiness, and both of those are now better–BUT I'm feeling so fatigued!!! I know this is also a side-affect, but does that also get better? I can't stand this dragging around!!!

It certainly has helped with the desire to drink and the obsession of thinking about it all the time. I did have a few drinks one evening when with friends–more out of habit than really craving a drink. And I could stop after a few–which was a major improvement!!

•••

I have been on Acamprosate a few times this year. It takes 4-5 days to works and it works really well. The longer you stay on it the better it seems to work. I could watch a beer commercial and I didn't have any desire for one at all!

•••

I decided to try the medication, Acamprosate, instead of Topa (reasons for side effects). This drug is great! I have decided that abstinence is the better choice for me. Within I week it takes effect. No more cravings! The best thing is that there are virtually no side effects (at least none that I have experienced).... I do not go to AA for reasons of shame. I work as a Professional in my community and have not been able to go public w/ my drinking problem.

•••

Acamprosate is a very good medication—it's for people who are aiming for abstinence, not moderation, so you should not drink for 5-7 days before you begin taking it. Topamax is used primarily for people who are looking to moderate, although some (like me) use it with abstinence as their goal. Quite a few people are using Acamprosate with great success, and if Topamax were to become a problem for me, for any reason, I wouldn't hesitate to use Acamprosate. Why not work with your doctor and see how it goes.

BACLOFEN (HIGH DOSE)

INTRODUCTION TO BACLOFEN

Baclofen has been FDA-approved since 1977 for its use in treating muscle spasticity associated with spinal cord injury and seizures.

It has been researched for its properties in relation to alcoholism for over 39 years.

Some researchers believe that "baclofen may inhibit the earliest type of drug cue-induced motivational processing–that which occurs outside of awareness–before it evolves into a less manageable state."[214]

There are a few important things to be aware of in regards to baclofen.

First, unlike other medications for alcohol dependence, baclofen is taken in increasingly high doses until the patient reaches a switch point.

At this point, the patient stays at the switch level for several weeks, and then extremely gradually tapers down their dose to a maintenance dose.

Despite the enormous amount of evidence that doses must be as high as 300mg/day (10 times the often-prescribed level), and that high doses are safe, some doctors refuse to prescribe the drug at appropriate levels.

There is no evidence that the medication works at (the low) levels that it is sometimes prescribed at.

To achieve success with baclofen, it is, therefore, critical to find a physician that is familiar with the research and willing to work with you to customize the dosing.

Second, at very high doses, baclofen may become quite intolerable–making you very sleepy.

It's important to remember that the objective is not to stay at the maximum dose permanently–that it is a period of 8-10 weeks or so where high dosage amounts are necessary to reach the switch point.

If the side effects are intolerable, try to taper up more slowly or have patience while your body adjusts.

If you do decide to reduce your dosage or stop taking baclofen altogether, do so very slowly.

In one doctor's self-case report published in the journal 'Progress in Neurology and Psychiatry', Dr. Phillip Thomas (an alcoholic who was successful with baclofen), discusses how when his entire supply of medication was stolen, he was forced to go into abrupt withdrawal, which resulted in limb spasms, paranoia, and suicidal thoughts.[108]

In addition to the book by Dr. Amiesen book ('The End of My Addiction')[22], a very useful information journal article (published in the British Journal of Medicine) called 'Prescribing Guide for Baclofen in the Treatment of Alcoholism—for Use by Physicians'[215] has been written by some of the most important researchers involved with baclofen (including Dr. R. Beaurepaire, and P. Jaury), and has been translated from French into English.

It is available at this book's website.

THE BACK-STORY

Baclofen is available in generic form, which means that there is little interest from pharmaceutical companies in marketing the medication to doctors or the general public.

Dr. Oliver Amiesen was a French-American cardiologist and a severe alcoholic who experimented on himself with numerous medications to help him find a way out of alcoholism.

It was through Amiesen's tireless work that baclofen has become a drug that is available for the treatment of alcoholism, and funded by the public health care system for this purpose, in France.

After reading research about baclofen, and taking it at high doses, Amiesen was able to find what he described as the 'switch.'

When he reached this switch, Amiesen realized that he no longer felt the inexorable craving to drink that he had felt for so long.

Previously crippled by alcoholic binges, after his discovery Amiesen spent the rest of his life abstaining or drinking at a normal social level. Amiesen attributed baclofen to saving his life.

Amiesen wrote a self-published case study about his experiences[216], as well as a book[22]. The book 'The End of My Addiction' is both moving and informative and is a highly recommended resource for anyone (doctors, patients, family members and others) wishing to learn a great deal more about baclofen.

Baclofen was recently granted authorization in France for the on-label treatment of Alcohol Use Disorder. (Previously it was widely available for the treatment of AUD in France in an off-label format). Patients in France will now receive reimbursement for its cost.[217]

BACLOFEN MEDICATION FAQ

MEDICATION OVERVIEW

What is the medication called?

Baclofen

What are common brand names and generic names for this medication?

Baclofen oral, Liquid Baclofen, Lioresal, Remular, Lioresal Oral, Gablofen, Chlorophenibut, Kemstro, Liofen, Gablofen, Lyflex, Beklo, Baclosan. (Not Intrathecal Baclofen or (R-S) baclofen, or arbaclofen)

What 'type' of medication is this?

GABAB agonist

What is it usually prescribed for?

Neuromuscular Agents, Skeletal Muscle Relaxant

How is it described?

- Baclofen is a centrally acting muscle relaxant commonly prescribed for spasticity in patients with multiple sclerosis.

- Baclofen is a gamma-amino-butyric acid (GABA) derivative used as a skeletal muscle relaxant. Baclofen stimulates GABA-B receptors leading to decreased frequency and amplitude of muscle spasms. It is especially useful for treating muscle spasticity associated with spinal cord injury.

- In alcoholism, baclofen "may inhibit the earliest type of drug cue-induced motivational processing–that which occurs outside of awareness–before it evolves into a less manageable state."[214]

AVAILABILITY & FDA APPROVAL STATUS

A prescription for alcoholism is usually:

Off-Label except for in France where it is on-label

Is it FDA approved in the USA? When?

Yes—FDA Approved in 1977

Is it HC approved in Canada? When?

Yes—Health Canada Approved in 1978

Is it EMA approved in Europe? When?

Yes—EMA Approved Approved–date unknown;

How is it available?

By prescription in USA, Canada and parts of Europe

RESEARCH FOR ITS USE IN ALCOHOLISM

How many years has this medication been researched specifically for the treatment of alcoholism?

39+ years (since 1976)

What is the strength of the supporting research?

"The majority of clinical surveys conducted to date–including case reports, retrospective chart reviews, and randomized placebo-controlled studies–suggest the ability of baclofen to suppress alcohol consumption, craving for alcohol, and alcohol withdrawal symptomatology in alcohol-dependent patients."[43]

What credentials does the researcher making the statements above have?

Dr. Roberta Agabio–Researcher at Dept. of Neuroscience, University of Cagliari, Italy; Head of the Centre for the Study of Adolescent Alcohol Dependence; Editorial Board Member, Journal of Studies on Alcohol and Drugs; Alcohol Medical Scholars Program; Published more than forty articles on peer-reviewed international scientific journals and several chapters in scientific books. Former President of the Sardinian section of the Italian Society of Alcoholism (SIA) and a member of the Research Society on Alcoholism (RSA), the International Society on Biomedical Research on Alcoholism (ISBRA) and the European Society for Biomedical Research on Alcoholism (ESBRA).

RESEARCH FINDINGS ABOUT EFFECTIVENESS IN TREATMENT FOR ALCOHOLISM

How many patients need to be treated to see one true medication responder? (Known as the 'Number Needed to Treat–NNT)

The NNT for baclofen is three[35]. This means that on average three patients need to be treated to see one true medication responder.

How effective is this medication for the treatment of alcoholism?

- Addiction researcher Dr. Renault De Beaurepaire describes the results of his 2012 study: All patients were rated 'at high risk' at the start of the study. Approximately half of them were rated "at low risk" at 3, 6, 12, and 24 months. The number of patients at "low risk" and at "moderate risk" (improved patients) was 84% at 3 months, 70% at 6 months, 63% at 1 year, and 62% at 2 years.[44]

- "The constancy of improvement over the 2-years was remarkable...ninety-two percentage of patients reported that they experienced the craving-suppressing effect of baclofen."[44]

In research, how did this medication compare to other medications for the treatment of alcoholism?

- Baclofen's NNT of three is lower than any other known medications for the treatment of alcoholism including naltrexone (with an NNT of 7-10)[78]. However, medications work differently for different people depending upon their specific gene variations and the type of alcoholism they have. NNT's also differ by treatment goal. For example, NNT's for 'abstinence' will differ than that for 'reduction of drinking'.

- In comparison to other medications prescribed by doctors, Baclofen's NNT is similar or lower than the treatment of depression with any given antidepressant medication.[37]

TREATMENT CANDIDATES FOR THIS MEDICATION

Note: this section highlights study findings that have identified some characteristics that may increase odds of effectiveness. This does not mean it won't help individuals without these characteristics.

What treatment goals might this medication help achieve?

Decrease or complete suppression of alcohol craving; maintain abstinence; lower anxiety; decrease number of drinks per day; increase number of alcohol-free days.

What are some typical feelings and motivators of people this medication tends to help?

By targeting the inhibition system of the "Relief Pathway," baclofen may help treat alcoholism that is motivated by anxiety and/or depression. It may help the brain to re-implement inhibition systems that allow individuals to avoid alcohol even once craving is triggered.

Has this medication been shown to be more successful in early-onset or late-onset alcoholics?

Research has not yet provided insight on this answer.

Is this medication typically more effective in people with a strong family history of alcoholism?

Research has not yet provided insight on this answer.

Are there specific genetic markers that have been found to be relevant in treatment with this medication?

Research has not yet provided insight on this answer.

Do Alcoholics Have Difficulty Taking this Medication as Prescribed? (i.e. Are there "Compliance" Issues?)

No known compliance issues. Discontinuation may occur due to side effects.

Are there other characteristics (gender, taste sensitivity, alcoholism type, co-morbid disorders, smoker status) that may be related to success with this medication?

Research has not yet provided insight on this answer.

DIRECTIONS FOR USE & HOW IT WORKS

At what dose and for how long does research suggest the medication should be taken?

- This medication is often prescribed at far too low a dose to be effective. Much evidence shows that treatment is most successful with no superior limit of dose and that impact is tied to dosage size.[218][44]

- At doses of 30mg/day, Baclofen is unlikely to change drinking outcomes.[219]

- Titrate up from 30mg daily (10mg taken 3 times per day) to 150 to 300mg daily (divided throughout day);

- Maximum dose is dependent upon individual results.

- Patients need to be able to work closely with a doctor to increase dosage even as high as 300mg/day to achieve the greatest effectiveness. Strong side effects (such as sleepiness) will likely be felt at the highest doses.

- Patients should maintain the highest dose for several weeks before reducing to a lower maintenance dose. Do not stop suddenly. If titrating down, do so at the same speed of initial increase in medication.[215]

- Specific and detailed dosing instructions are found in this document: 'Prescribing Guide for Baclofen in the Treatment of Alcoholism—for Use by Physicians'[215] (link available from book website).

Has this medication been tested with other medications for the treatment of alcoholism and found to be complimentary?

Baclofen has been found effective in combination with naltrexone in rats. A baclofen/naltrexone combination medication (PXT3003) was just given orphan drug approval by the FDA and EMA as a treatment for another medical condition, showing that the combination is safe in humans.[220]

What is known about how this medication actually works in alcoholics? What is the 'Mechanism of Action'?

According to researchers: "Baclofen is a GABA-B agonist and, through this mechanism, the dopaminergic response to alcohol may be inhibited."[192]

SAFETY CONCERNS

Is this medication addictive? Does it have abuse potential?

Baclofen is non-addictive.

How safe is this medication?

- Baclofen is "relatively safe, has little abuse potential, and can work in combination with other drugs."[221] High doses are safe and have been studied for treatment of diseases such as paraplegia for many years.

- One 1992 study indicated: "some patients, to experience adequate symptomatic relief, require dosages of baclofen that significantly exceed the conventional 80 mg daily maximum advocated by the 1992 Physicians' Desk Reference. In this pilot study of baclofen... the safety and efficacy of high-dose baclofen was confirmed."[222]

- And in 1991 an analysis of MS patients taking high-dose baclofen looking at the frequency with which baclofen was prescribed at doses greater than 80mg/day found, "about 20% of patients had taken high-dose baclofen, and 15% were still receiving a high dose. Taking a high dose was not associated with discontinuing treatment."[223]

- Do not stop suddenly. If titrating down, do so at the same speed of initial increase in medication so suicidal ideation does not occur.[108]

Can this medication be taken while drinking?

There is moderate interaction between alcohol and baclofen. While it is not recommended to take this medication while drinking, it can be initiated while the alcohol-dependent individual is still drinking. Side-effects may be enhanced if taken while drinking. If you do begin drinking while on Baclofen, try to maintain your pre-drinking dosage, as sudden discontinuation is not recommended.

What are the expected side effects of this medication?

At the highest dosages, sleepiness is expected.

What are other fairly common side effects?

Research has showed fairly common side effects include drowsiness, dizziness, weakness, upset stomach, confusion.

Where can I find a complete list of all side effects, precautions, and instructions in case of emergency or overdose?

You can find this on the US National Library of Medicine website. Search google for 'baclofen and National Library of Medicine' or visit:

http://bit.ly/baclofensides

What does the National Institute of Health (NIH) say about liver impact and where can I find further information on liver impact of this medication?

- A 2014 study specifically of patients with alcoholic hepatitis tested baclofen and liver impact and concluded: "Baclofen's safety and efficacy in improving the clinical condition patients with alcoholic liver disease has been supported."[224]

- 2013 research found, "baclofen is safe in patients with alcohol dependence, including those with moderate to severe liver cirrhosis."[225]

- Baclofen has not been convincingly linked to clinically significant liver injury.[226]

- Also visit this page on livertox.nlm.nih.gov:

http://bit.ly/livertoxbaclofen

What known drug interactions should I watch for and where can I find more information on drug interactions?

- Moderate interaction between baclofen and zonisamide, aripiprazole, levetiracetam, baclofen, gabapentin, topiramate, valproic acid.

- Known to interact with at least 709 other drugs.[227]

- Also visit the livertox.nih.gov site page:

http://bit.ly/livertoxbaclofen

Where can I find alerts and Black Box Warnings? (Black Box Warnings are cautions affixed to medications by the government)

- Visit the nlm.nih.gov site page:

http://bit.ly/baclofensides

Were there any known black box warnings at the time this book was written?

No—but you may still wish to visit the link above for up-to-date information.

OTHER USEFUL INFORMATION

Note: Links to all recommended information sources can be found on the book's website.

Recent Research:

- 2015: High-Dose Baclofen for the Treatment of Alcohol Dependence (BACLAD Study): A Randomized, Placebo-Controlled Trial[228]

- 2014: Utilization of Baclofen in Maintenance of Alcohol Abstinence in Patients with Alcohol Dependence and Alcoholic Hepatitis with or without Cirrhosis[224]

- 2012: Suppression of alcohol dependence using baclofen: A 2-year observational study of 100 patients[44]

- 2005: Complete and prolonged suppression of symptoms and consequences of alcohol dependence using high-dose baclofen: A self-case report of a physician[216]

Newspaper and Magazine Articles:

- Baclomania: The Cult Of A Cure For Alcoholism[229]

- Treating Alcohol Addiction: Can a Pill Replace Abstinence?[230]

- Can Alcoholism Be Treated?[231]

Books:

- The End of My Addiction[22]

- B4A Baclofen Handbook[232]

Other Useful Sources:

- 2014: Prescribing Guide for Baclofen in the Treatment of Alcoholism–for Use by Physicians[215]

- NHS Guide: Baclofen at a Tailored Dose Reduces Alcohol Use, Craving and Adverse Consequences of Drinking in Alcoholics with Medical Disease due to Alcohol Dependence [233]

Websites:

baclofen4alcoholism.com

baclofenalcoholusaforum.wordpress.com

baclofene.org (French)

baclofene.fr (French)

baclofen.wiki (German)

CONNECTING WITH OTHERS

Online Forum(s):

- The 'MyWayOut' community started out focused on topiramate but is now a good place to read about and connect with others regarding a variety of medications for the treatment of alcoholism.

- Visit MyWayOut at:

http://bit.ly/mywayoutforum

- A link to Google search results for a search within the MyWayOut forum for this specific medication:

http://bit.ly/mywaybac

- Baclofene Forum (French):

baclofene.com

- Baclofen Forum (German):

forum-baclofen.com

Reviews from others on Drugs.com:

- For baclofen and 'alcohol withdrawal':

http://bit.ly/drugsbac

- For brand name and 'alcohol withdrawal':

http://bit.ly/drugsbrandbac

Reviews from others on WebMD:

Reviews are not specifically for the use of drug with alcoholism;

- For 'baclofen':

http://bit.ly/webmdbac

- For brand name:

http://bit.ly/webmdbacbrand

Generic Wikipedia Link:

http://bit.ly/wikibaclofen

DrugBank.ca Link (Detailed Drug Data Including Pricing):

http://bit.ly/drugbankbaclofen

SIGNIFICANT BACLOFEN RESEARCH &

FINDINGS

2015–Muller–European Neuropsychopharmacology
High-Dose Baclofen for the Treatment of Alcohol Dependence (BACLAD Study): A Randomized, Placebo-Controlled Trial

- In a 12-week high-dose phase of a study, more patients given baclofen (68%) maintained total abstinence than those receiving placebo (23.8%).

- Cumulative abstinence duration was also significantly higher in patients given baclofen compared to patients given placebo.

- The study concluded, "No drug-related serious adverse events were observed during the trial. Individually titrated high-dose baclofen effectively supported alcohol-dependent patients in maintaining alcohol abstinence and showed a high tolerability, even in the event of relapse."[228]

2014–Agabio–Frontiers in Neuroscience
GABAB Receptor Ligands for the Treatment of Alcohol Use Disorder: Preclinical and Clinical Evidence

- Agabio stated, "the majority of clinical surveys conducted to date–including case reports, retrospective chart reviews, and randomized placebo-controlled studies–suggest the ability of baclofen to suppress alcohol consumption, craving for alcohol, and alcohol withdrawal symptomatology in alcohol-dependent patients."[43]

2014–de Beurepaire–The Use of Very High-Doses of Baclofen for the Treatment of Alcohol-Dependence: A Case Series

- "Baclofen, particularly high-dose baclofen, has recently emerged as a treatment of major interest for alcohol-dependence... the maximal dose of baclofen that may be used is a matter of discussion."

- In this report, de Beurepaire analysed the medical charts of the last 100 patients seen in his clinic, 17 of whom have been taking high dose of baclofen (over 300mg/day). His analysis of the charts shows that the "very high-doses of baclofen were justified in almost all the cases."[234]

- The author states, "to be effective, baclofen may need to be given at high or very high doses. An imposed limit to the dose of baclofen is a loss of the opportunity of being cured for many patients."

- "Baclofen is not more dangerous at high doses than at low doses when the treatment is well supervised by the physician. Side effects, even severe side effects, can occur at any dose. Most of the time, difficult to bear side effects present at low doses will vanish or change in nature when the baclofen dose is increased. Therefore, on the condition of a good therapeutic alliance between the patient and the physician, baclofen should be prescribed with no imposed upper limit of dosage.[234]

2014–Leggio–Psychopharmacology
A Preliminary Double-Blind, Placebo-Controlled Randomized Study of Baclofen Effects in Alcoholic Smokers

---

- "This study provides preliminary evidence suggesting a possible role of baclofen in the treatment of alcoholic smokers."[235]

2014–Lesouef–Thérapie
Efficacy of Baclofen on Abstinence and Craving in Alcohol-Dependent Patients: A Meta-Analysis of Randomized Controlled Trials

---

- A meta-analysis (analysis of multiple previous studies) found "compared to placebo baclofen was associated with a significant increase of 179% in the percentage of abstinent patients at the end of the trial."[236]

2014–Marsot–Alcoholism: Clinical and Experimental Research
High Variability in the Exposure of Baclofen in Alcohol-Dependent Patients

---

- A study designed to identify factors that lead to best dosage levels was unable to find an association between aspects such as age, gender, weight, and correct dosage.

- It was observed that there is a high variation in dosage levels to achieve effect and hypothesized that too-low doses given to some individuals resulted in lack of response.[237]

2014–Yamini–Alcohol and Alcoholism
Utilization of Baclofen in Maintenance of Alcohol Abstinence in Patients with Alcohol Dependence and Alcoholic Hepatitis with or without Cirrhosis

---

- This study analyzed the "effects of baclofen utilized over 12 months in patients with alcoholic hepatitis with or without cirrhosis and alcohol dependence on these liver parameters: aspartate aminotransferase (AST), alanine aminotransferase (ALT), total bilirubin (Tbili), prothrombin time (PT), international normalized ratio (INR), albumin and Model for End-Stage Liver Disease (MELD) score."

- Results showed that on average, "baclofen was used for 5.8 months. A significant decrease in (liver tests) AST, ALT, Tbili, INR, PT and MELD score was seen when comparing pre-baclofen use compared with post-baclofen use."

- Of the 35 patients who were started on baclofen, "34 (97%) remained abstinent and there were no serious adverse events."

- The study concluded, "Baclofen's safety and efficacy in improving the clinical condition patients with alcoholic liver disease has been supported."[224]

2014–Young–The Journal of neuroscience: the official journal of the Society for Neuroscience
Nipping Cue Reactivity in the Bud: Baclofen Prevents Limbic Activation Elicited by Subliminal Drug Cues

---

- The study tested whether Baclofen could block drug triggers and cues that activate the reward circuitry in addicts (even subliminally).

- The study found, "baclofen may inhibit the earliest type of drug cue-induced motivational processing—that which occurs outside of awareness—before it evolves into a less manageable state."[214]

2013–Brennan–Clinical Pharmacology: Advances and Application
Clinical Effectiveness of Baclofen for the Treatment of Alcohol Dependence: A Review

---

- The literature review indicated, "Patients randomized to baclofen experience higher rates of abstinence from alcohol than those taking placebo in two of the trials."

- "Secondary analyses indicate that baclofen is safe in patients with alcohol dependence, including those with moderate to severe liver cirrhosis, and may provide beneficial anxiolytic effects."[225]

2013–Padula–OA Alcohol
Novel Anticonvulsants for Reducing Alcohol Consumption: A Review of Evidence from Preclinical Rodent Drinking Models

---

- A review focusing on anticonvulsants (Baclofen is an anticonvulsant) found they are "relatively safe, have little abuse potential, and can work in combination with other drugs."

- The study concluded, "the results from these preclinical and clinical studies provide compelling evidence that anticonvulsants are a promising class of medication for the treatment of AUDs."[221]

2012–De Beaurepaire–Frontiers in Psychiatry
Suppression of Alcohol Dependence Using Baclofen: A 2-Year Observational Study of 100 Patients

---

- The study stated that "while all patients were rated "at high risk" at baseline, approximately half of them were rated "at low risk" at 3, 6, 12, and 24 months. The sum of patients who were at "low risk" and at "moderate risk" (improved patients) was 84% at 3 months, 70% at 6 months, 63% at 1 year, and 62% at 2 years. The constancy of improvement over the 2-years was remarkable. The average maximal dose of baclofen taken was 147 mg/day."

- Ninety-two percentage of patients reported that they experienced the "craving-suppressing effect of baclofen."

- Significant relationships were found between the amount in grams of alcohol taken before treatment and the maximal dose of baclofen required, and between the existence of a mental disorder and a lesser effect of baclofen.

- "Conclusion: Baclofen produces an effortless decrease or suppression of alcohol craving when it is prescribed with no superior limit of dose."[44]

2012–Muzyk–CNS Drugs
Defining the Role of Baclofen for the Treatment of Alcohol Dependence: A Systematic Review of the Evidence

---

- A review of previous Baclofen trials concluded: "subjects ... experienced higher rates of abstinence and lower anxiety scores; the effect of baclofen was statistically significant in two trials assessing patients with more severe alcohol dependence...Baclofen appeared to be safe, well tolerated and to have low addiction liability even in the setting of moderate-to-severe liver cirrhosis."[238]

2012–Rigal–Alcohol and Alcoholism
Abstinence and 'Low-Risk' Consumption I Year after the Initiation of High-Dose Baclofen: A Retrospective Study among 'High-Risk' Drinkers

---

- In Rigal's study, "after 1 year, 80% ...were either abstinent or drinking at low-risk levels in their 12th month of treatment. The mean baclofen dose at 1 year was 129 ± 71 mg/day."

- Rigal concluded, "High-dose baclofen should be tested in randomized placebo-controlled trials among high-risk drinkers."[239]

2012–Thomas–Progress in Neurology and Psychiatry
Suppression of Alcohol Dependence Using High-Dose Baclofen: A Self-Case Report

---

- As with Dr. Olivier Ameisen before him, Dr. Thomas published a journal article describing how "his own alcohol dependence and the severe chronic anxiety at the root of it were both successfully suppressed by taking high-dose baclofen."[108]

- Dr. Thomas noted suicidality upon unplanned and sudden discontinuation.

2011–Addolorato–Alcohol and Alcoholism
Dose-Response Effect of Baclofen in Reducing Daily Alcohol Intake in Alcohol Dependence: Secondary Analysis of a Randomized, Double-Blind, Placebo-Controlled Trial

---

- Published research showing the importance of dosage size in the treatment of alcoholism with Baclofen. Addolorato concluded that greater dosage sizes resulted in better results.[218]

2010–Garbutt–Alcoholism: Clinical and Experimental Research
Efficacy and Safety of Baclofen for Alcohol Dependence: A Randomized, Double-Blind, Placebo-Controlled Trial

---

- Published results of a human study which showed that at a very low dose (30mg/day) Baclofen was not able to change drinking outcomes.[219]

2009–Evans–Alcoholism: Clinical and Experimental Research
Acute Interaction of Baclofen in Combination with Alcohol in Heavy Social Drinkers

---

- Published results of a study showing "Baclofen alone has minimal abuse liability in heavy social drinkers, and baclofen is relatively well tolerated and safe when given in combination even with intoxicating doses of alcohol."[240]

2007–Addolorato–Lancet
Effectiveness and Safety of Baclofen for Maintenance of Alcohol Abstinence in Alcohol-Dependent Patients with Liver Cirrhosis: Randomised, Double-Blind Controlled Study

---

- Published results of an investigation that found, "Baclofen is effective at promoting alcohol abstinence in alcohol-dependent patients with liver cirrhosis."

- "The drug is well tolerated and could have an important role in treatment of these individuals."[35]

2006–Bucknam–Alcohol and Alcoholism
Suppression of Symptoms of Alcohol Dependence and Craving Using High-Dose Baclofen

---

- Published report about a patient who had taken up to 140mg/day of high dose baclofen and been successful in finding a "complete and prolonged suppression of symptoms and consequences of alcohol dependence."[241]

2005–Ameisen–Alcohol and Alcoholism
Complete and Prolonged Suppression of Symptoms and Consequences of Alcohol-Dependence Using High-Dose Baclofen: A Self-Case Report of a Physician

---

- French cardiologist, Dr. Olivier Ameisen (who had tested high-dose baclofen on his own severe alcoholism after reading the earlier Krupitsky and Roberts' research) published a self-report of his successful treatment.

- He stated that after reaching the dose of 270 mg/day of Baclofen he "became and have remained free of alcohol dependence symptoms effortlessly for the ninth consecutive month. Anxiety is well controlled."

- He wrote, "High-dose baclofen induced complete and prolonged suppression of symptoms and consequences of alcohol dependence, and relieved anxiety."[216]

2005–Colombo–Drug and Alcohol Dependence
Effect of the Combination of Naltrexone and Baclofen, on Acquisition of Alcohol Drinking Behavior in Alcohol-Preferring Rats

---

- Published results of further rat studies with naltrexone and baclofen: "the drug combination resulted in a significant reduction in daily alcohol intake and retardation in the acquisition of alcohol drinking behavior."[242]

2004–Flannery–Alcoholism
Baclofen for Alcohol Dependence: A Preliminary Open-Label Study., Alcoholism, clinical and experimental research

---

- Another baclofen study in humans found that "there were statistically significant reductions in the number of drinks per drinking day and the number of heavy-drinking days, and there was an increase in the number of abstinent days."

- Significant decreases in anxiety and craving were also shown."[243]

2004–Stromberg–Pharmacology Biochemistry and Behavior
The Effect of Baclofen Alone and in Combination with Naltrexone on Ethanol Consumption in the Rat

---

- Study with alcohol (ethanol) addicted rats showed that at high doses, both baclofen, and another drug, naltrexone, both reduced consumption of alcohol individually and even more so when tested together.[244]

2000–Addolorato–Alcoholism, clinical and experimental research
Ability of Baclofen in Reducing Alcohol Craving and Intake: II–Preliminary Clinical Evidence

---

- Conducted a study in alcoholics showing that both craving and alcohol intake were reduced.[245]

1999–Childress–The American Journal of Psychiatry
Baclofen blocks cue-induced cravings in cocaine users

- Baclofen was found to block cue-induced cravings in cocaine users.[246]

1997–Roberts–Psychopharmacology
Baclofen Suppression of Cocaine Self-Administration: Demonstration Using a Discrete Trials Procedure

---

- Research conducted at Ottawa's Carleton University showed that high dose Baclofen suppressed cocaine addiction in cocaine-addicted rats.[247]

> **1993–Krupitsky–Drug and Alcohol Dependence**
> **Baclofen Administration for the Treatment of Affective Disorders in Alcoholic Patients**

- Research published by the Leningrad Regional Dispensary of Narcology in Russia about the effects of a drug called baclofen on 90 alcoholic patients. It found that baclofen was an effective drug in assisting the anxiety and depression that alcoholics often experience.[248]

> **1992–Aisen–The Journal of the American Paraplegia Society**
> **Clinical and Pharmacokinetic Aspects of High Dose Oral Baclofen Therapy**

- Regarding early high-dosing, Aisen found, "some patients, to experience adequate symptomatic relief, require dosages of baclofen that significantly exceed the conventional 80 mg daily maximum advocated by the 1992 Physicians' Desk Reference. In this pilot study of baclofen kinetics and dynamics in eleven patients, the safety and efficacy of high-dose baclofen was confirmed"[222]

> **1992–Smith–Neurology**
> **High-Dose Oral Baclofen: Experience in Patients with Multiple Sclerosis**

- The safety of high dose baclofen (prescribed for MS treatment at high doses) was illustrated in this research, which reviewed a "sample of charts from an outpatient clinic for multiple sclerosis to determine the frequency with which baclofen was prescribed for spasticity in high doses (greater than 80 mg/d).

- About 20% of patients had taken high-dose baclofen, and 15% were still receiving a high dose. Taking a high dose was not associated with discontinuing treatment."[223]

> **1987–Daoust**
> **(Journal and Article Name Unknown)**

- Daoust's study found the selective role of GABA-B in the modulation of alcohol intake.

1986–Gerkin–Annals of Emergency Medicine

- A research report about a woman who ingested and enormous amount–2000mg+ of baclofen–in a suicide attempt and made a full recovery. ('High' dose for AUD treatment is up to 300mg/day)[249]

1976–Cott–Naunyn-Schmiedeberg's Archives of Pharmacology
Suppression of Ethanol-Induced Locomotor Stimulation by GABA-like Drugs
---

- Showed that baclofen blocked alcohol-induced locomotion in mice and influenced dopamine metabolism. "These findings also indicate a potential interaction between GABA-like drugs and alcohol in man, and may be of heuristic value in the treatment of chronic alcoholism."[250]

1973–Ahlenius–Clinical Pharmacology and therapeutics
Antagonism by Alpha Methyltyrosine of the Ethanol-Induced Stimulation and Euphoria in Man
---

- Found dopamine mediates the neuphorogenic properties of alcohol in humans, reducing alcohol reward and consumption.[251]

PERSONAL EXPERIENCES WITH BACLOFEN

I couldn't. Not for lack of trying. The only thing that ever worked was baclofen, and that only because I could keep drinking while it worked. Because every decision I've made for more than a decade had to do with drinking...No act of God was going to stop that madness in my brain chemistry. Again, not for lack of trying.

•••

In all respects, I believe alcoholism to be a disease—a tangible misfiring of brain activity. I am no scientist or chemist, just a laymen alcoholic who tried every known approach to recovery. How much of this miswiring is pre-alcohol or occurs during active alcoholism is not known and does not much matter.

The fact for me is this:"You cannot cure a physical problem with talk therapy"....Period...End of Story

You can delay the perceived reality (using talk therapy), but in the end, you still have a defect. Many times, pre-baclofen, I felt like I should have been on the island of broken toys-forever. Nothing worked. Finally, a medication that addresses the part of my brain that is responsible for the onslaught of recurring thoughts (baclofen) is brought to my attention. It not only works for the alcohol but for so many other cyclical thoughts. You can fix mechanical problems with mechanical solutions.

TOPIRAMATE

INTRODUCTION TO TOPIRAMATE

Topiramate is an FDA-approved medication that has been widely prescribed for epilepsy and migraines. It has never been FDA-approved for the treatment of alcoholism (it must be prescribed off-label) and, therefore, was never marketed to physicians or the general public as a treatment for AUD.

Because of this, few doctors have heard of its use for the treatment of alcoholism.

Don't let the fact that it must be prescribed off-label dissuade you from learning more about it though–topiramate is, in fact, a very promising medication that research shows may be much more effective for some than any of the medications that are FDA-approved for the treatment of alcohol use disorder.

The main side effects that are widely-reported by those who take topiramate include types of cognitive impairment, described as mental slowing, reduced verbal fluency, and memory issues.

Some people struggle to find specific words in their memory when taking topiramate.

There does not seem to be evidence that any of these side effects are in any way permanent and it is suggested that tapering up to the correct dosage very gradually and slowly may help to minimize some of the side effects.

Very occasionally, some individuals have experienced serious possibly irreversible eye damage from topiramate due to Acute Angle-Closure Glaucoma (AACG). Seek immediate treatment if taking topiramate and experiencing any eye-related side-effects.

There has also been research that shows that topiramate can contribute to kidney stone formation.

One other possible side-effect of topiramate is weight loss. It has been tested in individuals with obesity and found to be an effective weight-loss aid in some cases.

As has been shown in other medications (acamprosate, naltrexone, ondansetron, sertraline and disulfiram), topiramate is more effective in the treatment of individuals with specific genetic markers.

In the case of topiramate, it was shown in 2014 and 2009 by both Kranzler et al., and Ray et al., that those with the genetic variant GRIK1 (rs2832407) may have fewer heavy drinking days and side effects when treated with topiramate than those without the variant.

THE BACK-STORY

10 years ago, Alaskan author Roberta Jewell (a pseudonym) published her book '*My Way Out: One Woman's Remarkable Journey in Overcoming Her Drinking Problem…*'

Published before Amiesen's 2008 book, Jewell's book is the first book I am aware of that was directed at a non-medical audience about a medication that could effectively treat alcoholism.

The author also started a thriving online community that has become a lifeline for thousands of people who are trying to find medical solutions to treat their own alcoholism. Both the book and the website are good reference sources for anyone considering taking topiramate for alcoholism.

While the community that Jewell founded, (at http://www.mywayout.org/community) was initially focused only on topiramate, it has organically expanded its focus to include many of the other medications as well as non-medical approaches.

Because of this, it is both an excellent resource and support group not only for individuals trying topiramate but also for several of the other medications in this book.

There are thousands of people who have visited the MyWayOut site and posted their experiences with topiramate over many weeks and months of use. If you are interested in reading about others' experiences, there are very few places online that can compare with this site.

TOPIRAMATE MEDICATION FAQ

MEDICATION OVERVIEW

What is the medication called?

Topiramate

What are common brand names and generic names for this medication?

Topomax, Topiramate, Topamax, Topiragen, Topimax, Epitomax, Topiramat-Cilag, Topiramat-Janssen, Topamax Migräne and Topamac, Qudexy (Do NOT confuse with Toprol, a different med)

What 'type' of medication is this?

Anti-seizure

What is it usually prescribed for?

Anticonvulsants, Anti-Obesity Agents, Neuroprotective Agents / Dioxolopyrans

How is it described?

Topiramate is a unique anti-seizure medication that is used in the treatment of partial and generalized seizures. It is often prescribed for migraines. Although not well understood, topiramate is thought to reduce craving for alcohol by targeting the glutamate brain pathways and inhibiting dopamine release. Topiramate reduces brain levels of the neurotransmitter dopamine (which is believed to create the pleasurable sensations alcoholics get from drinking), potentially resetting the brain's chemistry.

AVAILABILITY & FDA APPROVAL STATUS

A prescription for alcoholism is usually:

Off-Label

Is it **FDA** approved in the USA? When?
Yes–FDA Approved in 1996

Is it **HC** approved in Canada? When?
Yes–HC Approved in 2006 (generic)

Is it **EMA** approved in Europe? When?
Yes–EMA Approved, date unknown

How is it available?
By prescription in USA, Canada and parts of Europe

STRENGTH AND CREDIBILITY OF RESEARCH FOR ITS USE IN ALCOHOLISM

How many years has this medication been researched specifically for the treatment of alcoholism?
12+ years (2003)

What is the strength of the supporting research?
"Topiramate, within the dosage range of 75-300mg/day, could be considered as a first-line treatment option for the management of Alcohol Use Disorders. Its use appears to be safe and well-tolerated, especially in light of very recent findings."[252]

What credentials does the researcher making the statements above have?
Bankole Johnson: One of top alcohol addiction researchers in the world; Chair of the Department of Psychiatry, University of Maryland School of Medicine; Appointed to the National Advisory Council for NIDA, 2004-7; Member, Medications Development Subcommittee of NIDA's Advisory Council on Drug Abuse, 2004-7; Member, Extramural Advisory Board for NIAAA, 2004-present; Member, Medications Development Scientific Advisory Board for NIDA, 2005-9; Distinguished Psychiatrist Lecturer Award, American Psychiatric Association (APA), 2006

RESEARCH FINDINGS ABOUT EFFECTIVENESS IN TREATMENT FOR ALCOHOLISM

How many patients need to be treated to see one true medication responder? (Known as the 'Number Needed to Treat–NNT)

The NNT Number for topiramate is unknown. (The NNT number is the number treated before it is effective in one individual)

How effective is this medication for the treatment of alcoholism?

- "Topiramate can be a useful tool in the treatment of Alcohol Use Disorder [alcoholism]. Its efficacy, based on the current sample of studies, seems to be of somewhat greater magnitude than that of the most commonly prescribed medications for AUDs (naltrexone and acamprosate)."[253]

- "Topiramate, within the dosage range of 75-300mg/day, could be considered as a first-line treatment option for the management of AUDs. Its use appears to be safe and well-tolerated, especially in light of very recent findings."[252]

In research, how did this medication compare to other medications for the treatment of alcoholism?

- "Two trials suggested that topiramate is also more efficacious than naltrexone, and one open-label study reported better results for disulfiram than for topiramate."[254]

- Graphs from this 2015 research clearly and vividly illustrate superiority of topiramate versus levetiracetam and zonisamide in testing.[255]

TREATMENT CANDIDATES FOR THIS MEDICATION

Note: this section highlights study findings that have identified some characteristics that may increase odds of effectiveness. This does not mean it won't help individuals without these characteristics.

What treatment goals might this medication help achieve?

Reduce frequency of drinking; Reduce amount of alcohol use; Reduce cravings; Increase length of abstinence; Decrease potential of relapse

What are some typical feelings and motivators of people this medication tends to help?

By targeting the 'Relief Pathways' of the brain, it may help treat alcoholism that is motivated by anxiety, tension.

Has this medication been shown to be more successful in early-onset or late-onset alcoholics?

Research has not yet provided insight on this answer.

Is this medication typically more effective in people with a strong family history of alcoholism?

Research has not yet provided insight on this answer.

Are there specific genetic markers that have been found to be relevant in treatment with this medication?

The presence of the genetic marker rs2832407 (C-allele homozygote) may indicate a strong possibility the medication will be effective.

Do Alcoholics Have Difficulty Taking this Medication as Prescribed? (i.e. Are there "Compliance" Issues?)

Inability to tolerate the side effects may lead to discontinuation.

Are there other characteristics (gender, taste sensitivity, alcoholism type, co-morbid disorders, smoker status) that may be related to success with this medication?

May help individuals with PTSD symptoms.

DIRECTIONS FOR USE & HOW IT WORKS

At what dose and for how long does research suggest the medication should be taken?

- Increase dose gradually and slowly.

- For Efficacy: topiramate (up to 300 mg/d) was superior to placebo at not only improving drinking outcomes but increasing overall well-being and quality of life and lessening dependence severity and its harmful consequences."[256]

- For Liver Safety: The recommended starting dose for adults is 25 mg twice daily, escalating at weekly intervals to a maximum of 200 mg twice daily. (http://livertox.nlm.nih.gov/Topiramate.htm)

- After 3-6 months, patients may reduce dose; discontinue or remain at current dosage. If dosing down or discontinuing, taper down slowly.

- Side effects usually disappear when medication is discontinued.

Has this medication been tested with other medications for the treatment of alcoholism and found to be complimentary?

Yes—topiramate his has been shown effective in research with naltrexone and ondansetron.[257]

What is known about how this medication actually works in alcoholics? What is the 'Mechanism of Action'?

Researchers indicate: Topiramate has at least six important mechanisms of action. These include: 1) facilitation of inhibitory GABA-mediated currents on the GABAA receptor 2) antagonism of AMPA and kainate glutamate receptors; 3) inhibition of L-type calcium channels and limitation of calcium-dependent second messenger systems; 4) limitation of activity-dependent depolarization and excitability of voltage-dependent sodium channels; 5) activation of potassium conductance, and 6) weak inhibition of carbonic anhydrase isoenzymes — CA-II and CA-IV, which are found in both neuronal and peripheral tissues.[45]

SAFETY CONCERNS

Is this medication addictive? Does it have abuse potential?

Topiramate is non-addictive.

How safe is this medication?

- Researchers have found, "no serious side effects of topiramate were recorded throughout the study. Conclusions: Low-dose topiramate ... is well tolerated and effective."[258]

- "Topiramate is safe and well tolerated."[259]

- In rare cases, topiramate has caused irreversible damage to eyes. For information see the patient.info link:

http://bit.ly/acuteangle

- Development of kidney stones has been reported and confirmed in research.

Can this medication be taken while drinking?

"Topiramate treatment can be initiated while the alcohol-dependent individual is still drinking."[45] There is a moderate interaction between this drug and alcohol. While it is not recommended to take this medication while drinking, it can be taken while the alcohol-dependent individual is still drinking though side-effects if taken while alcohol is in one's system may be enhanced.

What are the expected side effects of this medication?

These include cognitive impairment, mental slowing, reduced verbal fluency and memory issues.

What are other fairly common side effects?

Dizziness, Weight loss, pins and needles, somnolence, nausea, diarrhea, fatigue, nasopharyngitis, depression, forgetting words, slowed thinking, memory impairment. (http://en.wikipedia.org/wiki/Topiramate)

Where can I find a complete list of all side effects, precautions, and instructions in case of emergency or overdose?

You can find this on the US National Library of Medicine website. Search google for 'topiramate and National Library of Medicine' or visit:

http://bit.ly/topiramatesides

What does the National Institute of Health (NIH) say about liver impact and where can I find further information on liver impact of this medication?

- Topiramate has been rarely associated with hepatic injury and largely when used in combination with other anticonvulsant medications.

- Also visit the livertox.nih.gov site link:

http://bit.ly/livertoxtop

What known drug interactions should I watch for and where can I find more information on drug interactions?

- Major interactions between topiramate and aripiprazole, zonisamide. Moderate interactions between topiramate and alcohol, valproic acid, baclofen.

- Known to interact with at least 575 other drugs.

- Also visit the drugs.com drug-interaction checker:

http://bit.ly/drugstopiramate

Where can I find alerts and Black Box Warnings? (Black Box Warnings are cautions affixed to medications by the government)
Visit:

http://bit.ly/topiramatesides

Were there any known black box warnings at the time this book was written?
No—but you may still wish to visit the link above for up-to-date information.

OTHER USEFUL INFORMATION

Note: Links to all recommended information sources can be found on the book's website at APrescriptionForAlcoholics.com

Recent Research:

- 2010: Topiramate in the New Generation of Drugs: Efficacy in the Treatment of Alcoholic Patients[45]

- 2010: Medication Treatment of Different Types of Alcoholism[178]

- 2015: Zonisamide, Topiramate, and Levetiracetam[255]

- 2012: BAP updated guidelines: evidence-based guidelines for the pharmacological management of substance abuse, harmful use, addiction and comorbidity: recommendations from BAP[260]

Newspaper and Magazine Articles:

- Article: Targeting Addiction[84]

Books:

- My Way Out: One Woman's Remarkable Journey in Overcoming Her Drinking Problem[261]

CONNECTING WITH OTHERS

Online Forum(s):

- The 'MyWayOut' community started out focused on topiramate but is now a good place to read about and connect with others regarding a variety of medications for the treatment of alcoholism.

- Visit MyWayOut at:

  http://bit.ly/mywayoutforum

- A link to Google search results for a search within the MyWayOut forum for this specific medication:

  http://bit.ly/mywayouttopa

Reviews from others on Drugs.com:

Reviews are not specifically for Alcoholism

- For 'topiramate':

  http://bit.ly/drugscomtopiramate

- For brand name:

  http://bit.ly/drugstopbrand

Reviews from others on WebMD:

(Choose 'Filter by Condition' dropdown and select 'Habit of Drinking too Much Alcohol')

- For 'topiramate':

  http://bit.ly/webmdtopiramate

- For brand name:

  http://bit.ly/webmdtopirbrand

Generic Wikipedia Link:

   http://bit.ly/wikitopiramate

DrugBank.ca Link (Detailed Drug Data Including Pricing):

   http://bit.ly/drugbanktop

SIGNIFICANT TOPIRAMATE RESEARCH & FINDINGS

2015–Guglielmo–CNS Drugs
Topiramate in Alcohol Use Disorders: Review and Update

- This recent extensive review concludes that topiramate can now be considered a first-line treatment option for alcoholism and sheds light on the typology of the alcoholic who might benefit from topiramate.

- "Topiramate, within the dosage range of 75-300mg/day, could be considered as a first-line treatment option for the management of AUDs. Its use appears to be safe and well-tolerated, especially in light of very recent findings."[252]

- "In particular, topiramate shows a greater beneficial effect in subjects with a typology of craving characterized by drinking obsessions and automaticity of drinking."

2015–Knapp–Journal of Clinical Psychopharmacology
Zonisamide, Topiramate, and Levetiracetam

- A recent study concluded that "compared with placebo, both zonisamide and topiramate produced significant reductions in the drinks consumed per day, percent days drinking, and percent days heavy drinking."

- Topiramate showed significant mental slowing and affected verbal fluency and working memory.[255]

2014–Batki–Alcoholism: Clinical and Experimental Research
Topiramate Treatment of Alcohol Use Disorder in Veterans with Posttraumatic Stress Disorder: A Randomized Controlled Pilot Trial

- A study in veterans with PTSD concluded, "in veterans with co-occurring PTSD and AUD, topiramate may be effective in reducing alcohol consumption, alcohol craving, and PTSD symptom severity."[253]

2014–Blodgett–Alcoholism: Clinical and Experimental Research
A Meta - Analysis of Topiramate's Effects for Individuals with Alcohol Use Disorder

- A systematic search identified seven trials, which included 1125 participants that compared topiramate to placebo for the treatment for Alcohol Use Disorder (AUD).

- The review concluded, "Topiramate can be a useful tool in the treatment of AUDs. Its efficacy, based on the current sample of studies, seems to be of somewhat greater magnitude than that of the most commonly prescribed medications for AUDs (naltrexone and acamprosate)."[253]

2014–Kranzler–The American Journal of psychiatry
Topiramate Treatment for Heavy Drinkers: Moderation by a GRIK1 Polymorphism

- "Topiramate treatment significantly reduced heavy drinking days and increased abstinent days relative to placebo. Patients receiving topiramate also had lower concentrations of the liver enzyme γ-glutamyl transpeptidase and lower scores on a measure of alcohol-related problems than the placebo group."

- The study also found that for individuals who carried a specific genetic marker (rs2832407 C-allele homozygote) topiramate had a significantly greater reduction of heavy drinking days.[262]

2014–Moore–Pharmacology Biochemistry and Behavior
The Efficacy of a Low Dose Combination of Topiramate and Naltrexone on Ethanol Reinforcement and Consumption in Rat Models

- Alcoholic rat testing of topiramate alone, naltrexone alone and the combination together found, "with greater efficacy and fewer side-effects, the combination shows promise as a treatment for AUDs."[263]

2013–Del Re–Addiction science & clinical practice
Prescription of Topiramate to Treat Alcohol Use Disorders in the Veterans Health Administration

---

- The study stated that "the US Veterans Health Administration (VHA) monitors the proportion of patients with alcohol use disorders (AUD) who receive FDA-approved medications for alcohol dependence (naltrexone, acamprosate, and disulfiram)."

- "Evidence supporting the off-label use of the antiepileptic medication topiramate to treat alcohol dependence may be as strong as these approved medications."[32]

2013–Navarrete–Addiction Biology
Effects of Naltrexone plus Topiramate on Ethanol Self-Administration and Tyrosine Hydroxylase Gene Expression Changes

---

- "The administration of naltrexone significantly reduced ethanol consumption and the motivation to drink."

- In combining two medications, "the administration of naltrexone plus topiramate reduced ethanol consumption markedly compared with single-drug treatment."[257]

2012–Miller–The International Journal of Psychiatry in Medicine
Medical Treatment of Alcohol Dependence: A Systematic Review

- A review of 85 studies with 18,937 patients, done between 1960 and 2010 showed "evidence for oral naltrexone (6% more days abstinent than placebo in the largest study) and topiramate... (26.2% more days abstinent than placebo in a recent study) is positive but modest. Acamprosate shows modest efficacy with recently abstinent patients...Depot naltrexone [injection] shows efficacy (25% greater reduction in the rate of heavy drinking vs. placebo, in one of the largest studies) in a limited number of studies."

- The review also observed that some studies suggest patients do better with psychosocial treatments plus medication while others show that brief support can be equally effective.[199]

2011–Edwards–Current pharmaceutical design
Current and Promising Pharmacotherapies, and Novel Research Target Areas in the Treatment of Alcohol Dependence: A Review

---

- In a review of all current and promising medications for treatment of alcoholism: "Topiramate is likely the most promising new treatment for AD, however, further research is needed to determine the optimal dose and appropriate length of treatment."[264]

2011–Lynch–Psychopharmacology
Severity of Drinking as a Predictor of Efficacy of the Combination of Ondansetron and Topiramate in Rat Models of Ethanol Consumption and Relapse

---

- Research on alcohol-addicted rats to test topiramate and ondansetron independently and in combination found that in all three cases (only topiramate; only ondansetron; both together) produced a "similar modest but persistent reduction" in alcohol consumption.

- In heavy-drinking rats, the combination of topiramate and ondansetron worked best. In light-drinking rats, there was little difference in the effectiveness of the three variations (all three were effective, but the combination was not better).

- Researchers concluded that in heavy drinkers, the combination of drugs might be better than individual drugs alone.[265]

2011–Paparrigopoulos–BMC Psychiatry
Treatment of Alcohol Dependence with Low-Dose Topiramate: An Open-Label Controlled Study

---

- A study of individuals with alcoholism found "low-dose topiramate as an adjunct to psychotherapeutic treatment is well tolerated and effective in reducing alcohol craving, as well as symptoms of depression and anxiety, present during the early phase of alcohol withdrawal."

- "Furthermore, topiramate considerably helps to abstain from drinking during the first 16-week post-detoxification period."[258]

2010–Arbaizar–Actas Espanolas de Psiquiatria
Topiramate in the Treatment of Alcohol Dependence: A Meta-Analysis

---

- A review and analysis of previous trials showed that topiramate is more effective than placebo in reducing percentage of heavy drinking days (23.2%), and increasing the number of days of abstinence.

- Two trials suggested that topiramate is more effective than naltrexone.[254]

2010–Johnson–Current Pharmaceutical Design
Topiramate in the New Generation of Drugs: Efficacy in the Treatment of Alcoholic Patients

---

- Johnson states in his research: "there is now solid clinical evidence to support the efficacy of topiramate for the treatment of alcohol dependence."

- "Topiramate treatment can be initiated while the alcohol-dependent individual is still drinking…topiramate may have differential effects based on genetic vulnerability."[45]

2008–Baltieri–Addiction
Comparing Topiramate with Naltrexone in the Treatment of Alcohol Dependence

---

- Baltieri found "Topiramate was statistically superior to placebo on a number of measures including time to first relapse (7.8 versus 5.0 weeks), cumulative abstinence duration (8.2 versus 5.6 weeks), weeks of heavy drinking (3.4 versus 5.9) and percentage of subjects abstinent at 4 weeks (67.3 versus 42.6) and 8 weeks (61.5 versus 31.5)."

- The research also found that "naltrexone showed trends toward inferior outcomes when compared to topiramate."[266]

**2008–Florez–Alcoholism: Clinical and Experimental Research
Using Topiramate or Naltrexone for the Treatment of Alcohol-Dependent
Patients**

- In a comparison of topiramate or naltrexone, research found: "Both groups showed substantial reduction in their drinking."

- The study concluded that "topiramate was better at reducing alcohol-related cravings throughout the study…Both topiramate and naltrexone were efficacious in the treatment of alcohol dependence, and the treatment costs were similar."[267]

**2007–Johnson–JAMA the Journal of the American Medical Association
Topiramate for Treating Alcohol Dependence: A Randomized Controlled Trial**

- Research showed: "Topiramate was 8.44% better than placebo at reducing the percentage of heavy drinking days over 14 weeks; 16.19% better at decreasing the percentage of heavy drinking days and better than placebo at all other drinking outcomes."

- "Conclusion: Topiramate is a promising treatment for alcohol dependence."[268]

**2004–Johnson–Archives of General Psychiatry
Oral Topiramate Reduces the Consequences of Drinking and Improves the Quality
of Life of Alcohol-Dependent Individuals: A Randomized Controlled Trial**

- Research showed, "Topiramate, compared with placebo, improved the odds of overall well-being; reported abstinence and not seeking alcohol; overall life satisfaction; and reduced harmful drinking consequences."

- Johnson concluded that "topiramate (up to 300 mg/d) was superior to placebo at not only improving drinking outcomes but increasing overall well-being and quality of life and lessening dependence severity and its harmful consequences."[256]

2004–Rubio–Pharmacopsychiatry
Effects of Topiramate in the Treatment of Alcohol Dependence

- In a 12-week study, patients received topiramate (262 mg/day) plus the psychoactive drugs they were taking for the other disorders.

- The research found that amount and frequency of craving and alcohol use decreased significantly by week 2 and that "Topiramate is safe and well tolerated, and may be beneficial in the treatment of alcohol dependence."[259]

2003–Johnson–Lancet
Oral Topiramate for Treatment of Alcohol Dependence: A Randomized Controlled Trial

---

- Lancet research reported "At study end, participants on topiramate, compared with those on placebo, had 2.88 fewer drinks per day, 3.10 fewer drinks per drinking day, 27.6% fewer heavy drinking days, 26.2% more days abstinent...differences in craving were also significantly greater than those of placebo."[269]

PERSONAL EXPERIENCES WITH TOPIRAMATE

Short Forms Used Below:

- AF–Alcohol-Free (A day when no alcohol is consumed)
- Bac–Baclofen
- SEs–Side Effects
- RJs Story–the 'My Way Out' book written about topiramate

•••

*I wish I could have tried this years ago. The 8th day I went to 50 mg, where I have been for 11 days, and have been AF for 11 days without any struggle. I haven't had ANY cravings. It was literally like a switch. I feel like going out and getting a bottle of booze right now about as much as I feel like getting a can of pinto beans. I keep waiting for the honeymoon to end, the placebo effect to wear off, but it hasn't! You all know that alcoholic mindset where a certain time of the day comes and it's like a ticking time bomb, you have to fight and struggle against yourself to not drink? GONE. I don't give it a second thought, there just are NO CRAVINGS. No desire. I have had some VERY stressful days this last week when in the past nothing would have stopped me from drinking away my frustrations, and while my mind automatically *thought* about alcohol, it just as quickly didn't WANT alcohol. I don't know if that makes sense, but as far as I'm concerned it's a Christmas freakin' miracle.*

My Doctor has made it clear that we will adjust my dose ... so I know I can go up to 75, 100mg or higher if I feel cravings...but I feel good on 50 mg so I hope I can stay here.

*Side effects: 1) I've seen others complain this makes them dopey and tired. My doctor said take it at bedtime for that reason. I can't take it at bedtime because it keeps me up all night thinking as sharp as a tack, so I take it at around 5 p.m. I do get a *bit* tired a few hours later. Not fall asleep tired, just yawning a bit. 2) Any carbonated beverage tastes [bad].*

And THAT'S IT. I am 100% functional on Topiramate, it's like being on nothing at all. Except I don't drink!

I will update this as time goes on, but for now, I just wanted to say if you've struggled with Bac don't overlook alternatives. I was so convinced Bac was the only way that when it didn't work for me I was in despair. Turns out Topiramate (knock on wood) is 1000 times more suited for me. On paper the SE's are as scary as Bac, but at least in my reality, they are minuscule and relief came in 8 short days. Maybe I am the exception, but damn, I wish I would have tried this years ago!

•••

I asked my doctor to prescribe Topiramate and she agreed. I am currently at 100 mg and I have to say I do not want to drink. I still have psychological urges, but I have actually tried having a drink and I can't finish it. Alcohol just does not really appeal to me. Also, I was a big beer drinker and the Topiramate makes it taste downright nasty to me.

I plan on continuing to titrate up to 300 mg and see what dose works best for me. As far as negative side effects, I have been a little spaced-out, typing can be a little difficult, and I have a problem getting the right words out sometimes (sometimes I actually feel like I HAVE been drinking :) . All in all, the positives have outweighed the negatives for me and I'm glad I am taking it.

When I drank, I always felt like an "on" switch was flipped in my brain and I had no "off". Once I started drinking, I just could not stop. I feel like Topiramate has given me the "off" switch that I have been lacking my whole life.

Whatever you decide to do, good luck on your journey."

•••

Yes, I too have been on Topiramate for approx. 4 1/2 months. Same results. Cravings reduced almost immediately. Weight was not an issue, but have lost additional lbs. Have to be careful not to get too thin. Don't want my Doctor to take me off the Topiramate.

When I went to my doctor, I took the Lancet medical study, a copy of RJ's story, the book, my supplements, and told my doctor that I had struggled & used alcohol as a way of self-medicating my stress for year and that I had allowed it to get out of hand. I was honest with him about how much I was drinking.

I explained to him how hard it was for me to come to him and how ashamed I felt. I was crying and embarrassed. He knows me as a successful type A over-achiever who puts too much stress on herself. He was very empathetic. After looking things over, he, who is over weight said, "I use food—and you use alcohol, as a way of handling our stress. Let's see if we can get you some help."

I don't mean to oversimplify, but I think the presentation is very important. Find the right doctor, who you feel comfortable with. Someone who will listen to you and cares."

•••

I'm so frustrated and sick and tired of trying to help myself. I really gave a good presentation myself, so I thought. I brought the book, and the Lancet report and tried to explain it basically the same way. I even had pages bookmarked so I could keep my thoughts together. I don't know if it is because I am in California or not but it seems like the doctors here are ultra-sensitive to you if you have a drinking problem, it's like it raises a red flag or something and they automatically want you to go through the 12 step program and quit right away! It's so close-minded.

I'm so frustrated and sick and tired of trying to help myself with something only to get shut down, I am seriously considering going to a new doctor and flat out lie and say I have migraines just to get the prescription. It's really hard on me to get turned away, I feel like some kind of freak or something!"

Naltrexone (Daily Dosage, As Needed or Injection)

"In honor of David's life, his family requests that you learn about The Sinclair Method of alcohol treatment and then help others become educated about it."[109]
—Obituary of Dr. David Sinclair

Introduction to Naltrexone

Naltrexone is one of the three medications (including acamprosate and disulfiram) for alcohol use disorder that is FDA-approved for the treatment of alcohol use disorder in many countries.

For this reason, doctors may be more open to prescribing it than other treatments that are off-label (and insurance programs may be more likely to cover its costs).

As has been shown in other medications (acamprosate, topiramate, ondansetron, sertraline and disulfiram), naltrexone is more effective in the treatment of individuals with specific genetic markers.

As discussed elsewhere in the book, it is extremely likely that genetic variations determine both how you respond to alcohol as well as how you respond to naltrexone.

Methods

There are three 'methods' for taking naltrexone. There is research available that supports all three of these methods. While each method has its advocates and detractors, one has not been clearly proven more effective than another. The methods are:

1) Daily Dose

2) Monthly Injection (also known as Vivitrol, Extended Release, XR, depot, XR-NTX, or long-acting intramuscular)

3) As Needed (also known as targeted, TSM or The Sinclair Method)

Daily Dose

Doctors who are familiar with naltrexone and agree to prescribe it typically prescribe a 50mg pill to be taken on a daily basis with abstinence from alcohol. This is called the 'Daily Dose' method.

Monthly Injection

Monthly naltrexone injection is also known by the brand name Vivitrol.

It is also called Extended Release, XR, depot, XR-NTX, 'once-monthly extended release' or long-acting intramuscular.

The injection method is basically the same as the 'Daily Dose' method (in that there is a constant level of naltrexone in ones' system whether you are drinking or not).

The biggest advantage to the injection is that there is no daily commitment to taking medication (which can be very difficult for some alcoholics). Instead, only a monthly commitment to a single injection must be made.

Vivitrol is sometimes balked at given the cost of injection which can be around $1000. However, drug plans and other co-pay options exist that may lower this cost significantly. Don't rule this medication out due to costs until you look into options. You can find an application at this link that may help cover the cost of Vivitrol:

http://bit.ly/vivitrolcopay

As Needed

The 'as needed' method is also known as targeted, TSM or The Sinclair Method.

The 'As Needed' method involves taking a 50-100mg pill one hour before drinking and *only* on days when there is a risk of drinking.

The 'As Needed' method was championed and even patented by Dr. David Sinclair.

Sinclair hypothesized that if the positive reinforcement effects of alcohol-triggered endorphins were blocked each time an alcoholic drank, (and not when they didn't drink) then eventually the conditioned reaction would weaken, and alcoholics would drink progressively less and experience significant craving reductions.

Recently, pharmaceutical company Lundbeck gained FDA-approval and launched nalmefene (a substance very similar to naltrexone and also patented early on by Dr. Sinclair) in Europe, and has heavily promoted the fact that nalmefene is to be taken by patients 'as needed' (similar to naltrexone).

Lundbeck's marketing of nalmefene in this way has created stronger validity and credibility for this method than it experienced in the past and has helped doctors take a second look at naltrexone or nalmefene 'as needed'.

Because naltrexone has been researched for alcoholism for over 20 years, not only does it have extensive research on its effectiveness, but it is also probably the medication with the most research providing clues to who it may and may not work best for.

Research shows that people with the following traits are more likely to respond favorably:

- male gender;
- strong sweet-liking;
- high craving;

- those highly susceptible to alcohol-cue triggers;

- those motivated by the pleasure and 'high' of alcohol (rather than as an escape from anxiety and depression);

- early-onset alcoholics;

- those with a strong family history of alcoholism;

- those with certain specific gene variations.

Many of these characteristics are associated with the 'Type-B Alcoholic' (early-onset) profile.

Anecdotally there is also some indication that individuals that show or feel an immediate initial response to naltrexone (versus those that experience very little initial reaction) are more likely to be strong responders.

Please note, however, that these attributes are only 'clues' and not absolutes. For example, Claudia Christian, who is a high-profile naltrexone advocate and a 'strong responder' (having a fast and successful response to naltrexone) has very few of those characteristics. She is female, had late-onset alcoholism and no known family history of alcoholism.

Christian wrote about how this method helped her overcome alcoholism in her autobiography and she has also produced and appeared in the documentary 'One Little Pill' which is an excellent movie about naltrexone.

[Caution: Abstinent individuals who are very reactive to alcohol imagery cues may wish to avoid watching the documentary as it can trigger strong cravings.]

For those interested in the 'as needed' method an additional excellent resource is a book called 'The Cure for Addiction: The Medically Proven Way to Eliminate Alcohol Addiction' which focusses exclusively on the 'as needed' method.

Despite the name of Dr. Eskapa's book, naltrexone taken 'as needed' is not a cure for alcoholism for everyone.

As with most medications, it does not work for everyone.

Eskapa's book cites rates around 60-70% for the effectiveness of this method. In reality, his estimate may be on the high side. However, there is research indicating that it may be effective in as few as one in seven individuals.

THE BACK-STORY

The 'as needed' method provided one of the first medication options for alcoholics which enabled them to focus on easily decreasing alcohol intake, instead of trying to achieve immediate long-term abstinence (as AA, disulfiram and acamprosate do).

This method has been called 'paradoxical' because the notion that one has to drink alcohol to decrease its hold seems counterintuitive, and doctors may have struggled with the ethics of prescribing a pill to an alcoholic that must be taken with alcohol.

Also, historically society has been so focused on the AA-way (i.e. that the only solution to alcoholism is abstinence), that a solution that doesn't enforce abstinence has been questionable for some with this mindset.

There is research that shows that those with the most severe alcoholism are also the ones who may have the most difficulty in compliance—or in other words, they are likely to stop taking it prior to drinking. In this case, the injection version of the medication may be an excellent option.

For individuals who do wish to try naltrexone via the 'as needed' method, the forum, 'TheSinclairMethod.net' is an excellent resource both for support from others and for many years' worth of information posted by thousands of members about their experiences with this method, which is usually referred to as TSM on the site.

For individuals who wish to try naltrexone via injection or via Daily Dose, the 'MyWayOut.org/community' forum may be a more supportive and informative place.

Naltrexone & Gene Variation

Interactions

Dr. Raymond Anton is a psychiatrist and director of Medical University of South Carolina's Center for Drug and Alcohol Programs, and Dr. Lara Ray is a Ph.D. and Associate Professor at the University of Colorado.

Anton and Ray have been conducting research on two of the numerous genes linked to alcoholism, seeing the impact of the presence of these genes on how alcoholics respond to both alcohol and medications like naltrexone.

Their work has shown that it is not just single gene variations that are important, but the interaction of multiple variations in multiple genes that determine both alcohol and medication response.

OPRM1 is a gene related to how opioid receptors work, and SLC6A3 is a gene related to how dopamine works in the brain. Variations of these two genes seem to increase one's risk of developing alcoholism.

Together, these two genes probably have something to do with how enjoyable and ultimately addictive alcohol is when it enters the brain and becomes part of a chain reaction triggering their expression.

For OPRM1, researchers looked at alcoholics with two genetic variations: either the OPRM1 A variation (A-Allele) or the OPRM1 G-Variation (G-Allele). ('Allele' is just another word for variation.)

Scientists have seen that alcoholics with these two OPRM1 variations respond differently to both alcohol and to the medication naltrexone. And several studies have shown that approximately 23% of treatment-seeking alcoholics carry the OPRM1 G-Allele.[270]

Studies have also shown that G-Allele carriers seem to respond better to naltrexone, and several studies in both primates and humans have shown that the effect of both alcohol and alcohol cues in the brains of G-allele carriers is stronger and more profound than in A-allele carriers.

Studies also showed that G-allele carriers respond to alcohol with a different effect (blunting the alcohol) than those without the G-allele.

But other studies have been contradictory—showing no impact on naltrexone treatment in G-allele carriers.

Dr. David Oslin commented on his 2015 study, published in JAMA Psychiatry, saying, "Some patients are very strong responders to naltrexone, and other patients don't seem to benefit whatsoever. And unfortunately, we don't have a way of predicting that still, right now. This study doesn't take away from naltrexone as a treatment option, we just can't personalize it yet."[271]

Do contradictory studies disprove earlier studies?

Not necessarily. Sometimes they simply point to another factor or factors at play. While inconclusive research is frustrating—who doesn't just want cut-and-dry clarity—it also helps reveal that there are more variables at work.

The variable that some researchers felt might be at work with contradictory G-allele studies is related to the gene described earlier: SLC6A3.

Researchers believed that two variations of this gene—one called 'A9' and another called 'A10'—might be interacting with the effect of alcohol and naltrexone on the G-allele carriers.

Researchers had already seen that SLC6A3 'A9' carriers exhibit greater impulsivity and reward seeking—probably because of a difference in how their brains process dopamine.

So in several studies of alcoholics, these genes were observed. With two variations of each gene, alcoholics with the following variations were looked at:

- Group 1: OPRM1 G-Allele with SLC6A3 A9

- Group 2: OPRM1 G-Allele with SLC6A3 A10

- Group 3: OPRM1 A-Allele with SLC6A3 A9

- Group 4: OPRM1 A-Allele with SLC6A3 A10

The results of one study showed that Group 2—people with both OPRM1 G-Allele and SLC6A3 A10—reacted very differently to alcohol than other groups. They experienced significant increases in stimulation, vigor, and positive mood when drinking.

The same study showed that whether they carried the A9 or A10 variation or not, G-Allele carriers felt the effect of alcohol much more quickly than A-Allele carriers and had a greater response in measures of positive mood.[138]

This strong positive reaction to alcohol connects the presence of these genes to the increased risk of developing alcoholism during the early phases of disease development.

And another study showed that Group 3–people with the OPRM1 A-Allele and the SLC6A3 A9 variation (the opposite combination to Group 2) showed a significant reduction in drinking when treated with naltrexone.

And, most importantly, aside from Group 3, no other group (not even the G-Allele carriers) in this small study showed a reduction in drinking when treated with naltrexone.[270]

This type of research illustrates both the complexity of the genetic component of alcoholism, and the complex interactions with medications like naltrexone. And it reminds us that if medications don't work for someone, it doesn't mean they 'don't work'; it just means they don't work for that particular individual.

The bottom line for naltrexone users is this though: the best way to learn whether naltrexone (in its varying methods) will work for you, is to try it.

If it is not effective for you, then simply move on to the next medication option. Many medications work on different targets, with different genetic variations, you may need to keep trying before you find the one that works for your DNA.

NALTREXONE MEDICATION FAQ

MEDICATION OVERVIEW

What is the medication called?

Naltrexone (NTX)

What are common brand names and generic names for this medication?

- Pill Form: Revia, Depade, Nalorex, Opizone (Do not confuse with Naloxone, or Nalorphine, a different med).

- Injection Form: Vivitrol Injection, Vivitrol Implant, Vivitrex, Depot injectable naltrexone, Nalexone Injection. Also see methylnaltrexone (Relistor)

What 'type' of medication is this?

Opioid Receptor Antagonist

What is it usually prescribed for?

Alcohol use disorder, Appetite Depressants, Narcotic Antagonists, Central Nervous System Depressants, Alcohol Antagonists, Opioid Receptor Antagonist / Morphinans

How is it described?

Naltrexone is a synthetic opioid antagonist used in the prevention of relapse of opiate addiction and alcoholism. It can help reduce the frequency and severity of relapse to drinking.

AVAILABILITY & FDA APPROVAL STATUS

A prescription for alcoholism is usually:

On-Label

Is it FDA approved in the USA? When?

Yes–FDA Approved pill form in 1994; (Injection FDA approved in 2006)

Is it HC approved in Canada? When?

Yes–HC Approved pill form in 1997; (injection not yet approved)

Is it EMA approved in Europe? When?

Yes–EMA Approved pill form in 1996 (later in some areas); (injection not yet approved)

How is it available?

Europe Pill form available by prescription in USA, Canada and parts of Europe (injection only by prescription in USA)

STRENGTH AND CREDIBILITY OF RESEARCH FOR ITS USE IN ALCOHOLISM

How many years has this medication been researched specifically for the treatment of alcoholism?

23+ years (1992)

What is the strength of the supporting research?

- "Meta-analyses of available trials, even when the negative study is included in the analysis, unequivocally support NTX efficacy."[1]

- "There is abundant evidence supporting the use of naltrexone for treatment of alcohol dependence (Level A)."[41]

- As early as 2002, one report showed that up to 2001 there had already been 14 trials assessing the effectiveness of naltrexone compared with placebo for treating alcoholism, enrolling 2127 subjects, in five countries. It stated, "there is strong evidence that naltrexone significantly reduces alcohol relapses to heavy drinking, the frequency and quantity of alcohol consumption in those who do drink, and alcohol craving."[46]

What credentials does the researcher making the statements above have?

- Markus Heilig: One of top alcohol addiction researchers worldwide; former NIAAA Clinical Director; active medical practitioner; author of more than 200 peer-reviewed journal articles, including papers in

Science, PNAS, Lancet, Archives of General Psychiatry. Research work has 8000+ citations.

- Michael Soyka: Respected researcher and Medical Director located in Switzerland. Numerous peer-published papers and extensive credentials.

RESEARCH FINDINGS ABOUT EFFECTIVENESS IN TREATMENT FOR ALCOHOLISM

How many patients need to be treated to see one true medication responder? (Known as the 'Number Needed to Treat–NNT. The lower the NNT, the better.)

- Naltrexone's NNT has been found to be between 7 and 10.[136] This means that seven to ten people must take naltrexone for it to work in one individual. (This number is similar to treatment with most antidepressants, and lower than many other commonly prescribed medications).

How effective is this medication for the treatment of alcoholism?

- "Naltrexone is one of the most evaluated medications in clinical research for reducing craving. It was superior to placebo in lessening craving, preventing relapse to heavy drinking, and in increasing the percentage of abstinent days."[47]

- "Oral and long-acting injectable naltrexone... are approved for treatment of alcohol dependence. Their availability and consideration of their use in treatment are now standards of high-quality care...."[48]

In research, how did this medication compare to other medications for the treatment of alcoholism?

- "In the trial reported in this issue, the number needed to treat (NTT) for gabapentin on the key outcome of abstinence from heavy drinking is five. Similar NNT estimates apply to naltrexone for alcohol dependence."[78]

- A review of 64 trials from 1970 to 2009 found: "Acamprosate had a significantly larger effect size than naltrexone on the maintenance of abstinence, and naltrexone had a larger effect size than acamprosate on the reduction of heavy drinking and craving.[195]

- "Naltrexone showed trends toward inferior outcomes when compared to topiramate."[266]

TREATMENT CANDIDATES FOR THIS MEDICATION

Note: this section highlights study findings that have identified some characteristics that may increase odds of effectiveness. This does not mean it won't help individuals without these characteristics.

What treatment goals might this medication help achieve?

- Oral naltrexone reduces heavy drinking, but is less consistent as an abstinence promoter, whereas once-monthly extended-release naltrexone (XR-NTX) also maintains abstinence; both have been shown to decrease relapse risk and diminish craving.

- "Naltrexone may represent a pharmacotherapy to help patients at the initial state of recovery, when craving is at its most intense."[47]

What are some typical feelings and motivators of people this medication tends to help?

By targeting the opioid system of the "Reward Pathway," naltrexone may help treat alcoholism that is motivated by a craving for the 'pleasure' and 'high' of alcohol. Heavy drinking (bingeing) is associated with high cravings that are related to this system.

Has this medication been shown to be more successful in early-onset or late-onset alcoholics?

Research indicates this medication may be more likely to be helpful for individuals with early-onset alcoholism.

Is this medication typically more effective in people with a strong family history of alcoholism?

Research indicates this medication may be more likely to be helpful for individuals with early-onset alcoholism.

Are there specific genetic markers that have been found to be relevant in treatment with this medication?

There is strong evidence that naltrexone response is related to specific genetic markers, such as the OPRM1 Asn40Asp polymorphism and SLC6A3 variants.[138272]

Do Alcoholics Have Difficulty Taking this Medication as Prescribed? (i.e. Are there "Compliance" Issues?)

Some alcoholics (not all) struggle to comply with the 'daily dose' and 'as needed' methods. The injection format can overcome this problem. Those with difficulty complying may also be the ones that the drug is most effective with if compliance is achieved (individuals with higher severity of alcoholism; high craving; early-onset; strong family history).

Are there other characteristics (gender, taste sensitivity, alcoholism type, co-morbid disorders, smoker status) that may be related to success with this medication?

- Research has shown these characteristics may be related to success: male gender, sweet-liking, high craving, individuals who are highly susceptible to alcohol-cue triggers.

- It has also been shown effective in adolescents and young adults, as well as older adults.

- Regarding sweet preference, "Higher sweet preference was significantly related to successful treatment measures in the naltrexone group but not in the placebo group."[161]

DIRECTIONS FOR USE & HOW IT WORKS

At what dose and for how long does research suggest the medication should be taken?

- There are three ways to take naltrexone. It is very important to consider which way may work best for you. Each method may have markedly different results for the same individual.

- "Daily Dose Method"–50-100 mg per day, every day; higher dose has been shown to impact effectiveness (positively).

- "Targeted" (also known as "As Needed" or "TSM" or "The Sinclair Method")–50-100mg 1 hour before drinking, only on days when there is a risk of drinking.

- "Injection" (also known as "Extended Release" or "XR" or "depot", or "long-acting intramuscular")–380mg injection given intramuscularly once per month. For Monthly Injection, higher dose (380 mg) has been shown as more effective than a smaller injection dose (190mg).

- "The length of treatment with naltrexone has not been well studied though many clinicians recommend one year of treatment."[273]

Has this medication been tested with other medications for the treatment of alcoholism and found to be complimentary?

- Yes, naltrexone has been widely tested with other medications and found complimentary. These include: acamprosate, topiramate, ondansetron, prazosin, sertraline.

- Antidepressant citalopram was also well tolerated with naltrexone but did not show a complimentary effect.

- Baclofen has been found effective in combination with naltrexone in rats. A baclofen/naltrexone combination medication (PXT3003) was just given orphan drug approval by the FDA and EMA as a treatment for another medical condition, showing that the combination is safe in humans.[274]

What is known about how this medication actually works in alcoholics? What is the 'Mechanism of Action'?

- Researchers indicate: "efficacy of naltrexone is believed to be mediated through interactions between dopamine and the endogenous opioid neuropeptide systems."

- "The endogenous opioids are involved in the expression of alcohol's reinforcing effects and may promote drug-seeking behaviors. Naltrexone functions as a competitive antagonist at opioid receptors."

- "In animal models, alcohol administration was shown to promote beta-endorphin release in regions of the brain that are involved in reward. Relief of the tonic inhibiting effects of GABA neurons by beta-endorphins in the VTA (Ventral Tegmental Area of brain) promotes dopaminergic signaling from this area of the brain to the nucleus accumbens."[192]

- Naltrexone seems to work by altering subjective responses to alcohol. Studies have shown that it alters the subjective response by dampening feelings of alcohol-induced stimulation, and alcohol 'high', decreasing ratings of liking and enjoyment of intoxication and increasing fatigue, tension, and confusion.[134] Sinclair has theorized that over time the conditioned response to alcohol is broken.

SAFETY CONCERNS

Is this medication addictive? Does it have abuse potential?

Naltrexone is non-addictive.

How safe is this medication?

In a study where alcohol dependent outpatients received high dose naltrexone at a dose of 150 mg/day (3 times the dosage typically recommended), "liver function tests were obtained at weeks 0, 3, 5, 7, and 9. High-dose naltrexone was safe and well tolerated using the procedure described. No serious adverse effects were reported. Liver markers were stable or showed improvement."[275]

Can this medication be taken while drinking?

- There is a moderate interaction between this drug and alcohol.

- It can be initiated while the alcohol-dependent individual is still drinking without causing harm, and, in fact, is sometimes recommended this way (using the 'as needed' method).

What are other fairly common side effects?

Nausea, headache, constipation, dizziness, anxiety, daytime sleepiness, and insomnia.

Where can I find a complete list of all side effects, precautions, and instructions in case of emergency or overdose?

You can find this on the US National Library of Medicine website. Search google for 'naltrexone and National Library of Medicine' or visit:

http://bit.ly/nalsides

What does the National Institute of Health (NIH) say about liver impact and where can I find further information on liver impact of this medication?

- Naltrexone has been associated with low rates of serum enzyme elevations during therapy and with rare instances of clinically apparent liver injury.

- While often considered hepatotoxic, naltrexone has not been definitively linked to cases of clinically apparent liver injury.

- Also visit the livertox.nlm.nih.gov site at:

http://bit.ly/livertoxnal

What known drug interactions should I watch for and where can I find more information on drug interactions?

- Interactions with opioid analgesics. Moderate interaction between valproic acid, disulfiram, alcohol.

- Known to interact with at least 470 other drugs.

- Also visit the drugs.com drug interaction checker:

http://bit.ly/nalinteraction

Where can I find alerts and Black Box Warnings? (Black Box Warnings are cautions affixed to medications by the government)

Visit:

http://bit.ly/nalblackbox

Were there any known black box warnings at the time this book was written?

YES: naltrexone may cause liver damage if taken in large doses. Check the url above for other more recent black box warnings.

OTHER USEFUL INFORMATION

Note: Links to all recommended information sources can be found on the book's website at APrescriptionForAlcoholics.com

Recent Research:

- 2014: Clinical and biological moderators of response to naltrexone in alcohol dependence: A systematic review of the evidence[276]

- 2002: Evidence for the Efficacy of Naltrexone in the Treatment of Alcohol Dependence (Alcoholism)[46]

- 2012: BAP updated guidelines: evidence-based guidelines for the pharmacological management of substance abuse, harmful use, addiction, and comorbidity: recommendations from BAP[260]

- 2010: Medication treatment of different types of alcoholism.[178]

Documentary:

- Highly recommended 'One Little Pill' documentary at:

  http://bit.ly/onelittlepill

- Please use caution if you are highly sensitive to alcohol-image triggered relapses.

Newspaper and Magazine Articles:

- Article: Targeting Addiction[84]

Books:

- The Cure for Alcoholism[277]

- Babylon Confidential[114]

Websites:

cthreefoundation.org

cthreeeurope.com/about

CONNECTING WITH OTHERS

Online Forum(s):

- The 'MyWayOut' community started out focused on topiramate but is now a good place to read about and connect with others regarding a variety of medications for the treatment of alcoholism.

- Visit MyWayOut at:

http://bit.ly/mywayoutforum

- A link to Google search results for a search within the MyWayOut forum for this specific medication:

http://bit.ly/mywaynal

- The 'OptionsSaveLives' forum (CThree Foundation):

optionssavelives.freeforums.net

Reviews from others on Drugs.com:

- For 'naltrexone':

http://bit.ly/drugsnal

Reviews from others on WebMD:

(Choose 'Filter by Condition' dropdown and select 'Habit of Drinking too Much Alcohol')

- For 'naltrexone':

http://bit.ly/webmdnal

- For pill format brand name:

http://bit.ly/webmdpillnal

For injection format brand name:

http://bit.ly/webmdnalxr

Wikipedia Link:

http://bit.ly/wikinal

DrugBank.ca Link (Detailed Drug Data Including Pricing):

http://bit.ly/drugbanknal

SIGNIFICANT NALTREXONE RESEARCH & FINDINGS

Which Methods for Research Findings?

For each piece of research highlighted below, the following terms are included under the name of the Journal article, ('Applies to') to highlight which method or methods the research may be relevant to.

- Non-Specific: It is unclear which method the research used; or the research could apply to all three methods;

- Daily Dose: Research specifically used a method where naltrexone is taken every day whether drinking or not;

- Injection: Research specifically used a method where naltrexone injection taken once per month;

- As Needed: Research specifically used a method where naltrexone was taken one hour before drinking only on drinking days;

In some regards, research conclusions for the 'Daily Dose' method may also apply to the 'Injection' method since in both cases (where compliance is 100%), the same medication is consistently in the patient's body whether drinking or not.

2015–Crowley–Australian Prescriber
Long-Term Drug Treatment of Patients with Alcohol Dependence Research
Applies to: Non-Specific method

- Crowley states, "Naltrexone and acamprosate have well-established efficacy and are first-line treatments."

- "Naltrexone is recommended for patients aiming to cut down their alcohol intake who do not have severe liver disease or an ongoing need for opioids."[278]

2015–Donoghue–Addiction
The Efficacy of Acamprosate and Naltrexone in the Treatment of Alcohol
Dependence, Europe versus the Rest of the World: A Meta-Analysis
Applies to: Daily Dose method

- A review of multiple trials with a total of 2649 participants showed, "both acamprosate and naltrexone appear to reduce the risk of individuals returning to drinking alcohol in those who are alcohol-dependent."[197]

2015–Harris–Alcoholism: Clinical and Experimental Research
Extended Release Naltrexone for Alcohol Use Disorders: Quasi-Experimental
Effects on Mortality and Subsequent Detoxification Episodes
Applies to: Injection method

- "Among patients with AUDs [Alcohol Use Disorder or alcoholism], those receiving XRN [Extended Release Naltrexone Injection] had lower 1-year mortality and fewer detoxifications compared to similar patients not receiving XRN."

- "These results…support the use of XRN, especially among patients with high rates of psychiatric comorbidities and previous addiction treatment who are still struggling with AUDs and/or facing a period of vulnerability to relapse."[48]

2015–Mason–Journal of Clinical Psychiatry
Acamprosate, Alcoholism, and Abstinence
Applies to: Non-Specific

- "Some studies have found a lack of naltrexone efficacy in women with alcohol dependence."[193]

2015–O'Malley–The Journal of Clinical Psychiatry
Reduction of Alcohol Drinking in Young Adults by Naltrexone
Applies to: Daily Dose; As Needed

- A trial with participants ages 18-25 with more than 4 heavy drinking days in the last month found: "Naltrexone did not reduce the frequency of drinking or heavy drinking days, but reduced secondary measures of drinking intensity."

- "While effects were modest, the risk-benefit ratio favors offering naltrexone to help young adult heavy drinkers reduce the amount of alcohol they drink."[279]

2015–Verplaetse–Psychopharmacology
Low-Dose Prazosin Alone and in Combination with Propranolol or Naltrexone: Effects on Ethanol and Sucrose Seeking and Self-Administration in the P Rat
Applies to: Non-Specific

- "In rats, "Prazosin in combination with propranolol or naltrexone was more effective than either drug alone."[280]

2014- Garbutt–Addiction
Clinical and Biological Moderators of Response to Naltrexone in Alcohol Dependence: A Systematic Review of the Evidence
Applies to: Non-Specific

- A report looked at 622 trials between 1990 and 2012 to determine what characteristics are most likely to lead to success with naltrexone.

- The most significant characteristics were: family history of alcohol problems, the existence of a specific gene variation (OPRM1 Asn40Asp polymorphism), male gender, sweet-liking, strong craving.[276] (Note: another trial showed that strong craving also may lead to low ability to comply.)

2014–Haass-Koffler–CNS Drugs
Pharmacological Approaches to Reducing Craving in Patients with Alcohol Use Disorders
Applies to: Daily Dose; As Needed

- A review of data from multiple clinical trials showed "naltrexone-treated patients drink less both in terms of quantity and frequency when compared with placebo-treated subjects and craved less alcohol compared to acamprosate-treated subjects."[47]

- The review also showed naltrexone to decrease relapse and reduce craving. Studies showed that naltrexone is more effective for heavy drinking alcoholics and in patients with a strong family history of alcoholism.

- The study referenced 'Type A' (late-onset alcoholics), and 'Type B' alcoholics, which are those with the following characteristics: Heavy drinking; early onset; tend to crave alcohol more intensely than moderate drinking late-onset alcoholics.[47]

- The study found naltrexone more successful in reducing relapse when patients experienced a high level of alcohol craving and hypothesized it would be helpful at the initial state of recovery when craving may be at its most intense.

- The author also referenced "targeted naltrexone" data showing that naltrexone taken only when craving occurs was effective in maintaining alcohol reduction by heavy drinking alcoholics.

- Haass-Koffler also referenced the finding that naltrexone as an anti-craving medication is more effective in individuals with certain opioid receptor genes and variations, and not as effective in individuals without these variations.[47]

2014–Moore–Pharmacology Biochemistry and Behavior
The Efficacy of a Low Dose Combination of Topiramate and Naltrexone on Ethanol Reinforcement and Consumption in Rat Models
Applies to: As Needed

- Alcoholic rat testing of topiramate alone, naltrexone alone and the combination together found, "with greater efficacy and fewer side-effects, the combination shows promise as a treatment for AUDs [Alcohol Use Disorder or Alcoholism]."[263]

2014–Nunes–JAMA Internal Medicine
Gabapentin: A New Addition to the Armamentarium for Alcohol Dependence?
Applies to: Non-Specific

- Nunes argues that because the NNT [Number Needed to Treaat] for gabapentin is five, and the NNT for naltrexone is seven, medications for alcohol use disorder are now as effective as antidepressants are for the treatment of depression.

- He also points out the importance of trying more than one: "the treatments act by different mechanisms, and if 1 fails another may work. The key is to keep trying different approaches, or combinations. We are arguably now in a position with respect to alcohol dependence similar to our position for other chronic conditions like depression or hypertension, with a number of different treatment options, both psychosocial and pharmacological."[78]

2014–Vuoristo-Myllys–The American Journal of Drug and Alcohol Abuse
Outcome Predictors for Problem Drinkers Treated with Combined Cognitive Behavioral Therapy and Naltrexone
Applies to: As Needed

- Targeted use (TSM) of naltrexone was tested on patients to test compliance. The study found that patients with more severe alcohol problems had more difficulty in adhering to taking the medication.[281]

2013–Arias–American Journal on Addictions
Pharmacogenetics of Naltrexone and Disulfiram in Alcohol Dependent, Dually Diagnosed Veterans
Applies to: Daily Dose

- This study looked at the genetic variants that influence whether naltrexone and disulfiram are effective.

- Two different variations of a single gene led to very different outcomes from medical treatment. Carriers of the gene with variation 1 ("T") had more abstinence on naltrexone than carriers of the variation 2 ("CC"). Variation 1 ("T") carriers had extremely high rates of abstinence (greater than 90%). Individuals with variation 2 ("CC"), were much more successful with disulfiram–with less drinking on disulfiram for these carriers. This study shows that effectiveness of naltrexone is highly dependent on ones' genetic make-up.[282]

2013–Laaksonen–Journal of Addiction Research and Therapy
Predictors of Self-Reported Adherence to Naltrexone Medication in an Outpatient Treatment for Problem Drinking
Applies to: As Needed

- This study using the TSM method (take one tablet on days when they perceived a risk of drinking) found that patients with very high cravings for alcohol may have more difficulty taking naltrexone 'as needed' than those who do not.

- "In clinical trials the reported medication adherence has often been poor, being one of the key problems associated with naltrexone treatment." Average naltrexone adherence in this study was 78% (high compared to trials requiring daily dosing).

- Poor adherence with naltrexone was associated with unemployment and high craving for alcohol at treatment entry.[283]

2013–Lukas–NeuroImage
Extended-Release Naltrexone (XR-NTX) Attenuates Brain Responses to Alcohol Cues in Alcohol-Dependent Volunteers: A Bold FMRI Study
Applies to: Monthly Injection

- This study looked at brain activation 2 weeks before and 2 weeks after receiving naltrexone injection.

- Brain activation was significantly altered in the patients after receiving naltrexone injection (XR). The affected brain regions are associated with the integration of emotion, cognition, reward, punishment, and learning/memory, suggesting that "XR-NTX helps to modify a patient's response to alcohol-related cues/triggers."

- "Such an effect on brain function may interrupt the processes associated with "slips" and relapse, which may account for XR-NTX's ability to maintain abstinence." The study also stated, "oral naltrexone reduces heavy drinking, but is less consistent as an abstinence promoter, whereas once-monthly extended-release naltrexone (XR-NTX) also maintains abstinence."[145]

2013–Maisel–Addiction
Meta-Analysis of Naltrexone and Acamprosate for Treating Alcohol Use Disorders: When Are These Medications Most Helpful?
Applies to: Non-Specific

- A review of 64 trials from 1970 to 2009 found: "Acamprosate had a significantly larger effect size than naltrexone on the maintenance of abstinence, and naltrexone had a larger effect size than acamprosate on the reduction of heavy drinking and craving.[195]

- For naltrexone, requiring abstinence before the trial was associated with better abstinence maintenance and reduced heavy drinking compared with placebo. For acamprosate, detoxification before medication administration was associated with better abstinence compared with placebo."[195]

2013–Miranda–Addiction Biology
Effects of Naltrexone on Adolescent Alcohol Cue Reactivity and Sensitivity: An Initial Randomized Trial
Applies to: Daily Dose

- "This study provides the first experimentally controlled evidence that naltrexone reduces drinking and craving, and alters subjective responses to alcohol in a sample of adolescent problem drinkers...Naltrexone was generally well tolerated by participants."[284]

2013–Navarrete–Addiction Biology
Effects of Naltrexone plus Topiramate on Ethanol Self-Administration and Tyrosine Hydroxylase Gene Expression Changes
Applies to: Non-Specific

- This study looked at treatment with topiramate and naltrexone individually and together on mice. It measured their effects on alcohol drinking and also looked at gene expression in one part of their brains.

- It found naltrexone significantly reduced alcohol consumption and the motivation to drink. Topiramate had a lower effect. However, both given together had a much more significant effect on reduction in drinking and the expression of the gene than any single drug alone did.[257]

2013–Orrico–Journal of Psychopharmacology
Improved Effect of the Combination Naltrexone/D-Penicillamine in the Prevention of Alcohol Relapse-like Drinking in Rats
Applies to: Monthly Injection

- Alcohol Deprivation Effect (ADE) was found by Sinclair and Senter in 1968.[150] It is an increase in alcohol consumption and preference after a period of forced abstinence.

- This novel 2013 research looked at the effect of naltrexone XR (injection) and D-penicillamine (DP) in delaying alcohol deprivation effect. It found XR-treated "animals displayed a delayed ADE. However, XR+DP treatment prevented this delayed effect. Our present data indicate that this combination therapy shows an adequate anti-relapse preclinical efficacy that overcomes the preclinical limitations of XR alone."[285]

2012–Rubio–Alcohol and Alcoholism
Naltrexone versus Acamprosate: One Year Follow-up of Alcohol Dependence Treatment
Applies to: Daily Dose

- In Rubio's study, "time to first relapse (five or more drinks in a day) was 63 days (naltrexone) versus 42 days (acamprosate). At the end of one year, 41% receiving naltrexone and 17% receiving acamprosate had not relapsed.

- The cumulative number of days of abstinence was significantly greater, and the number of drinks consumed at one time and severity of craving were significantly less, in the naltrexone group compared to the acamprosate group."[286]

2012–Harris–Psychiatric Services
Extended Release Naltrexone for Alcohol Use Disorders: Quasi-Experimental Effects on Mortality and Subsequent Detoxification Episodes
Applies to: Monthly Injection

- "Acamprosate, oral and long-acting injectable naltrexone, and disulfiram are approved for treatment of alcohol dependence. Their availability and consideration of their use in treatment are now standards of high-quality care…."[48]

2011–Anton–The American Journal of Psychiatry
Gabapentin Combined with Naltrexone for the Treatment of Alcohol Dependence
Applies to: Daily Dose

- This clinical trial looked at whether gabapentin, combined with naltrexone, was better than naltrexone alone and/or placebo during the early drinking cessation phase (first six weeks).

- It found that the naltrexone/gabapentin group had 1) a longer delay to heavy drinking than the naltrexone-alone group; 2) less heavy drinking days than the naltrexone-alone group; and 3) less drinks/drinking day than the naltrexone-alone group.

- Poor sleep was associated with more drinking in the naltrexone-alone group, but not in the naltrexone/gabapentin group.

- It concluded "the addition of gabapentin to naltrexone improved drinking outcomes over naltrexone alone during the first six weeks after cessation of drinking."[287]

2011–Bryson–The American Journal of Managed Care
Extended-Release Naltrexone for Alcohol Dependence: Persistence and Healthcare Costs and Utilization
Applies to: Monthly Injection, Daily Dose

- Research looked at patients submitting healthcare cost claims to an insurance company. "Patients taking acamprosate and disulfiram were more likely to discontinue treatment than patients taking naltrexone, and oral naltrexone patients were more likely to discontinue treatment than XR-NTX patients."

- It also found that "Non-pharmacy healthcare costs and utilization of inpatient and emergency services decreased in the XR-NTX group relative to other study groups."[288]

2011–Laaksonen–Alcohol and Alcoholism
Predictors for the Efficacy of Naltrexone Treatment in Alcohol Dependence: Sweet Preference
Applies to: Non-Specific

- High sweet taste preference has a genetic linkage. This study showed that this genetic marker can also correlate to effectiveness of naltrexone.

- It found that higher sweet preference was significantly related to successful treatment outcomes in the naltrexone group.

- It concluded, "sweet preference has a strong correlation to treatment outcomes with naltrexone, and sweet preference might be used as a predictor for better treatment results in alcoholics."

- Our study offers one possible new explanation of the clinical observation that naltrexone is not effective for every patient.[161]

> **2011–Yoon–Human Psychopharmacology**
> **Safety, Tolerability, and Feasibility of High-Dose Naltrexone in Alcohol Dependence: An Open-Label Study**
> **Applies to: Daily Dose**

- This study showed that giving alcoholic patients doses three times higher than the standard dose (150mg/day instead of 50mg/day) and performing liver function testing at weeks 0, 3, 5, 7, 9 resulted in positive outcomes.

- "High-dose naltrexone was safe and well tolerated…no serious adverse effects were reported. Liver markers were stable or showed improvement. High-dose naltrexone significantly reduced alcohol consumption and number of drinks per drinking day."

- It concluded that high-dose naltrexone may be a viable treatment option for alcohol-dependent patients with strong alcohol cravings.[275]

> **2010–Garbutt–Current Pharmaceutical Design**
> **Efficacy and Tolerability of Naltrexone in the Management of Alcohol Dependence**
> **Applies to: Non-Specific; Monthly Injection**

- In a major review of trials, Garbutt stated, "By 2010 about 4,000 individuals had been studied."

- Meta-analyses of these trials revealed that "oral naltrexone is effective in reducing relapse to heavy drinking but less effective in enhancing abstinence."

- Garbutt also stated that naltrexone injection has also shown effectiveness. Regarding safety, "the tolerability of naltrexone is reasonable with the most common side effect being nausea. Hepatotoxicity with naltrexone has not emerged as a clinical problem at the standard 50 mg dose though at higher doses hepatoxicity is of concern."

- It was also pointed out that optimum length of treatment is not well studied, though many doctors recommend one year of treatment."[273]

2010–Pettinati–American Journal of Psychiatry
A Double-Blind, Placebo-Controlled Trial Combining Sertraline and Naltrexone
for Treating Co-Occurring Depression and Alcohol Dependence
Applies to: Daily dose

- Most studies have not found that antidepressants are helpful in reducing excessive drinking in alcoholics with depression. However, in a study looking at sertraline and naltrexone, it found that in patients combining both medications there was a complimentary effect.

- It found, "the sertraline plus naltrexone combination produced a higher alcohol abstinence rate (53.7%) and demonstrated a longer delay before relapse to heavy drinking (median delay=98 days) than the naltrexone (abstinence rate: 21.3%; delay= 29 days), sertraline (abstinence rate: 27.5%; delay=23 days), and placebo (abstinence rate: 23.1%; delay=26 days) groups".

- It concluded that more patients with depression and alcoholism receiving the sertraline plus naltrexone combination improved abstinence rates, delayed relapse to heavy drinking, had serious adverse events, and tended to not be depressed by the end of treatment.[289]

2010–Rosner–Cochrane Review
Opioid Antagonists for Alcohol Dependence
Applies to: Non-Specific

- In a large Cochrane Review of 50 previous trials with 7793 patients, naltrexone reduced the risk of heavy drinking and decreased drinking days.

- It found that the main side effects were mainly gastrointestinal problems (e.g. nausea) and daytime sleepiness.

- The review found naltrexone to be "an effective and safe strategy in alcoholism treatment," and stated, "Naltrexone does not have serious side effects."[290]

> **2009–Kranzler–Journal of Clinical Psychology**
> **Targeted Naltrexone for Problem Drinkers**
> **Applies to: Daily Dose, As Needed**

- In a study comparing 'Daily Dose' to 'TSM' it was found that "at week 12, men in the targeted naltrexone group drank significantly less than patients in the other groups did.

- On a secondary outcome measure, drinks per drinking day, during week 12, the targeted naltrexone group drank significantly less than the other groups did."[291]

> **2008–Baltieri–Addiction**
> **Comparing Topiramate with Naltrexone in the Treatment of Alcohol Dependence**
> **Applies to: Daily Dose**

- In a 2008 comparison, "Naltrexone showed trends toward inferior outcomes when compared to topiramate."[266]

> **2008–Florez–Alcoholism: Clinical and Experimental Research**
> **Using Topiramate or Naltrexone for the Treatment of Alcohol-Dependent Patients**
> **Applies to: Daily Dose**

- "Naltrexone patients had higher nicotine consumption throughout the study. Topiramate was better at reducing alcohol-related cravings throughout the study."[267]

> **2008–Kuzmin–European Journal of Pharmacology**
> **Memantine Enhances the Inhibitory Effects of Naltrexone on Ethanol Consumption**
> **Applies to: Daily Dose**

- A rat study showed that the combination of low doses of memantine and naltrexone may have therapeutic value in the treatment of alcoholism "particularly in a subgroup of alcoholic patients who have high sensitivity to the adverse side effects of naltrexone [at standard doses.]"[292]

2008–Myrick–Archives of General Psychiatry
Effect of Naltrexone and Ondansetron on Alcohol Cue-Induced Activation of the Ventral Striatum in Alcohol-Dependent People
Applies to: Daily Dose

- Study compared naltrexone and ondansetron on alcohol cue-activated activation of the ventral striatum part of the brain.

- "The study found evidence that these medications, alone or in combination, could decrease alcohol cue–induced activation of the ventral striatum."[293]

2008–Rosner–Journal of Psychopharmacology
Acamprosate for Alcohol Dependence
Applies to: Non-Specific

- "Naltrexone was found to have a significant effect on the maintenance of abstinence as well as the prevention of heavy drinking. Acamprosate was shown only to support abstinence; it did not influence alcohol consumption after the first drink... acamprosate was found to be more effective in preventing a lapse, whereas naltrexone was better in preventing a lapse from becoming a relapse. The superiority of either one drug or over the other one cannot be determined as a general rule, it rather depends on the therapeutic target."[201]

2008–Soyka–World Journal of Biological Psychiatry
World Federation of Societies of Biological Psychiatry (WFSBP) Guidelines for Biological Treatment of Substance Use and Related Disorders, Part I: Alcoholism
Applies to: Non-Specific

- "There is abundant evidence supporting the use of naltrexone for treatment of alcohol dependence (Level A)."[41]

2007–Krishnan–Biological Psychiatry
Family History of Alcoholism Influences Naltrexone-Induced Reduction in Alcohol Drinking
Applies to: Daily Dose; As Needed

- Men with a family history of alcoholism receiving a 100mg/day of naltrexone significantly decreased drinking compared with variations of: family history at lower dose, and no family history at high and lower doses.

- Conclusion: Family history of alcoholism might be a significant predictor of response to naltrexone and that men with this family history "are more likely to benefit from naltrexone therapy for alcohol drinking."[294]

2007–O'Malley–Journal of Clinical Psychopharmacology
Efficacy of Extended-Release Naltrexone in Alcohol-Dependent Patients Who Are Abstinent before Treatment
Applies to: Monthly Injection

- O'Malley's study stated that Extended-release naltrexone (once-a-month injection also known as XR-NTX) is a Food and Drug Administration-approved treatment for alcohol dependence.

- It found the rate of abstinence was several times higher for XR-NTX 380 mg compared with placebo: median time to first drink was 41 days versus 12 days; rate of continuous abstinence at end of the study was 32% versus 11%. XR-NTX at a 380 mg dose substantially increased time to first heavy drinking event (>180 days vs 20 days), decreased the median number of any drinking days per month by 90% (0.7 vs 7.2) and decreased heavy drinking days per month by 93% (0.2 days vs 2.9 days).

- The XR-NTX 380 mg group also had more than twice as many responders compared with placebo (70% vs 30% where 'responder' is defined as having no more than 2 heavy drinking days in any consecutive 28-day period.)

- Outcomes for those at a lower dose (190 mg) were not as good, demonstrating the importance of dose size.

- The study stated, "In conclusion, XR-NTX 380 mg prolonged abstinence and reduced the number of heavy drinking days and drinking days in patients who were abstinent for as few as 4 days before treatment initiation."[295]

2007–Ooteman–European Neuropsychopharmacology
The Effect of Naltrexone and Acamprosate on Cue-Induced Craving, Autonomic Nervous System and Neuroendocrine Reactions to Alcohol-Related Cues in Alcoholics
Applies to: Daily Dose

- Ooteman hypothesized that "naltrexone exerts its effects primarily on cue-induced craving and neuroendocrine cue reactivity, whereas acamprosate exerts its effect primarily on autonomic nervous system reactions to alcohol-related cues."

- The study showed that consistent with the hypotheses, naltrexone reduced craving more than acamprosate, and acamprosate reduced heart rate more than naltrexone."[204]

2006–Anton–JAMA
Combined Pharmacotherapies and Behavioral Interventions for Alcohol Dependence: The COMBINE Study: A Randomized Controlled Trial
Applies to: Daily Dose

- A large 1-year trial with 1383 recently alcohol-abstinent volunteers with AUD [Alcohol Use Disorder or Alcoholism] found that patients receiving medical management with naltrexone, CBI, or both fared better on drinking outcomes, whereas acamprosate showed no evidence of efficacy, with or without CBI.

- No combination produced better efficacy than naltrexone or CBI alone in the presence of medical management...naltrexone with medical management could be delivered in health care settings, thus serving alcohol-dependent patients who might otherwise not receive treatment."[296]

2006–Morley–Addiction
Naltrexone versus Acamprosate in the Treatment of Alcohol Dependence: A Multi-Centre, Randomized, Double-Blind, Placebo-Controlled Trial
Applies to: Daily Dose

- "The results of this study support the efficacy of naltrexone in the relapse prevention of alcoholism amongst those with low levels of clinical depression and alcohol dependence severity. No effect of acamprosate was found in our sample."[297]

2005–Anton–Journal of Clinical Psychology
Naltrexone Combined with Either Cognitive Behavioral or Motivational Enhancement Therapy for Alcohol Dependence
Applies to: Daily Dose

- Anton found that because cognitive behavioral therapy (CBT) and naltrexone share common mechanisms of action, such as craving reduction and relapse prevention, these therapies are likely to be well suited to use in combination."[298]

2005–Colombo–Drug and Alcohol Dependence
Effect of the Combination of Naltrexone and Baclofen, on Acquisition of Alcohol Drinking Behavior in Alcohol-Preferring Rats
Applies to: Daily Dose; As Needed

- Rat testing compared naltrexone in combination with baclofen. "The drug combination resulted in a significant reduction in daily alcohol intake... These results suggest that combination of naltrexone plus baclofen may result in a synergistic reduction in alcohol intake in rats. The researcher hypothesized that the two drugs work in a complimentary way."[242]

2005–Garbutt–JAMA: the journal of the American Medical Association
Efficacy and Tolerability of Long-Acting Injectable Naltrexone for Alcohol Dependence: A Randomized Controlled Trial
Applies to: Monthly Injection

- An extensive trial was run with 624 individuals across 24 hospitals and clinics focusing on the extended release (injected) form of naltrexone.

- It found that compared with placebo, 380 mg of long-acting naltrexone resulted in a 25% decrease in the event rate of heavy drinking days; 190 mg of naltrexone resulted in a 17% decrease.

- Gender and pre-treatment abstinence each showed significant impact on the treatment outcome, with men and those with abstinence before the trial both showing better results of treatment.

- Discontinuation due to adverse events occurred in 14.1% in the 380-mg and 6.7% in the 190-mg group and 6.7% in the placebo group.

- Conclusion: "Long-acting naltrexone was well tolerated and resulted in reductions in heavy drinking among treatment-seeking alcohol-dependent patients during 6 months of therapy. These data indicate that long-acting naltrexone can be of benefit in the treatment of alcohol dependence.[299]

> **2004–Kim–Psychiatry and Clinical Neurosciences**
> **Effect of the Combination of Naltrexone and Acamprosate on Alcohol Intake in Mice**
> **Applies to: Daily Dose; As Needed**

- Mice tests found that naltrexone, at the higher dose, but not the lower dose, significantly reduced alcohol consumption, but a high dose of naltrexone combined with the high dose of acamprosate achieved the greatest reduction.[207]

> **2004–Stromberg–Pharmacology Biochemistry and Behavior**
> **The Effect of Baclofen Alone and in Combination with Naltrexone on Ethanol Consumption in the Rat**
> **Applies to: Daily Dose; As Needed**

- This research was an experiment combining baclofen and naltrexone on rats. It evaluated "the effect of three doses of baclofen (2.5, 5.0, or 7.5 mg/kg)... administered alone or in combination with a single dose of naltrexone (1.0 mg/kg)."

- Individually both naltrexone and baclofen, at the two higher doses significantly reduced ethanol consumption. Even greater decrease in ethanol consumption was found when both were combined.[244]

> **2002–Leavitt–Addiction Treatment Forum**
> **Evidence for the Efficacy of Naltrexone in the Treatment of Alcohol Dependence (Alcoholism)**
> **Applies to: Daily Dose; As Needed**

- Leavitt's easy to read report concludes that up to 2001 fourteen trials assessed the effectiveness of naltrexone compared with placebo for treating alcoholism, enrolling 2127 subjects, in five countries.

- It stated, "There is strong evidence that naltrexone significantly reduces alcohol relapses to heavy drinking, the frequency and quantity of alcohol consumption in those who do drink, and alcohol craving."

- "Naltrexone is significantly beneficial in helping those patients who cannot remain abstinent to reduce their drinking behaviors, breaking the vicious, self-destructive cycle in alcoholics whereby one drink leads to another...Longer-term naltrexone therapy extending beyond three months may be most effective, and naltrexone might be used on an as needed, "targeted," basis indefinitely".[46]

2001–Sinclair–Alcohol and Alcoholism
Evidence about the Use of Naltrexone and for Different Ways of Using It in the Treatment of Alcoholism
Applies to: As Needed

- Sinclair found that naltrexone, naloxone, and nalmefene were "effective when paired with drinking but ineffective when given during abstinence."

- He recommended that: (1) naltrexone should be administered to patients who were still currently drinking; (2) the instructions should be to take naltrexone only when drinking was anticipated; (3) this treatment should continue indefinitely.[300]

1999–Anton–American Journal of Psychiatry
Naltrexone and Cognitive Behavioral Therapy for the Treatment of Outpatient Alcoholics: Results of a Placebo-Controlled Trial
Applies to: Non-Specific

- Early research found: "Naltrexone-treated subjects drank less, took longer to relapse, and had more time between relapses...over the study period, 62% of the naltrexone group did not relapse into heavy drinking, in comparison with 40% of the placebo group."[301]

1999–Garbutt–JAMA
Pharmacological Treatment of Alcohol Dependence
Applies to: Non-Specific

- An early but very extensive review of previous trials looked at 41 studies and 11 follow-up or subgroup studies. The quality of research findings was rated 'grade A, B, C'.

- The review found, "Naltrexone (grade A) reduces the risk of relapse to heavy drinking and the frequency of drinking compared with placebo but does not substantially enhance abstinence, i.e., avoidance of any alcohol consumption."[210]

1997–Oslin–American Journal on Addictions
Tolerability of Naltrexone in Treating Older, Alcohol-Dependent Patients
Applies to: Non-Specific

- Naltrexone found to be well tolerated by alcohol addicted older adults.[302]

1990–Sinclair–Annals of Medicine
Drugs to Decrease Alcohol Drinking
Applies to: As Needed

- Sinclair publishes his hypothesis that naltrexone is only effective if used while the patient is drinking. (Later known as TSM–The Sinclair Method).

- He stated, "learned responses are extinguished if they are made repeatedly while the reinforcement is blocked, and opiate antagonists appear to block the reinforcement from alcohol. A series of experiments support the hypothesis that drinking alcohol while an antagonist is present extinguishes the alcohol-drinking response in rats."[303]

1986–Volpicelli–Life Sciences
Naltrexone Blocks the Post-Shock Increase of Ethanol Consumption
Applies to: Daily Dose; As Needed

- Research shows that naltrexone blocks ethanol consumption in rats.[304]

1976–Ross–Proceedings of the Western Pharmacology Society
Ethanol Preference in the Hamster: Effects of Morphine Sulfate and Naltrexone, a
Long-Acting Morphine Antagonist
Applies to: Daily Dose; As Needed

- First known research on alcohol, naltrexone and rodents.[305]

PERSONAL EXPERIENCES WITH NALTREXONE

Short Forms Used Below:

- AF–Alcohol-Free (A day when no alcohol is consumed)
- TSM–The Sinclair Method ('As Needed' Method)
- Targetted Method–('As Needed' Method)
- Nal–Naltrexone
- Pre-nal–Before starting naltrexone medication
- The Book–Dr. Roy Escapa's The Cure For Addiction: The Medically Proven Way...' (considered to be the 'how to' guide for the 'as needed' method).

•••

Here is a run-down of my first day of taking Nal using 'as needed' (targeted) method.

Took my first drink—a shot of citrus vodka about an hour after taking the Nal (1/4 dose—intend to quickly titrate up to 50mg). Typically, when I take the shot, it gives me this burn that starts in my mouth and follows down my throat and I get a tingle. I took the shot and—nothing—I felt—nothing—it was just like drinking a glass of water. Wow! It was really a weird sensation. And soon after I would expect to be preparing for my next one. I walked into the pantry (out of habit to get a shot or a maybe glass of wine instead) and walked out twice without anything. My habit was saying "what the heck" but my mind felt somewhat comfortable without it. I have had no side effects.

A bit later, I still did not have a craving to drink, but I did anyway...having two more drinks before dinner for a total of three. After I ate dinner, I felt very satisfied and decided not to drink any further. You gotta know....THIS NEVER HAPPENS! WHEN I START DRINKING IT IS ON!

Interesting Observations:

* Until I took the Nal, I could intellectually understand what a craving was, but the Nal showed me PHYSICALLY what the relief of the craving FELT like through the absence of it. That was very interesting to not feel that usual sensation that almost immediately makes me start thinking of the next one.

* With the craving factor removed, I realized how much of this is equally habitual and I need to work on that. From a physical standpoint, it would have been fairly easy not had the other two drinks, but I chose to do so, just like I chose to do so by not continuing after three drinks.

* After two drinks, I had to walk downstairs to get the dog. I felt a little off balance and light headed and my mind said "Whoa, you are a bit tipsy, maybe you need to slow down" I had to laugh out loud at this voice in my head because I have no

recollection of EVER feeling tipsy. I am sober to drunk at Mach 5 and I always feel "in control" (not) until I black out. Just keeping it real!

* I was very, very tired early in the evening, but when I went to bed I could not make myself fall asleep. I honestly laid there with my eyes closed feeling tired and unable to sleep and it was weird, because I felt so relaxed overall. I did not take any sleep aid and by the time I figured I needed one, it was too late. I had to get up at 6 am to get the kids off to school. I tossed and turned, sleeping only very briefly, and had terrible battles with hot flashes and night sweats (to me, it is hard to tell what is due to drinking and what is due to menopause because some of the symptoms are the same).

* I woke up without a hangover (yeah buddy!) but I was understandably very tired.

Tonight I have back-to-back meetings from 4:30 pm to 10:00 pm, so it is going to be a necessary, but grateful AF evening (hopefully).

I am going to enjoy the honeymoon phase for sure and will hope for success as the longer journey continues!

•••

I have only had one thought of not taking nal. I just wanted to finish one beer in my fridge last night and I thought "Well, crap. I have to take Naltrexone and wait an hour before having one beer??" I had a thought of just not taking it for just the one beer. But my better thinking won and I didn't have that beer without naltrexone. The thought of intermittent reinforcement and ruining the good thing I got going on here really stopped me from breaking that golden rule.

People say "alcoholics will just skip the pill, it's so easy." No, many of us won't. Because we don't want to go back and start over again. We are proud of ourselves for drinking less than we used to. We are happy that we can finally feel 'normal'! People may slip up and not take the pill, but they usually regret it. And how is that any different than those trying to abstain who fall off the wagon over and over?

•••

I leveled out at a certain level and drank every day like that for a long time. I am at about 1 year exactly and tonight is my second AF Monday in a row, and things are getting a tiny bit better every day, with setbacks that I decided to just roll with.

I know it is tough on the family and there is lots of self-doubt, but I would say my life is 80-85% better than the pre-nal. It has taken me a long time and I am still drinking way too much, but my progress continues and everyone in my family has stopped worrying about me. I can actually choose not to drink on a night like tonight. That is a miracle from where I was at. As well, I can safely attend a function where booze is served and have 2 or 3 in 2 or 3 hours and stop. Never before.

When I checked into rehab 2 years ago, I was falling apart. Now, my biggest problem is that I want to lose some weight. That is the only thing bothering me right now.

•••

Yesterday I got my 4th naltrexone injection. I have had no adverse side effects, and I love that I don't have to remember to take the pill and wait an hour. I am drinking every day, but at a much lower level. I don't drink until I have to stumble to bed and pass out for the night. I drink 3-4 drinks and stop drinking after dinner. This fall, I have a couple of meetings/conventions to attend which involve a lot of cocktail parties and dinners. I know that I can handle it. I am going to try to push an alcohol free day and see how it feels.

•••

"I was a DAILY BINGE drinker, that's daily blackouts, who was physically addicted. ...Anyway, I still have not been back to any meetings and am back to getting joy out of life doing the things I love. No offense to meetings and if they work then do them please, but I have over 10 years of going in and out of the rooms and for me I could not do a single thing in life other than focus on things related to 12 steps 24/7... and now I feel free where I can do what I want and do things I enjoy but still not drink ... this is the first time in close to 20 years that I felt free and in control! And guess what? Even though I drank once while on Naltrexone injection and things could have gotten ugly, even when I have given 150% in a 12 step program only one time have I done better than only drinking 1 time in 100 days like I am now! So I am doing as good or better than my best effort at a 12 step program, BUT I'M NOT A ZOMBIE and reporting my life to others constantly and am able to do what I want to do! I love it!"

•••

So long as I follow the Golden Rule for the rest of my life and always take NAL before consuming any alcohol, I will remain cured...Should I disregard the Golden Rule, I will return in a matter of days (and certainly not more than a few weeks) to my previous wretched, alcoholic, self. A small price to pay, that little pill, for all the pain, suffering, and horror it has rid from my life. I am grateful, not burdened, by my knowledge of my dependence on that pill.

My cure happened rather quickly. In my first month...I observed encouraging signs, and around the 3-month mark I began believing that it was going to work and I was gaining good (and unheard of) control. Around month 4 or 5 I was free. For me, it was effortless. Or it least, so it seems in retrospect. Take the pill, drink as you normally would. That was all. At 6 months max, I lost all interest in alcohol. I read the book in its entirety, and I was a textbook example of how TSM works.

•••

I bought and read the book [Dr. Roy Escapa's The Cure For Addiction: The Medically Proven Way...']. Then I brought the book into my regular Doctor, confessed to my addiction, and produced a copy of the letter for one's Physician from the book. My Doc seemed a bit skeptical and left the office to do a few minutes research. He then returned with a prescription for Naltrexone. Of course, he told me not to drink while taking it, but we both understood that I would. A month's supply cost me $36 at Walmart. My journey had begun.

I didn't start out to be abstaining of course. But by the end of June I became curious to experience life without my endorphins being blocked, so I quit both NAL and drinking for the next 7 months...

The good news, in a way, is TSM takes 4 to 12 months to work, which gives us the time we need to slowly adjust and say our good-byes. Don't worry if at first you cannot picture a life without alcohol, or all of your alcohol-related activities. I couldn't either. Just take your pill and drink as you normally would for 3 or 4 months and don't worry about anything else. After a couple of months, it will be time to start peering into the future and figuring out how you intend to fill the vacuum.

Nalmefene

Introduction to Nalmefene

Nalmefene is an opioid antagonist that is structurally similar to naltrexone but thought to have some advantages over naltrexone.

The list of suggested benefits of nalmefene over naltrexone are usually stated as: "no dose-dependent association with toxic effects to the liver, greater oral bioavailability, longer duration of antagonist action, and more competitive binding with opioid receptor subtypes that are thought to reinforce drinking."[112]

It is thought that these advantages may help to improve the tolerability of nalmefene over naltrexone for some patients.

It may be important to remember that because naltrexone has lost any patent protection and nalmefene (Selincro) is still protected in Europe, the actual distinctions between the two drugs may be less significant than the importance of the *perception of a distinction.*

This is because pharmaceutical company Lundbeck is now heavily marketing Selincro as a new medication to treat aspects of alcohol use disorder in Europe and elsewhere (and now-generic naltrexone, in its pill form anyways, is not profitable for any company to invest marketing dollars in).

While there is a great deal of data on nalmefene's sister naltrexone, to date nalmefene itself has not been widely studied. More studies have been initiated in Japan and will be run by Lundbeck's partner Otsuka Pharmaceuticals.

THE BACK-STORY

The launch of Selincro is much more important than simply the fact that a new drug is available for the treatment of addiction for the first time in more than a decade.

Its launch will set the tone for the next ten years of advancement (or stagnation) in drug development and marketing for medications for alcohol addiction.

Every pharmaceutical company, addiction drug research funding source and addiction researcher is watching carefully.

While Selincro is being marketed as new, it is not new at all, and actually has a very long history compared to many of the medications discussed in this book.

NALMEFENE HISTORY

In 1988, Dr. John Sinclair filed a patent in the US Patent Office for a "Method for treating alcohol-drinking response."

In the patent, Sinclair identifies what will later be called "The Sinclair Method," a method of taking medication for alcoholism "as needed" with opiate antagonists including naltrexone.

The patent was assigned to Alko Limited of Helsinki Finland, the country's national alcoholic beverage retailing monopoly which reports into the Finnish Ministry of Health and Social Affairs.

Later in 1990, Sinclair filed a second US patent application for the same method, but this time "with nalmefene."

Thus began a grinding, 25-year process that nalmefene took on the road from drug discovery to launch.

Sinclair's patent was finalized in 1992. Between 1992 and 2001 Contral Pharma began development of the drug and planned to complete phase III trials quickly in 2003 or 2004.

But before they could complete this expensive process they needed risk capital. So in 2002 Contral, and another firm, Finland's BioTie (which had gone public in 2000), merged, becoming BioTie Therapies and combining operations to save costs and receive new capital. 2002 financial filings show both Sinclair and the Finnish Ministry held shares in the new BioTie, though it is not clear if they still own shares today.

Management seemed to lose focus on nalmefene's clear benefits at this point and phase III clinical trials were conducted and assessed poorly—so that nalmefene's phase III results were not statistically significant enough to receive marketing approval.

BioTie revisited the strategy and initiated marketing authorization for nalmefene in 2006, but in 2008 Lundbeck began to slowly buy up global marketing rights to Selincro, region by region, starting by buying UK and Ireland rights that it is presumed BioTie had sold to Britannia Pharmaceuticals (Subsidiary of Stada).

BioTie's phase 3 setback cost them dearly because instead of launching in the mid-2000s and potentially capitalizing in the US, they lost IPR protection in the US market (which expired in 2011).

Lundbeck probably would have passed on the nalmefene opportunity completely except that nalmefene was considered a 'new chemical entity' (NCE) in Europe and thus, while its patent in Europe expired in 2012, it gained another 10 years of marketing exclusivity.[306]

Biotie's initial marketing application was put on ice while a new global launch strategy was developed and Lundbeck initiated new Phase 3 studies.

This time, with a new study design, the results looked promising.

Lundbeck acquired an equity stake in Biotie and then acquired the North-American and Mexican rights for nalmefene from Somaxon Pharmaceuticals. This series of masterful acquisitions and investment moves gave Lundbeck near-worldwide rights to nalmefene, excluding only Turkey and South-Korea.

In 2013, nalmefene (under the brand name Selincro) was finally launched in Europe by Cipralex-rights owner Lundbeck.

It was the first pharmaceutical approved for the treatment of alcohol dependence launched in Europe for at least 13 years.

While nalmefene and the 'as needed' approach that Lundbeck is marketing was the same approach that Sinclair had first patented in 1988, at some point Lundbeck made the strategic marketing decision to distance itself from using the phrase, 'The Sinclair Method'.

Neither TSM nor Dr. David Sinclair is mentioned in carefully crafted research, write-ups, press releases and presentations surrounding Selincro.

While unfortunate given Sinclair's major contributions, this is a wise move for Lundbeck as it allows the company to present nalmefene in a fresh new way.

Sometimes inventors and innovators are so ahead of their time that they are considered to be eccentric and misguided until eventually (often, unfortunately, many generations later), their discoveries gain the credibility and respect they deserve.

Sinclair's research was disruptive (in the way that disruptive technology is often, ultimately, the catalyst for major change).

By distancing themselves from TSM, Lundbeck has been able to paint the picture of 'Selincro–as needed' as both novel and new, as well as spinning a shiny, professional scientific and pharmaceutical aura around its launch and marketing. (An aura that the kind but quirky Dr. Sinclair could never really pull off).

Instead of the late Dr. Sinclair, the figurehead and lead researcher on much of the Lundbeck-sponsored studies is the influential and well-connected Dr. Wim Van Den Brink.

In Lundbeck's move to create in Selincro a treatment for alcoholism equivalent to what Lundbeck's Cipralex has been to the treatment of mental illness, Lundbeck is taking huge calculated risks.

Lundbeck's launch of Selincro is a signal that they are willing to bet millions that public and medical opinion on alcoholism treatment is prime for change.

Regardless of whether or not the drug is effective or the launch is successful, Lundbeck is a powerhouse—a company both wealthy and credible enough to educate and change attitudes–something that has been sorely needed in the world of addiction treatment.

The Selincro launch is not just about launching a drug, but about changing a paradigm.

In launching Selincro, they have needed to address and replace the idea that 'AA is the gold standard of treatment for alcoholism', and that reducing drinking levels (not just ultimate abstinence) is a worthwhile goal for alcoholics. They will need to help the medical community put aside its stigma to see that alcoholism is not only a brain disease, but one treatable with medication.

This paradigm change is truly the biggest challenge Lundbeck will face in marketing the drug.

One clinician, embodying the type of old guard that needs to change, published an editorial in The BMJ (formerly the British Medical Journal), calling nalmefene 'Bad Medicine', and protesting, "we now have a sponsored educational bandwagon promoting nalmefene in Scotland and a gathering army of salespeople."

Spence argued that Lundbeck had used "the dark art of subgroup analysis" to try to improve their study results and stated, "surely these resources would be better spent improving alcohol counseling services?"[307]

Despite the inevitable backlash that Lundbeck will continue to see, it seems to be making headway.

Lundbeck ran awareness and lobbying campaigns in countries including Belgium, France, Germany and the UK which subsequently decided to fund Selincro with their public health budgets.

Is nalmefene a great medication for the treatment of alcoholism? I can't say for sure, because it doesn't have the rich history of research that naltrexone and other drugs have. I suspect it will have both similar efficacy and challenges as naltrexone (the substances are similar in many regards).

Will it be a profitable and successful drug for Lundbeck? I certainly hope so.

Both BioTie and Lundbeck deserve both respect and any profit that they can earn from their venture.

There is no doubt that other drug companies are watching very closely. If Selincro is financially successful, Lundbeck will have paved the way for a new era of alcoholism treatment medications.

If they fail, then drug companies interested in drug development for alcoholism may close the door on alcoholism treatment advancements for another 10 years.

NALMEFENE MEDICATION FAQ

MEDICATION OVERVIEW

What is the medication called?

Nalmefene

What are common brand names and generic names for this medication?

Selincro, Nalmetrene, Nalmefene Hydrochloride, revex, nalmetrene. (Do not confuse with Nalmefene Injection)

What 'type' of medication is this?

Opioid Receptor Antagonist

What is it usually prescribed for?

Alcohol Use Disorder

How is it described?

- Nalmefene is an opiate receptor antagonist which is used to treat acute opioid overdose and in the management of alcohol dependence and addictive behaviors.

- Nalmefene is semi synthetic opiate receptor antagonist which is similar structurally to naltrexone and oxymorphone. It is for the reduction of alcohol consumption in adult patients with alcohol dependence who have a high drinking risk level, without physical withdrawal symptoms and who do not require immediate detoxification. Nalmefene attaches to certain opioid receptors in the brain. Opioid receptors play a role in addiction and, by attaching to them and modifying their activity, nalmefene helps reduce the urge to drink in people accustomed to large amounts of alcohol.

AVAILABILITY & FDA APPROVAL STATUS

A prescription for alcoholism is usually:

On-Label (where approved)

Is it FDA approved in the USA? When?

Not yet approved in pill form

Is it HC approved in Canada? When?

Not yet approved

Is it EMA approved in Europe? When?

Approved by the EMA in 2013

How is it available?

By prescription in parts of Europe

STRENGTH AND CREDIBILITY OF RESEARCH FOR ITS USE IN ALCOHOLISM

How many years has this medication been researched specifically for the treatment of alcoholism?

29+ years (1986)

What is the strength of the supporting research?

- Nalmefene has been less extensively researched than the structurally similar opioid antagonist naltrexone (which has been extensively researched.)

- Recently three large phase III trials were completed (two of 6-months duration and one of 12-month duration). It was on the basis of findings in these three studies that the drug received marketing authorization for the reduction of alcohol consumption in adults with alcohol dependence who have a high drinking risk level in Europe. The researcher heading all three trials was Dr. Wim van den Brink.

What credentials does above researcher hold?

- Wim van den Brink Ph.D.: Professor of Psychiatry and Addiction at the Academic Medical Center of the University of Amsterdam, co-author of 300+ peer-reviewed scientific publications, editor of European Addiction Research, Chair of the Scientific Program Committee of the European College of Neuropsychopharmacology.

RESEARCH FINDINGS ABOUT EFFECTIVENESS IN TREATMENT FOR ALCOHOLISM

How many patients need to be treated to see one true medication responder? (Known as the 'Number Needed to Treat–NNT)

- The NNT is seven for a 2-category downward shift in WHO Drinking risk level from 'Very High Risk' to 'Medium Risk'; NNT is nine for a 2-category shift from or 'High Risk' to 'Low Risk'. (Consistent with the NNT's found for Naltrexone, which is 10 for abstinence and 7 for Return to Heavy Drinking).

- This means that one in seven individuals who drink at a 'very high risk' level (based on alcohol quantity consumed), will be successful in lowering their consumption to place them in a 'medium risk' category. One in nine individuals who are in a 'high risk' category will be able to lower their consumption enough to place them in the 'low risk' category.

How effective is this medication for the treatment of alcoholism?

For individuals whose goal is 'reduced drinking' (not abstinence) and/or reduction in total alcohol consumption, some recent studies show a "significantly superior effect" in the number of heavy drinking days and total alcohol consumed, particularly among very heavy drinkers.[308]

In research, how did this medication compare to other medications for the treatment of alcoholism?

There is little research comparing nalmefene to other medications.

TREATMENT CANDIDATES FOR THIS MEDICATION

Note: this section highlights study findings that have identified some characteristics that may increase odds of effectiveness. This does not mean it won't help individuals without these characteristics.

What treatment goals might this medication help achieve?

Nalmefene may help patients reduce their total alcohol intake and number of heavy drinking days.

What are some typical feelings and motivators of people this medication tends to help?

Research has not yet provided insight on this answer.

Has this medication been shown to be more successful in early-onset or late-onset alcoholics?

No research available on this though there is some indication that heavy drinkers may benefit more significantly. Heavy drinkers may also be early-onset drinkers.

Is this medication typically more effective in people with a strong family history of alcoholism?

Research has not yet provided insight on this answer.

Are there specific genetic markers that have been found to be relevant in treatment with this medication?

The presence of the genetic marker rs2832407 (C-allele homozygote) may indicate a strong possibility the medication will be effective.

Do Alcoholics Have Difficulty Taking this Medication as Prescribed? (i.e. Are there "Compliance" Issues?)

As with naltrexone's 'Daily Dose' or 'As Needed' dosing (i.e. One hour before drinking), some individuals may have trouble taking nalmefene as prescribed.

Are there other characteristics (gender, taste sensitivity, alcoholism type, co-morbid disorders, smoker status) that may be related to success with this medication?

Research has not yet provided insight on this answer.

DIRECTIONS FOR USE & HOW IT WORKS

At what dose and for how long does research suggest the medication should be taken?

- The patient should take one Selincro 18mg tablet by mouth 'as needed', which means it should be taken when there is a chance that they will start drinking.

- Only one tablet can be taken on any given day and it should preferably be taken one to two hours before they are likely to start drinking. If the patient has started drinking without nalmefene, a tablet should be taken as soon as possible.

Has this medication been tested with other medications for the treatment of alcoholism and found to be complimentary?

Research has not yet provided insight on this answer.

What is known about how this medication actually works in alcoholics? What is the 'Mechanism of Action'?

Researchers indicate: "Nalmefene is an opioid receptor modulator ... It works in a similar fashion to naltrexone, as an opioid antagonist on the mu and delta receptors, and as an agonist at kappa receptors. It is hypothesized that the blockade of opioid receptors interferes with the reinforcing effects of alcohol, in turn reducing alcohol cravings."[192]

SAFETY CONCERNS

Is this medication addictive? Does it have abuse potential?

Nalmefene is non-addictive.

How safe is this medication?

Research "provides evidence for the long-term safety and efficacy of nalmefene as-needed in alcohol-dependent patients who continue to drink heavily, following a brief intervention."[308]

Can this medication be taken while drinking?

Can be initiated while the alcohol-dependent individual is still drinking without causing harm. Nalmefene is to be taken 'as needed' by the patient (1-2 hours before drinking).

What are the expected side effects of this medication?

Side effects are "mild or moderate, and transient."[309]

What are other fairly common side effects?

Common side effects include nausea, vomiting, tachycardia, hypertension.

430 · MEDICATIONS FOR ALCOHOLISM

Where can I find a complete list of all side effects, precautions, and instructions in case of emergency or overdose?
Visit:

http://en.wikipedia.org/wiki/Nalmefene#Side_effects

What does the National Institute of Health (NIH) say about liver impact and where can I find further information on liver impact of this medication?

- Therapy with nalmefene has not been linked to serum enzyme elevations or to idiosyncratic acute, clinically apparent liver injury.

- Nalmefene is extensively metabolized in the liver, but largely by glucuronidation rather than transformation to a different metabolite. Patients with opioid overdose often have underlying chronic liver diseases such as alcoholic liver disease, hepatitis B or C, but treatment with nalmefene does not appear to exacerbate those conditions.

- Read more at the livertox.nlm.nih.gov site link:

http://bit.ly/livertoxnalmef

What known drug interactions should I watch for and where can I find more information on drug interactions?

- Not known to interact with other drugs in the alcohol treatment medications database. Known to interact with at least eight drugs.

- Also see the drugs.com drug interaction tool:

http://bit.ly/nalfinteraction

Where can I find alerts and Black Box Warnings? (Black Box Warnings are cautions affixed to medications by the government)
Visit:

http://bit.ly/nalmefeneblack

Were there any known black box warnings at the time this book was written?

- Yes, this medication must not be used by patients taking opioids, or who have severe liver or kidney impairment or history of acute alcohol withdrawal syndrome. The drug carries a black-box warning tied to spikes in blood pressure.

- See also:

http://bit.ly/nalmefmore

OTHER USEFUL INFORMATION

Note: Links to all recommended information sources can be found on the book's website at APrescriptionForAlcoholics.com

Recent Research:

- 2015: Van den Brink, Expert Opinion on Drug Safety[310]

- 2010: Medication Treatment of Different Types of Alcoholism[178]

- 2014: Long-term efficacy, tolerability and safety of nalmefene as-needed in patients with alcohol dependence: A 1-year, randomised controlled study[308]

- 2013: A randomised, double-blind, placebo-controlled, efficacy study of nalmefene, as-needed use, in patients with alcohol dependence[311]

CONNECTING WITH OTHERS

Online Forum(s):

- The 'MyWayOut' community started out focused on topiramate but is now a good place to read about and connect with others regarding a variety of medications for the treatment of alcoholism.

- Visit MyWayOut at:

http://bit.ly/mywayoutforum

- A link to Google search results for a search within the MyWayOut forum for this specific medication:

  http://bit.ly/mywaynalmef

- US-based C Three Foundation Forum:

  optionssavelives.freeforums.net

- UK-based forum:

  http://bit.ly/uknalmefforum

- Germany-based forum (German):

  http://bit.ly/nalmefgermany

Generic Wikipedia Link:

http://bit.ly/wikinalf

SIGNIFICANT NALMEFENE RESEARCH &
FINDINGS

> 2015–Stevenson–PharmacoEconomics
> Nalmefene for Reducing Alcohol Consumption in People with Alcohol Dependence: An Evidence Review Group Perspective of a NICE Single Technology Appraisal

- "Therefore, the Appraisal Committee concluded that nalmefene in conjunction with psychosocial support was a cost effective use of NHS resources compared with psychosocial support alone for treating people with alcohol dependence drinking at a high risk level, without physical withdrawal symptoms and not requiring immediate assisted withdrawal from alcohol."[312]

> 2015–Van den Brink–Expert Opinion on Drug Safety
> Safety and Tolerability of as-Needed Nalmefene in the Treatment of Alcohol Dependence: Results from the Phase III Clinical Programme

- Van den Brink, the lead researcher on nalmefene, commented on tolerability and safety: "There was no difference in tolerability and safety if nalmefene was taken daily or intermittently; no signal of increased risk of suicide-related behavior with nalmefene."[310]

> 2014–Van den Brink–Journal of Psychopharmacology
> Long-Term Efficacy, Tolerability and Safety of Nalmefene as-Needed in Patients with Alcohol Dependence: A 1-Year, Randomised Controlled Study

- In a study of 422 (310 of them taking nalmefene) patients which examined long term safety and effectiveness, at month 13 there was a reduction in the number of heavy drinking days (HDDs) and a reduction in total alcohol consumption (TAC).

- In a subgroup analysis of patients with high/very high drinking risk levels (the target population), there was a significant effect in favor of nalmefene on total alcohol consumption at month 6, and on both heavy drinking days and total alcohol consumption at month 13.

- Improvements in liver enzymes were also greater with nalmefene. Most adverse events were mild or moderate, and transient. The study "provides evidence for the long-term safety and efficacy of nalmefene as-needed in alcohol-dependent patients who continue to drink heavily, following a brief intervention."[308]

2013–Gual–European Neuropsychopharmacology
A randomised, double-blind, placebo-controlled, efficacy study of nalmefene, as-needed use, in patients with alcohol dependence

---

- In a study of 718 patients (358 taking nalmefene) which examined effectiveness with alcohol dependence were given either placebo or 18mg/day of nalmefene.

- A significantly superior effect of nalmefene compared to placebo was seen by month 6 in heavy drinking days.

- A subanalysis showed that patients who did not reduce their drinking (in other words, those that used the 'as needed' approach) benefited more from nalmefene.

- A reduction in liver enzymes was also seen in the nalmefene group. This study "provides evidence for the efficacy of nalmefene, in terms of treatment goal (reduced drinking) and dosing regimen (as-needed), in alcohol dependent patients unable to reduce alcohol consumption on their own."[311]

2013–Sinclair–European Psychiatry
1613–As-Needed Use of Nalmefene in the Treatment of Alcohol Dependence

---

- In a study that looked at adherence to nalmefene in an "as-needed" dosing regimen, 68% of the nalmefene treated patients (78% of the study completers) adhered to the as-needed treatment regimen on at least 80% of the study days.

- Sinclair pointed out that patients were given instructions to take a tablet 1-2 hours before drinking. He stated, "as-needed use is a patient-centered approach engaging patients in active and responsible management of their illness. It should be seen as an integral part of disease management, increasing awareness of drinking amount and patterns, facilitating identification of at-risk situations."[313][175]

2013–Van Den Brink–European Psychiatry
1105–Long-Term Efficacy of Nalmefene as-Needed in Alcohol Dependent Patients with High Drinking Risk Levels: Results of a Subgroup Analysis

---

- In a study of severe alcoholics that looked at 187 patients (145 taking nalmefene), with a mean heavy drinking days of 19 ± 6.3/month, mean heavy drinking days decreased significantly to 7 days/month at 1 year.

- Improvements in clinical status and in liver enzymes were larger in the nalmefene compared to the placebo group.[314]

2013–Van den Brink–Alcohol and Alcoholism
Efficacy of As-Needed Nalmefene in Alcohol-Dependent Patients with at Least a High Drinking Risk Level: Results from a Subgroup Analysis of Two Randomized Controlled 6-Month Studies

---

- In a study of 667 patients (with 334 taking nalmefene), there was a superior effect of nalmefene compared with placebo in reducing the number of heavy drinking days and total alcohol consumption.[315]

2013–Van den Brink–European Psychiatry
1108–Esense 2–Randomized Controlled 6-Month Study of as-Needed Nalmefene: Subgroup Analysis of Alcohol Dependent Patients with High Drinking Risk Level

---

- In a study of 317 severe alcoholics (155 taking nalmefene), with mean heavy drinking days of 22 ± 6.2/month, this number was decreased to 10 days/month and mean total alcohol consumed also decreased significantly at month 6.

- Improvements in clinical status and alanine amino transferase were greater in the nalmefene group compared to the placebo group.[316]

> **2012–Mann–European Psychiatry**
> **Extending the Treatment Options in Alcohol Dependence: A Randomized Controlled Study of As-Needed Nalmefene**

- In a study of 605 patients (306 on nalmefene), there was a significantly superior effect of nalmefene compared to placebo in reducing the number of heavy drinking days and total alcohol consumed per day.

- The study found that "nalmefene was safe and well tolerated and dosing on an as-needed basis was feasible."[317]

- It also stated, "nalmefene provides clinical benefit, constitutes a potential new pharmacological treatment paradigm in terms of the treatment goal and dosing regimen, and provides a method to address the unmet medical need in patients with alcohol dependence that need to reduce their alcohol consumption."[318]

> **2008–Arias–Alcoholism: Clinical and Experimental Research**
> **Effects of Opioid Receptor Gene Variation on Targeted Nalmefene Treatment in Heavy Drinkers**

- The study found that "nalmefene significantly reduced the number of heavy drinking and very heavy drinking days per week, compared with placebo."[319]

> **2008–Soyka–Current Drug Abuse Reviews**
> **Opioid Antagonists for Pharmacological Treatment of Alcohol Dependence**

- Soyka stated that "although the number of clinical studies conducted with naltrexone by far exceeds the number conducted with nalmefene, the four studies on nalmefene published so far may indicate a role of this opioid antagonist in the treatment of alcoholism."[176]

> **2007–Karhuvaara–Alcoholism: Clinical and Experimental Research**
> **Effects of opioid receptor gene variation on targeted nalmefene treatment in heavy drinkers**

- A study where subjects were instructed to take nalmefene 10 to 40 mg when they believed drinking to be imminent found Nalmefene to be "effective and safe in reducing heavy drinking, even when accompanied by minimal psychosocial support."[319]

2004–Anton–Journal of Clinical Psychopharmacology
A Multi-Site Dose Ranging Study of Nalmefene in the Treatment of Alcohol Dependence

---

- A multisite trial showed that nalmefene was "reasonably well tolerated in recently abstinent alcoholics."[320]

2004–Drobes–Alcoholism, clinical and experimental research
Effects of Naltrexone and Nalmefene on Subjective Response to Alcohol among Non-Treatment-Seeking Alcoholics and Social Drinkers

---

- Participants were given either naltrexone or nalmefene for seven days before being given alcohol in a bar-like setting.

- Alcoholics reported higher levels of craving than social drinkers before and after the drink as well as higher levels of alcohol-induced stimulation.

- Both nalmefene and naltrexone suppressed initial increases in craving and stimulation amongst alcoholics who are not actively attempting to reduce drinking."[321]

2001–Sinclair–Alcohol and Alcoholism
Evidence about the Use of Naltrexone and for Different Ways of Using It in the Treatment of Alcoholism

---

- In discussing one study, Sinclair states, "These results are consistent with our pre-clinical studies in which naltrexone, naloxone, and nalmefene were effective when paired with drinking but ineffective when given during abstinence."

- He states, "This supported the hypothesis that the primary mechanism involved is extinction (as had been concluded earlier for the effects of naltrexone in opiate addiction treatment) because extinction only weakens responses that are made while reinforcement is blocked."[300]

1999–Mason–Archives of General Psychiatry
A Double-Blind, Placebo-Controlled Study of Oral Nalmefene for Alcohol Dependence

- In a study that measured relapse, Mason found that "significantly fewer patients treated with nalmefene than patients given placebo relapsed to heavy drinking through 12 weeks of treatment."

- The odds were 2.4 times greater that relapse would occur with placebo than with nalmefene.

- Mason concluded, "Treatment with nalmefene was effective in preventing relapse to heavy drinking relative to placebo in alcohol-dependent outpatients and was accompanied by acceptable side effects."[322]

1994–Mason–Alcoholism, Clinical and Experimental Research
A Double-Blind, Placebo-Controlled Pilot Study to Evaluate the Efficacy and Safety of Oral Nalmefene HCl for Alcohol Dependence

- Mason found that "nalmefene can be safely given to alcoholics, and that nalmefene may have a role in reducing alcohol consumption and preventing relapse, particularly at the 40 mg level."[323]

1992–Sinclair–United States Patent Database
Method for Treating Alcoholism with Nalmefene–Patent

- Sinclair's patent stated, "Nalmefene is a newer opioid antagonist that is structurally similar to naltrexone but with a number of potential pharmacological advantages for the treatment of alcohol dependence, including no dose-dependent association with toxic effects to the liver, greater oral bioavailability, longer duration of antagonist action, and more competitive binding with opioid receptor subtypes that are thought to reinforce drinking... Outcomes did not differ between the 20- and 80-mg dose nalmefene groups. Significantly fewer patients treated with nalmefene than patients given placebo relapsed to heavy drinking through 12 weeks of treatment ($P<.02$), with a significant treatment effect at the first weekly study visit ($P<.02$). The odds ratio of relapsing to heavy drinking was 2.4 times greater with placebo compared with nalmefene (95% confidence interval, 1.05-5.59). Patients treated with nalmefene also had fewer subsequent relapses (P<.03) than patients given placebo."[112]

1986–Gal–Clinical Pharmacology and Therapeutics
Prolonged Blockade of Opioid Effect with Oral Nalmefene

- "Findings suggest that nalmefene could provide prolonged effectiveness in limiting emergence of opioid effects during addiction therapy."[324]

PERSONAL EXPERIENCES WITH NALMEFENE

Short Forms Used Below:

- AF–Alcohol-Free (A day when no alcohol is consumed)
- SEs–Side Effects
- TSM–The Sinclair Method ('As Needed' Method)
- IMHO–'In my humble opinion'

•••

I used Naltrexone for TSM when I was drinking.

I have also tried Nalmefene more recently to try and put myself off the food binges which seem to have replaced the alcohol.

Nalmefene seems to be stronger and has more side effects than Naltrexone.

Nalmefene is in theory easier to get hold of in the UK than Naltrexone, and that is the reason I used it. Nalmefene is licensed on the NHS for use with alcoholics, while Naltrexone is not and there is a UK website which will issue a prescription and deliver within 24 hours.

I would guess that because of the licensing anyone in the UK approaching their GP (personal Dr) would probably be issued with Nalmefene these days. It is also approximately triple the cost of Naltrexone.

•••

Mid-forties guy here, history of heavy social evening drinking back to university days. Have got 15-year history of drinking after work to 'calm down' which has become an ingrained pattern.

Currently drinking nearly two bottles of wine per night. Feeling so very down about it, it's obviously unhealthy and wrong; so stuck. Aaaaah!!! A functional alcoholic.

Recently tried nalmefene twice. Side effects first time were severe: spaced-out, empty, robot-like, didn't sleep for 20 hours. Second time felt better, but sleep disturbance is a serious issue. Strange drifting through vivid tortured, exhausting nightmares while aware of being half-awake. It's taken me 10 days to get back to a normal sleep pattern, though still have terrible, detailed 'missions' of dreams. It's like a cross between severe jet-lag, flu and what I imagine an LSD 'bad trip' would be. It's not withdrawal phenomena–I don't really get that, or if I do, I'm aware of what it's like.

Anyone know whether naltrexone is better for the sleep disturbance?"

•••

I'm 4 weeks on nalmefene and side effects have long passed. Your explanation of what happened to you last night has made me remember just how bad the first few days were.

I remember thinking that anyone starting nalmefene should plan to be at home for the 1st three days at least. If you are out tonight you probably should stay af and not take nalmefene.

My SEs were nausea, extreme tiredness, flu-like symptoms and loss of appetite. These passed by day four.

I initially reduced my drinking quite a lot but they say there's a honeymoon period before one's alcohol consumption can go back to pre TSM levels.

All this seems daunting, however trust me it does pass and it's worth it.

•••

I hate to count my chickens before they hatch, but I finally feel like something is beginning to happen here! I mentioned that in the past few weeks I haven't 'craved' alcohol but seem to be almost mentally forcing it on myself. Even when I haven't felt like a drink, I've taken my pill at 5 pm anyway because I believe that I will get to 6.30pm and the craving will be so bad I will be tempted to crack open a bottle. Then, because I've taken the pill, I think 'what the hell, I've taken it, I might as well drink now.'

Last night, I really didn't want a drink. I don't mean that I simply wasn't craving, but the thought of having a glass of wine repulsed me. Stupidly (I know, I know), I went with my usual pattern and took my pill and then opened the wine anyway. I thought this is probably just a one off. However, today I feel the same. I really don't want a glass of wine. It's now 5 pm and I really do not want a drink tonight. I have no feelings of craving, no feelings of loss (what will I be missing). I just sniffed the half-empty bottle of red wine left from last night–just to make sure I'm not imagining things–and I really don't fancy drinking it.

So for the first time–I am having an AF day because I really do not want to drink.

I have deliberately not forced AF days as there were split opinions as to whether it helps move things forward or not and I was feeling utter despair that nothing seems to be happening.

As I say–I'm not counting my chickens, but this is the first time in years that I have felt this way. Fingers crossed that this will continue.

•••

I am making no progress at all. I feel that I should make excuses–but that's what addiction does and I want to be totally honest.

I have now been taking Nalmefene almost every day for 6 months. I have said that I feel less of the physical 'craving' I don't obsess about drinking all day long like I used to, however, having an AF day is near impossible. For some reason I just can't do it. I have had days when I'm adamant I won't drink. I will get to 7 pm and then think—Oh I'm going to take a Nalmefene and have just a glass of wine. But I simply can't have one glass of wine. I still feel compelled to drink the whole bottle (and sometimes more).

Nalmefene is making me feel 'blaahhh' most of the time. I don't feel so much joy in life anymore. I feel tired and depressed and could quite happily stay in bed all day. Six months!

I must admit, I am beginning to wonder if this will ever work for me. I can't image at this point in time being able to go an evening without drinking wine. On the very odd occasion that I have managed an AF day, all I can think about is the following day when I can have wine.

I'm not giving up yet—but I am seriously praying for a miracle here.

•••

Well of course it's far too early but since I started TSM I've not forced anything just followed the 1 hour before + drink as normal. Unlike others who are far more resilient I've never forced AF days, in fact I've had just one AF day since I started this. It was years before this that I had a break from drinking, I think I tried to stop in January 2013. Lasting just a few weeks.

So what's happened, over the past few days it has got increasingly difficult to drink, as if the appeal was when I was a kid and sipped my dads beer just to think yuck.

Last night I lazily opened my first can but it was really not enjoyable and as normal I just tried to push through this stage and usually I would get some pleasure in the end.

Last night really was different, by the end of the night I went to bed totally unsatisfied.

Today being a Sunday I would normally have a beer just before dinner around 4 pm. Today I just didn't want to have that drink. I'm sitting here now and of course I'm focusing on drinking because I'm writing this but I'm just not interested in having one. Believe me this is a first.

I wanted to write this now before I forget what it feels like, this isn't something I have done, I've made no effort what so ever. However what I feel today is a change from deep within, a switch has been thrown.

I'll have to see if it lasts but today I feel normal, I'm not sitting here thinking how a first cold beer might taste. No I'm not interested. I'm a bit bored to be honest but that's because I've been numbing my senses for so long, it was always going to be the case that I have a hole to fill but that's not the point here, what I'm feeling tonight at least is indifference to drink I guess.

•••

Recently a friend reminded me of the place I had been to with alcohol.

Until then and until I started to access memories of him begging me not to drink, me pushing my way past him, past someone who loved me to then go drink with a load of bums in a rough bar, him coming to my house and me drunk and confused at all times of day, behaving badly being sick, unable to attend a really important exam because I didn't have the strength to get out of my flat without passing out........and that is just the tip of the iceberg, I had 8 years of really serious stuff and alcohol was a problem from the age of 16.

I had my first blackout at 17, first drunk vomit at that age. Always blackouts, always ill, crying, hiding cans because my recycling was overflowing, waking up paranoid, abusive in drink, deciding to drink instead of going to work even when I was under an attendance warning. Waking up not knowing where I was, on nights out being picked up by the police asleep/passed out on benches in a summer dress. Falling down the stairs, falling onto the fire, overdoses, walking in front of lorries because I was drunk and didn't care, waking up with a smashed nose because I think I tripped and bust my nose on the doorstep, collapsing in a supermarket hungover. All sorts of things and I tried all sorts of things to quit.

Sheer miracle that I am here and alive.

Ten years ago I was told by a hospital consultant that I would not make it, that because of my drinking I would not live to the age I am now. 18 years of problematic drinking, final 8 years out and out alcoholic.

I also know of someone who drank very differently to me, no binges, daily drinker for 30 years who has used TSM and experienced the same miracle. Their life like their drinking was very different to mine, but they experienced a very similar effect.

I don't care whether it's a cure all, I do care that it's made available for those who wish to try and it is being made available as Nalmefene in the UK on the NHS (state health service). If it saves one life that is good enough for me—it has saved mine.

GABAPENTIN & PREGABALIN

INTRODUCTION TO GABAPENTINOIDS

Gabapentin (marketed under the brand name Neurontin) is one of three clinically used drugs known as gabapentinoids.

The other two drugs include pregabalin (brand name Lyrica) and newer gabapentin enacarbil (brand name: Horizant or Gralise).

Most of the research around gabapentinoids for the treatment of alcohol dependence is related to the oldest of the three drugs—gabapentin.

However, it is logical to conclude that gabapentin's effectiveness for this purpose may also be relevant to later gabapentinoids. (And clinical trials are currently underway to test gabapentin encarbil's effectiveness in alcohol dependence.)

For this reason, while most of the research we have is regarding gabapentin and alcohol dependence, information about both pregabalin and gabapentin encarbil are covered together in this section.

Gabapentin is a widely used medication with more than 18 million prescriptions filled yearly.

Gabapentinoids are analogs of gamma-aminobutyric acid (GABA), a neurotransmitter that slows down the activity of nerve cells in the brain.

Gabapentin and pregabalin were approved for the treatment of conditions such as partial seizures and nerve pain. The extended-release version of gabapentin (gabapentin enacarbil) is FDA-approved to treat restless legs syndrome.

Gabapentin (and to a lesser extent, pregabalin) is prescribed off-label for the treatment of alcohol dependence.

Gabapentin enacarbil is simply a slower-release version of the original gabapentin. Instead of taking several gabapentin pills throughout the day, only one of the extended-release enacarbil pills needs to be taken.

Gabapentin and pregabalin are structurally and pharmacologically related compounds. They share similar mechanism of action, but also differ in some characteristics. Gabapentin encarbil turns into gabapentin in the body but has twice the bioavailability of the original gabapentin (meaning it may be effective at lower doses, and, therefore, have fewer side effects.)

Pregabalin is considered to be more 'bioavailable' than gabapentin. This is seen as a benefit because it may achieve the same results as gabapentin in lower doses (thus theoretically also reducing the side effects seen with higher doses).

There are also several similarities–both drugs can be given without regard to meals; neither drug binds to plasma proteins; neither drug is metabolized by nor inhibits hepatic enzymes that are responsible for the metabolism of other drugs; both drugs are excreted renaly, with elimination half-lives of approximately six hours; both are used to treat nerve-related pain and partial seizures.

Because they have similar mechanisms of action and properties, there is little reason to take both together, however, if one is effective, but side-effects are unreasonable, it is possible that trying the other one may also be effective against alcoholism, and perhaps have more tolerable side effects.[325][326]

Gabapentinoids may help to reduce anxiety (and have also been known to be effective against depression). They have also been helpful in individuals that have trouble with insomnia, which can be a problem for many alcoholics.

Other research has shown two additional pieces of information about gabapentinoid of note for the treatment of alcohol dependence: first, there may be a potential benefit when combined with naltrexone; and second, there is evidence that gabapentinoids impact drinking outcomes up to six weeks after cessation of drinking.

One other very important element to be aware of in regards to gabapentinoids is their potential role in abuse.

Gabapentin is NOT an addictive substance. The United States federal government *has not* identified gabapentin as a 'Controlled Substance' (that is, one with potential for addiction).

However, pregabalin is a Schedule V Controlled Substance. Schedule V drugs have a low potential for abuse and the Schedule V list includes, for example, cough suppressants which contain small amounts of codeine.

Recent 2014 research indicates that pregabalin, in particular, can be used as a booster for other opioids and have been found as secondary substances in fatal poisonings for the following drugs: buprenorphine, codeine, fentanyl, methadone, oxycodone, tramadol. (A booster is a substance that makes another substance more potent).

Because of this booster potential, gabapentin may not be advisable for any alcoholic also using opioids or with the potential to do so.[327]

THE BACK-STORY

Gabapentin was first marketed in 1993 by Pfizer. Pfizer had both enormous success and substantial penalties for Gabapentin—it was one of the company's top performing drugs, but a subsidiary of the company was also fined 2.3 billion for promoting four drugs, including Lyrica, for uses not approved by the FDA. (This does not mean that the drugs don't work for many off-label uses—only that by promoting them for off-label uses, Pfizer was breaking laws).

Pregabalin received both European and FDA approval in 2004. Enacarbil gained approval in 2011.[328]

Once a successful drug has lost its marketing protection and becomes available generically, many drug companies will try to develop a 'similar but different' version of the drug. They seek to develop one that is effective or more effective than the first version for similar conditions, but is different enough to obtain patent and marketing protection from the FDA.

For Pfizer, pregabalin (and more recently, gabapentin enacarbil) are Pfizer's follow-up versions of gabapentin and given gabapentin's enormous profitability and potential it is not surprising that Pfizer should look for profitable next-generation versions of the drug.

Gabapentin is considered something of a 'wonder drug' by many, due to its broad effectiveness across a myriad of conditions. Despite being developed for its use in seizure prevention, today epilepsy and seizures are in fact its smallest market.

It is prescribed off-label for a multitude of uses, including treatment of bipolar disease, neuropathic pain, diabetic neuropathy, complex regional pain syndrome, attention deficit disorder, restless legs syndrome, trigeminal neuralgia, periodic limb movement disorders of sleep, premenstrual syndrome, migraine headache, drug and alcohol withdrawal seizures and alcohol dependence.[329]

Gabapentin is, in fact, one of the drugs prescribed most often for off-label uses—with 83% of all gabapentin prescriptions written for off-label uses, generating billions of dollars in off-label sales for this blockbuster drug.[329]

Because gabapentin has been used ubiquitously by many primary care physicians for many other indications (resulting in familiarity with the medication), it is hoped that gabapentin will be readily utilized by primary care givers for alcoholism. (As compared with less familiar treatments for alcohol dependence).

It is also extremely inexpensive—now that it is generic, one US-based researcher found that the 1800mg dose used in one study could cost less than $10/week.[330]

Gabapentin & Pregabalin Medication FAQ

Medication Overview

What is the medication called?

Gabapentinoids: Gabapentin, Gabapentin Enacarbil and Pregabalin

What are common brand names and generic names for this medication?

Neurontin, Lyrica, Horizant, Neurostil, Neurontin, Fanatrex, Gabarone, Gralise, Nupentin, Gabrion, Penral, Gabapin.

What 'type' of medication is this?

Gabapentinoid

What is it usually prescribed for?

Anti-Anxiety, antiparkinson, analgesics, anticonvulsants, calcium channel Blockers, antimanic agents, excitatory amino acid antagonists, epilepsy management, nerve pain management.

How is it described?

Gabapentin is a unique anticonvulsant that is used to manage epilepsy and nerve pain. The mechanism of action is unknown.

Gabapentin is structurally related to the neurotransmitter GABA, but it does not interact with GABA receptors, is not converted metabolically into GABA or a GABA agonist and is not an inhibitor of GABA uptake or degradation.

Gabapentin can also be used to assist with detoxification. Its activity in the GABA neurotransmitter pathway suggests it might alleviate alcohol craving, which is believed to involve GABA activation in a specific part of the brain (the amygdala). Previous studies have shown that gabapentin reduces this activity. This may increase rates of sustained abstinence and no heavy drinking and decrease alcohol-related insomnia and sad or anxious mood.

AVAILABILITY & FDA APPROVAL STATUS

A prescription for alcoholism is usually:

Off-Label

Is it FDA approved in the USA? When?

Yes—all three are FDA-approved: Gabapentin (1993); Pregabalin (2004); Gabapentin Encarbil (2011)

Is it HC approved in Canada? When?

Yes—all three are HC-approved: Gabapentin (1993); Pregabalin (2005); Gabapentin Encarbil (2013)

Is it EMA approved in Europe? When?

Yes—EMA Approved, date unknown

How is it available?

By prescription in USA, Canada and parts of Europe

STRENGTH AND CREDIBILITY OF RESEARCH FOR ITS USE IN ALCOHOLISM

How many years has this medication been researched specifically for the treatment of alcoholism?

15+ years (2000)

What is the strength of the supporting research?

- "The demonstration of the efficacy of gabapentin for relapse prevention among alcohol-dependent patients... is a significant development. This well designed and well-powered trial replicates the positive findings of several previous smaller trial...It would thus seem to have potential for widespread use for treatment of alcohol dependence in both specialty and primary care treatment settings."[78]

- In a review of six randomized controlled clinical trials lasting at least 4 weeks, the four largest trials showed "beneficial effects of gabapentin on at least one alcohol-related outcome measure."[49]

- A second, separate review of research found, "Gabapentin used to treat alcohol dependence was well tolerated with no severe adverse reactions reported in the extant literature... the current literature is promising for gabapentin in the treatment of alcohol"[331]

What credentials does the researcher making the statements above have?

- Dr. Edward Nunes: Former chair of the National Institute on Drug Abuse Treatment Research Review Committee, Member of Board of Directors of the Research Foundation for Mental Hygiene, Co-chair of New York State Psychiatric Institute Institutional Review Board; author of over 175 book chapters and peer-reviewed articles.

- Dr. Jonathan G. Leung PharmD, BCPS, BCPP: Psychiatric Clinical Pharmacist at the Mayo Clinic and Assistant Professor, Psychiatry and Pharmacy, Mayo Clinic College of Medicine.

RESEARCH FINDINGS ABOUT EFFECTIVENESS IN TREATMENT FOR ALCOHOLISM

How many patients need to be treated to see one true medication responder? (Known as the 'Number Needed to Treat–NNT)

- The Number Needed to Treat for gabapentin is 5-8.[37]

- This means gabapentin will be effective for one in five to eight patients. This is in the same range as the treatment of depression with any given antidepressant medication.

How effective is this medication for the treatment of alcoholism?

- The strongest evidence of effectiveness occurred in patients experiencing moderate to severe withdrawal when gabapentin was administered early in or concurrently during acute withdrawal and continued for up to 12 weeks.

- A large, well-managed 6-year study found gabapentin significantly improved rates of abstinence and no heavy drinking. Abstinence rate was 4.1% in the placebo group, 11.1% in the 900-mg group, and 17.0% in the 1800-mg group. The no heavy drinking rate was 22.5%

in the placebo group, 29.6% in the 900-mg group, and 44.7% in the 1800-mg group.[37]

- In another study, comparing pregabalin and naltrexone, pregabalin "resulted in better outcomes in patients reporting a comorbid psychiatric disorder."[332]

- The author stated, "results from this study globally place pregabalin within the same range of efficacy as that of naltrexone."[332]

In research, how did this medication compare to other medications for the treatment of alcoholism?

- Barbara Mason of the one of the top alcohol addiction research facilities in the world (Scripps Research Institute) states, "gabapentin's effect on drinking outcomes is at least as large or greater than those of existing FDA approved treatments...plus it's the only medication shown to improve sleep and mood in people who are quitting or reducing their drinking, and it's already widely used in primary care."[50]

TREATMENT CANDIDATES FOR THIS MEDICATION

Note: this section highlights study findings that have identified some characteristics that may increase odds of effectiveness. This does not mean it won't help individuals without these characteristics.

What treatment goals might this medication help achieve?

Abstinence, decrease in heavy drinking, decrease in craving, improved mood and sleep. A positive effect on drinking outcomes was also found after discontinuation of treatment.

What are some typical feelings and motivators of people this medication tends to help?

Gabapentin may work on the inhibition system, or the 'Relief Pathway,' which is the same system which baclofen works on. It may therefore help treat alcoholism that is motivated by anxiety and/or depression. It may help the brain to re-implement inhibition systems that allow individuals to avoid alcohol even once craving is triggered.

Has this medication been shown to be more successful in early-onset or late-onset alcoholics?

Research has not yet provided insight on this answer.

Is this medication typically more effective in people with a strong family history of alcoholism?

Research has not yet provided insight on this answer.

Are there specific genetic markers that have been found to be relevant in treatment with this medication?

Research has not yet provided insight on this answer.

Do Alcoholics Have Difficulty Taking this Medication as Prescribed? (i.e. Are there "Compliance" Issues?)

There are no known issues with compliance.

Are there other characteristics (gender, taste sensitivity, alcoholism type, co-morbid disorders, smoker status) that may be related to success with this medication?

Research has not yet provided insight on this answer.

DIRECTIONS FOR USE & HOW IT WORKS

At what dose and for how long does research suggest the medication should be taken?

- The recommended initial dose for adults is 300 mg three times daily increasing as needed to a maximum dose of 1800 mg daily.

- Studies show that effectiveness is dose dependent and, therefore, higher doses are more effective.

Has this medication been tested with other medications for the treatment of alcoholism and found to be complimentary?

Yes—gabapentin has been combined with naltrexone with complimentary outcomes.[287]

What is known about how this medication actually works in alcoholics? What is the 'Mechanism of Action'?

Researchers indicate: "its mechanism of pharmacological action remains unknown. Gabapentin increases the concentration and probably the synthesis of GABA in the brain... the GABAergic system in the central nucleus of the amygdala plays an important role in regulating voluntary ethanol intake."

SAFETY CONCERNS

Is this medication addictive? Does it have abuse potential?

- Gabapentinoids are not addictive, though a physical dependence can be developed, causing withdrawal syndrome upon discontinuation.

- These drugs have been known to be used as 'booster' drugs for other opioids in drug addicts.[333][327]

How safe is this medication?

"Gabapentin is a well-tolerated medication, with few adverse effects at low to moderate doses, although typical anticonvulsant adverse effects (e.g., sedation, dizziness) may occur at higher doses....it is already widely prescribed for treatment of chronic pain, mood, anxiety, and sleep problems, in addition to seizure prophylaxis."[78]

Can this medication be taken while drinking?

- There is moderate interaction between this drug and alcohol. While it is not recommended to take this medication while drinking, it can be taken while the alcohol-dependent individual is still drinking though side-effects if taken while alcohol is in one's system may be enhanced.

- Gabapentin can be used to assist with detoxification.

What are other fairly common side effects?

Can cause drowsiness, dizziness, headache, anxiety, and constipation.

Where can I find a complete list of all side effects, precautions, and instructions in case of emergency or overdose?

You can find this on the US National Library of Medicine website. Search google for 'gabapentin and National Library of Medicine' or visit:

http://bit.ly/gabalist

What does the National Institute of Health (NIH) say about liver impact and where can I find further information on liver impact of this medication?

- Topiramate has been rarely associated with hepatic injury and the apparent absence or low rate of significant hepatotoxicity from gabapentin may be due to its minimal hepatic metabolism and rapid urinary excretion.

- Also visit the livertox.nlm.nih.gov sitelink:

http://bit.ly/livertoxgabapentin

What known drug interactions should I watch for and where can I find more information on drug interactions?

- Moderate interaction between gabapentin and aripiprazole, baclofen and alcohol. Known to interact with at least 520 other drugs.

- Also see the drugs.com drug interaction checker:

http://bit.ly/interactgaba

Where can I find alerts and Black Box Warnings? (Black Box Warnings are cautions affixed to medications by the government)

Black Box warnings can be found here:

http://bit.ly/gabalist

Were there any known black box warnings at the time this book was written?

No–but you may still wish to visit the link above for up-to-date information.

OTHER USEFUL INFORMATION

Note: Links to all recommended information sources can be found on the book's website at APrescriptionForAlcoholics.com

Recent Research:

- 2015: The Role of Gabapentin in the Management of Alcohol Withdrawal and Dependence[331]

- 2010: Medication Treatment of Different Types of Alcoholism[178]

- 2014: Gabapentin: a new addition to the armamentarium for alcohol dependence?[78]

- 2014: Gabapentin Treatment for Alcohol Dependence A Randomized Clinical Trial[87]

- 2011: Gabapentin combined with naltrexone for the treatment of alcohol dependence[287]

Article:

- 2015: Drugs for Alcoholism Don't have to Lead to Sobriety, Bloomberg Business[334]

- 2013: Clinical Trial Indicates Gabapentin Is Safe and Effective for Treating Alcohol Dependence[50]

CONNECTING WITH OTHERS

Online Forum(s):

- The 'MyWayOut' community started out focused on topiramate but is now a good place to read about and connect with others regarding a variety of medications for the treatment of alcoholism.

- Visit MyWayOut at:

http://bit.ly/mywayoutforum

- A link to Google search results for a search within the MyWayOut forum for this specific medication:

http://bit.ly/mywaygaba

Reviews from others on Drugs.com:

- These links are not specifically for alcoholism, but you may find them useful anyways.

- For alcohol withdrawal:

http://bit.ly/drugsgaba

- General Information:

http://bit.ly/gababrand

Reviews from others on WebMD:

These links are not specifically for alcoholism, but you may find them useful anyways.

- About gabapentin:

http://bit.ly/webmdgaba

- Related to branded version:

http://bit.ly/webmdbrand

Generic Wikipedia Link:

http://bit.ly/wikigabapentin

DrugBank.ca Link (Detailed Drug Data Including Pricing):

http://bit.ly/drugbankgabapentin

SIGNIFICANT GABAPENTIN (AND PREGABALIN) RESEARCH FINDINGS

2014–Batki–American Journal of Psychiatry
Toward Personalized Medicine in the Pharmacotherapy of Alcohol Use Disorder:
Targeting Patient Genes and Patient Goals

- Batki found that in recent studies, "the antiepileptic drugs topiramate and gabapentin were found to be effective in improving several drinking-related outcomes."[2]

2014–Nunes–JAMA Internal Medicine
Gabapentin: a new addition to the armamentarium for alcohol dependence?

- Nunes' research found, "gabapentin is a well-tolerated medication, with few adverse effects at low to moderate doses, although typical anticonvulsant adverse effects (e.g.,sedation, dizziness) may occur at higher doses."

- "It is already widely prescribed for treatment of chronic pain, mood, anxiety, and sleep problems … it would thus seem to have potential for widespread use for treatment of alcohol dependence in both specialty and primary care treatment settings."[78]

- Nunes' writes, "In the trial reported in this issue, the number needed to treat (NTT) for gabapentin on the key outcome of abstinence from heavy drinking is 5. Similar NNT estimates apply to naltrexone for alcohol dependence (7), and, for that matter, for the treatment of depression with any given antidepressant medication. This means that, on average, five patients need to be treated to see 1 true medication responder. But, the treatments act by different mechanisms, and if 1 fails another may work. The key is to keep trying different approaches, or combinations. We are arguably now in a position with respect to alcohol dependence similar to our position for other chronic conditions like depression or hypertension, with a number of different treatment options, both psychosocial and pharmacological."[78]

2013–Mason–JAMA Internal Medicine
Gabapentin treatment for alcohol dependence a randomized clinical trial

---

- Mason's large, 6-year study found gabapentin significantly improved rates of abstinence and no heavy drinking. Positive effects were obtained with measures of mood, sleep, and craving. Abstinence rate was 4.1% in the placebo group, 11.1% in the 900-mg group, and 17.0% in the 1800-mg group.

- The 'no heavy drinking' rate was 22.5% in the placebo group, 29.6% in the 900-mg group, and 44.7% in the 1800-mg group.

- The study concluded: Gabapentin (particularly the 1800-mg dosage) was effective in treating alcohol dependence and relapse-related symptoms of insomnia, dysphoria, and craving, with a favorable safety profile. Increased implementation of pharmacological treatment of alcohol dependence in primary care may be a major benefit of gabapentin as a treatment option for alcohol dependence."[37]

- Also, "the drug also had a significant dose effect in increasing the rates of complete abstinence (p=0.04) and no heavy drinking (p=0.02) over the 12-week study period, the researchers say."[330]

2012–Guglielmo–Advances in Therapy
Pregabalin for Alcohol Dependence: A Critical Review of the Literature

---

- A critical review of existing research examined five studies: two trials for the treatment of alcohol relapse and three for the management of alcohol withdrawal syndrome with pregabalin. The review concluded "pregabalin could be a novel and effective treatment option for the management of alcohol relapse in detoxified patients ... in particular, pregabalin showed a greater beneficial effect on patients with comorbid conditions such as alcoholism and generalized anxiety disorders."[335]

> ### 2011–Anton–The American Journal of Psychiatry
> ### Gabapentin Combined with Naltrexone for the Treatment of Alcohol Dependence

- This clinical trial evaluated whether gabapentin and naltrexone, was better than naltrexone alone and/or placebo during the early drinking cessation phase (first six weeks).

- It found, "the naltrexone/gabapentin group had 1) a longer delay to heavy drinking than the naltrexone-alone ... 2) less heavy drinking days than the naltrexone-alone group ... and 3) less drinks/drinking day than the naltrexone-alone group ... These differences faded over the remaining study weeks."

- "Poor sleep was associated with more drinking in the naltrexone-alone group, but not in the combined group, while an alcohol withdrawal history was associated with better response in the combined group."

- "Conclusion—The addition of gabapentin to naltrexone improved drinking outcomes over naltrexone alone during the first six weeks after cessation of drinking."[287]

> ### 2010–Martinotti–Journal of psychopharmacology (Oxford, England)
> ### Pregabalin versus Naltrexone in Alcohol Dependence: A Randomised, Double-Blind, Comparison Trial

- In this study, comparing pregabalin and naltrexone, pregabalin "resulted in better outcomes in patients reporting a comorbid psychiatric disorder."

- "Results from this study globally place pregabalin within the same range of efficacy as that of naltrexone."[332]

> ### 2008–Brower–Alcoholism: Clinical and Experimental
> ### A Randomized Double-Blind Pilot Trial of Gabapentin Versus Placebo to Treat Alcohol Dependence and Comorbid Insomnia

- In a study with alcoholic patients, "Gabapentin significantly delayed the onset to heavy drinking, an effect which persisted for 6 weeks after treatment ended. Insomnia improved in both treatment groups during the medication phase, but gabapentin had no differential effects on sleep as measured by either subjective report or polysomnography."[336]

2008–Martinotti–Advances in Therapy
Efficacy and Safety of Pregabalin in Alcohol Dependence

- A small human study showed, "a significant progressive reduction of both craving and withdrawal symptomatology... pregabalin shows promise as a treatment for alcohol dependence."[337]

2008–Roberto–Journal of Neuroscience
Cellular and Behavioral Interactions of Gabapentin with Alcohol Dependence

- A study on rats provided insight into the mechanism behind gabapentin and concluded that gabapentin represents a potential medication for the treatment of alcoholism.[338]

2007–Furieri–Journal of Clinical Psychiatry
Gabapentin Reduces Alcohol Consumption and Craving: A Randomized, Double-Blind, Placebo-Controlled Trial

- "After 28 days of treatment, the gabapentin group showed a significant reduction in both number of drinks per day and mean percentage of heavy drinking, and an increase in the percentage of days of abstinence, compared to the placebo group..."

- "Conclusion: Gabapentin reduces alcohol consumption and craving, which may help patients to maintain abstinence. These results, together with the virtual absence of side effects and a favorable safety profile, support gabapentin as a potential drug for the treatment of alcohol withdrawal and dependence."[339]

2006–Bisaga–Drug and Alcohol Dependence
The Acute Effects of Gabapentin in Combination with Alcohol in Heavy Drinkers

- "Acute gabapentin administration was well tolerated in combination with alcohol, but did not alter the effects of alcohol.[340]

2003–Karam-Hage–Psychiatry and Clinical Neurosciences
Open Pilot Study of Gabapentin versus Trazodone to Treat Insomnia in Alcoholic Outpatients

- "Insomnia is common and may increase the risk of relapse in treated alcoholics, even after controlling for other clinical variables...Although the overall sleep of each medication group improved significantly over time, [abstinent alcoholic] patients who received gabapentin improved significantly more than did patients who received trazodone."[341]

2000–Karam-Hage–American Journal of Psychiatry
Gabapentin Treatment for Insomnia Associated with Alchohol Dependence

- "Gabapentin shows promise as a safe and effective treatment for alcohol-dependent patients with comorbid insomnia during early recovery."[342]

PERSONAL EXPERIENCES WITH GABAPENTIN

Short Forms Used Below:

- AF–Alcohol-Free (A day when no alcohol is consumed)
- SEs–Side Effects
- TSM–The Sinclair Method ('As Needed' Method)
- IMHO–'In my humble opinion'
- Bac–Baclofen
- AL–Alcohol
- Gaba–Gabapentin
- Naltrex–naltrexone

•••

I have continued to have dramatically reduced alcohol urges. My cravings are on par with say, ice cream. AND I can control my ice cream eating thus I can control my alcohol drinking. I don't even have to take the pill every day. I'm taking 300mg every other day unless I find myself struggling with not drinking.

For the record, gabapentin CAN be abused so it's best to use with caution. Also, tolerance can grow so going on and off it is best. I'm taking it "AS NEEDED" which is sometimes daily and then sometimes not. I have not experienced any "high" feeling except once, and I've taken it 15+ times.

I am also taking 25mg baclofen a day and 300-600mg gabapentin. I have been on the 20-25mg bac for months. The only difference to my being able to stop drinking was the adding of the gabapentin, and perhaps a personal revelation about my life.

Yesterday I caved and bought a bottle of wine. I believe it was because I was bored, and maybe because I forgot to take bac in the late afternoon. I took it at bedtime to help me sleep, though. The gabapentin alone did not help me avoid the AL enough to get me through. I was in the store and bought one bottle of chardonnay. I drank three glasses and felt I was white knuckling to not drink the rest.

However, the good news is I did NOT drink the rest and had no hangover...If I had been only on bac, my bottle of wine would have been gone based on my past six months on bac at this and higher levels so the gabapentin is working. AND I would have gone out for more or bought more to begin with. My mood is still elevated, and I feel great. I'm now exercising.

[note–the amount of baclofen being taken by this individual is far below the amount recommended for the treatment of alcohol dependence]

•••

Just thought I'd comment here. I have been alcohol-free going on 1 1/2 yrs. I will admit that the craving did not totally ebb. I was in a serious car accident some months ago. Luckily, I was able to ease off the narcotic pain meds w/o a problem. Last month my ortho prescribed gabapentin for my soft tissue and nerve pain. A very wonderful side effect of this med is absolutely NO craving for alcohol at all. Not sure if this med is used off-label for alcohol dependency, but it does work at least for me!!!

• • •

I was given gabapentin starting about a year ago for treatment-resistant depression. It actually seems to work which is a relief after trying virtually everything that seems to be available and none of it worked. I have noticed that I also really have no interest in drinking anymore! I even went on vacation and did drink a bit in moderation (something new for me having been a professional binge drinker for years) and after vacation I really just did not have any interest in drinking anything alcoholic. Very strange feeling, The only side effect that I have noticed (450 mg / day dosage taken in the evening) is that I sleep like the proverbial log. And, no desire to drink.

• • •

Baclofen removes cravings for alcohol, I've experienced it, but it doesn't really do much else now does it? Gabapentin, from what it sounds like, works in treating alcoholism by treating the SIDE EFFECTS of NOT DRINKING, the depression, anxiety, insomnia, etc. And so makes it easier to remain abstinent because the person is not feeling all the crap that generally leads to (re)lapse. So by removing some of the triggers that lead to drinking and the effects of not drinking, people don't drink so much, and if their goal is abstinence then that's all that much easier.

• • •

I'm taking 300mg gabapentin 3X's a day, naltrexone and 10mg aripiprazole. I've been on the gaba and the naltrex now for 6 days and find that this combo is working. I was on acamprosate w/ the gaba but didn't like the SE's from the acamprosate. The acamprosate does work though. I went from drinking 12-14 vodkas and or a combo of vodka and wine a night to having only 2. I feel as if I could take it or leave it, don't have that squirmy feeling anymore that the naltrexone alone didn't address. My Doc wants to titrate me up to 1800mg of the gabapentin per day, he is going for complete abstinence, hopefully one day I'll get there, but for right now this is a huge change for me. Tried rehab and AA didn't work for me, just wasn't my thing.

15 | B-LIST DRUGS – MEDICATIONS WORTH CONSIDERING TODAY

The medications included in this section are:

- Ondansetron

- Sertraline

- Prazosin

- Varenicline

- Zonisamide

- Olanzapine

- Sodium Oxybate

- Disulfiram

The medications in this section may be just as helpful to you, just as effective, just as useful and tolerable as those identified as 'most important'—so please don't confuse the fact that there is less information about each one as implying that they are 'not as good.'

I have not been as rigorous in including thorough, detailed information about each of these medications as I have for those in the previous section.

This is simply because, as I write this, there is no other resource that I know of that contains detailed, consolidated information about even the most important medications—and due to this, it has been my desire to make, at very least, the most important information available as quickly as possible.

Future editions of this book (if there are any), may fill the gaps here.

Ondansetron

Introduction to Ondansetron

Ondansetron is a medication that is often mentioned alongside A-List medications as part of the 'next wave' of promising medications for alcoholism.

For example, in a 2011 review, Edwards stated, "This review briefly summarizes research on currently approved medications for alcohol dependence, as well as promising medications like topiramate, baclofen, and ondansetron."[264]

With a little more research and the compilation of one or two additional critical reviews by respected journals (such as a Cochrane review), I would have included ondansetron on the A-List. And I predict that future editions of this book may include it there.

As it stands, the slightly limited research that does exist supporting ondansetron as a treatment for alcohol dependence is very positive and has shown a connection between its effectiveness in early onset alcoholics (those typically with a strong family background) with specific genetic markers.

As has been shown in other medications (acamprosate, topiramate, naltrexone, sertraline and disulfiram), ondansetron is more effective in the treatment of individuals with specific genetic markers.

In the case of ondansetron (as shown in 2011 by Johnson et al.), several genetic variants play a role in the effectiveness of treatment with ondansetron.

A region in a gene called SLC6A4 called the 5-HTTLPR region (which is short form for 'serotonin-transporter-linked polymorphic region) has been extensively researched for its connection with neuropsychiatric disorders.

One variation in this region is called 'LL genotype' and the medication ondansetron works better (or in scientist lingo–'exerts a preferential treatment effect') to reduce severe drinking in alcohol-dependent individuals with this variation.

In addition, there is a section of our DNA which is called the 'three prime untranslated region' (3'-UTR for short). Variations can also be found within this region, and one of them, called the 'TT allele' (or TT variation), further enhances the response of ondansetron in individuals who also carry the LL genotype variation.[343]

Dr. Bankole Johnson and his team (and other researchers) are working on tests which will identify carriers of these variations, allowing them to one day predict alcoholics for whom ondansetron will be successful.

ONDANSETRON MEDICATION Q & A

MEDICATION OVERVIEW

What is the medication called?

Ondansetron

What are common brand names and generic names for this medication?

Zofran, Zofran Oral, Ondansetron RapidFilm (better absorption)

What 'type' of medication is this?

Serotonin 5-HT3 receptor antagonist

What is it usually prescribed for?

Antipsychotic Agents / Indoles and Derivatives; used off-label to treat morning sickness; reduces nausea and vomiting caused by operations and chemotherapy

How is it described?

Ondansetron is usually described as a serotonin type 3 (5-HT3) receptor antagonists and potent antiemetic used for prevention of postsurgical or chemotherapy-induced nausea and vomiting and for some agents as therapy of diarrhea-predominant irritable bowel syndrome.

AVAILABILITY & FDA APPROVAL STATUS

A prescription for alcoholism is usually:

Off-Label

Is it FDA approved in the USA? When?

Yes—FDA Approved in 1991

Is it HC approved in Canada? When?

Yes—Health Canada Approved (date unknown)

Is it EMA approved in Europe? When?

Yes–EMA Approved (date unknown)

How is it available?

By prescription in USA, Canada and parts of Europe

STRENGTH AND CREDIBILITY OF RESEARCH FOR ITS USE IN ALCOHOLISM

How many years has this medication been researched specifically for the treatment of alcoholism?

Since at least 1993 (22+ years)

What is the strength of the supporting research?

- In a 2014 review, Wackernah states that Ondansetron has been studied in four blinded placebo-controlled trials comparing low doses for alcohol dependence, showing significantly reduced daily drinking. Other, additional studies using weight-based dosing found benefits in craving, abstinence, and total drinks.[192]

- Heilig finds that "ondansetron has a reasonably well-documented efficacy for early onset alcoholism."[1]

What credentials does the researcher making the statements above have?

- Robin Wackernah, Pharm.D., BCPP is an Assistant Professor at the Regis University School of Pharmacy;

- Markus Heilig: One of the top researchers of alcohol addiction worldwide; former NIAAA Clinical Director; active medical practitioner; author of more than 200 peer-reviewed journal articles, including papers in Science, PNAS, Lancet, Archives of General Psychiatry. Research work has 8000+ citations.

RESEARCH FINDINGS ABOUT EFFECTIVENESS IN TREATMENT FOR ALCOHOLISM

How many patients need to be treated to see one true medication responder? (Known as the 'Number Needed to Treat–NNT)

The NNT number for ondansetron is unknown.

How effective is this medication for the treatment of alcoholism?

"Clinical trials suggest that the drug is selectively effective in two clinical subgroups—early-onset alcoholics and those with a specific genetic variant of the serotonin transporter gene."[344]

In research, how did this medication compare to other medications for the treatment of alcoholism?

Research has not yet provided insight on this answer.

TREATMENT CANDIDATES FOR THIS MEDICATION

Note: this section highlights study findings that have identified some characteristics that may increase odds of effectiveness. This does not mean it won't help individuals without these characteristics.

What treatment goals might this medication help achieve?

Goals might include: reducing craving, reducing drinks per drinking day, increasing days abstinent.

What are some typical feelings and motivators of people this medication tends to help?

Research has not yet provided insight on this answer.

Has this medication been shown to be more successful in early-onset or late-onset alcoholics?

Ondansetron has been shown to reduce subjective craving in early onset (Type B), but not in late onset subjects (Type A), in whom the lowest ondansetron dose in fact increased craving somewhat.[1]

Is this medication typically more effective in people with a strong family history of alcoholism?

Yes–it is likely more effective for individuals with early onset alcoholism (which tends to have a strong genetic component.)

Are there specific genetic markers that have been found to be relevant in treatment with this medication?

Yes–the genetic variants LL/LS/SS (5-HTTLPR) (rs1042173) and SLC6A4 (5-HTTLPR) impact goals including the number of drinks per drinking day and the percentage of days abstinent.

Do Alcoholics Have Difficulty Taking this Medication as Prescribed? (i.e. Are there "Compliance" Issues?)

There are no known compliance issues.

Are there other characteristics (gender, taste sensitivity, alcoholism type, co-morbid disorders, smoker status) that may be related to success with this medication?

Research has not yet provided insight on this answer.

DIRECTIONS FOR USE & HOW IT WORKS

At what dose and for how long does research suggest the medication should be taken?

The dosage for ondansetron is 0.5/mg per day.

Has this medication been tested with other medications for the treatment of alcoholism and found to be complimentary?

- Yes, ondansetron has been shown complimentary to naltrexone in reducing cue-induced craving.[192]

- Research has also shown that ondansetron combined with topiramate may be more effective than either alone.[345]

What is known about how this medication actually works in alcoholics? What is the 'Mechanism of Action'?

Researchers indicate: "Ondansetron is an antiemetic medication that blocks 5-HT3 receptors. Due to alcohol's activity on 5-HT3, it is thought that ondansetron can be a useful medication in alcohol dependence"[192]

SAFETY CONCERNS

Is this medication addictive? Does it have abuse potential?

Ondansetron is non-addictive.

How safe is this medication?

Ondansetron has a safe profile in alcoholic patients.

Can this medication be taken while drinking?

While it is not recommended to take this medication while drinking, it can be taken while the alcohol-dependent individual is still drinking though side-effects if taken while alcohol is in one's system may be enhanced.

What are the expected side effects of this medication?

Well-tolerated with few side effects. Constipation, dizziness, headache.

Where can I find a complete list of all side effects, precautions, and instructions in case of emergency or overdose?

You can find this on the US National Library of Medicine website. Search google for 'ondansetron and National Library of Medicine' or visit:

http://bit.ly/nlmondansetron

What does the National Institute of Health (NIH) say about liver impact and where can I find further information on liver impact of this medication?

- The 5-HT3 receptor blockers are metabolized in the liver, largely via the cytochrome P450 system, but appear to have a low potential for causing liver injury.

- Also see the livertox.nlm.nih.gov site link:

http://bit.ly/livertoxondansetron

What known drug interactions should I watch for and where can I find more information on drug interactions?

- Known to interact with at least 360 other drugs.

- Also see the drugs.com drug interaction checker:

http://bit.ly/ondansetroninteract

Where can I find alerts and Black Box Warnings? (Black Box Warnings are cautions affixed to medications by the government)

Visit the nlm.nih.gov site to check black box warnings:

http://bit.ly/nlmondansetron

Were there any known black box warnings at the time this book was written?

No—but you may still wish to visit the link above for up-to-date information.

OTHER USEFUL INFORMATION

Note: Links to all recommended information sources can be found on the book's website at APrescriptionForAlcoholics.com

Recent Research:

- 2014: Pharmacological Approaches to Reducing Craving in Patients with Alcohol Use Disorders[47]

- 2014: Ondansetron Reduces Naturalistic Drinking in Nontreatment-Seeking Alcohol-Dependent Individuals with the LL 5'-HTTLPR Genotype: A Laboratory Study[346]

- 2014: Ondansetron and Sertraline May Interact with 5-HTTLPR and DRD4 Polymorphisms to Reduce Drinking in Non-Treatment Seeking Alcohol-Dependent Women: Exploratory Findings[347]

- 2013: Determination of Genotype Combinations That Can Predict the Outcome of the Treatment of Alcohol Dependence Using the 5-HT3 Antagonist Ondansetron[180]

CONNECTING WITH OTHERS

Online Forum(s):

- The 'MyWayOut' community started out focused on topiramate but is now a good place to read about and connect with others regarding a variety of medications for the treatment of alcoholism.

- Visit MyWayOut at:

http://bit.ly/mywayoutforum

- A link to Google search results for a search within the MyWayOut forum for this specific medication:

http://bit.ly/mywayondan

Generic Wikipedia Link:

http://bit.ly/wikiondansetron

DrugBank.ca Link (Detailed Drug Data Including Pricing):

http://bit.ly/drugbankondan

SIGNIFICANT ONDANSETRON RESEARCH & FINDINGS

2014–Haaas-Koffler–CNS Drugs
Pharmacological Approaches to Reducing Craving in Patients with Alcohol Use Disorders

---

- Haas-Koffler stated in her review that ondansetron has been found to reduce drinking behavior in early onset drinkers and that an fMRI study targeting part of the brain showed that naltrexone and ondansetron, alone or in combination, decreased alcohol cue-induced activation in the brain.[47]

2014–Kenna–Alcoholism: Clinical and Experimental Research
Ondansetron Reduces Naturalistic Drinking in Nontreatment-Seeking Alcohol-Dependent Individuals with the LL 5'-HTTLPR Genotype: A Laboratory Study

---

- Kenna's study provides "support that ondansetron may reduce drinking in non-treatment seeking individuals with the LL genotype."[346]

2014–Kenna–Alcohol
Ondansetron and Sertraline May Interact with 5-HTTLPR and DRD4 Polymorphisms to Reduce Drinking in Non-Treatment Seeking Alcohol-Dependent Women: Exploratory Findings

---

- A second 2014 study by Kenna found, "Women with the LL 5-HTTLPR genotype receiving ondansetron ... drank significantly fewer drinks per drinking day (DDD)."[347]

2014–Moore–Experimental and Clinical Psychopharmacology
Acute and Chronic Administration of a Low-Dose Combination of Topiramate and Ondansetron Reduces Ethanol's Reinforcing Effects in Male Alcohol-Preferring (P) Rats

---

- Moore showed in animals that a combination of ondansetron and topiramate was more efficacious than either alone."[345]

2014–Wackernah–Substance Abuse and Rehabilitation
Alcohol Use Disorder: Pathophysiology, Effects, and Pharmacologic Options for Treatment

- In a 2014 review, Wackernah states that ondansetron has been studied in four blinded placebo-controlled trials comparing low doses for alcohol dependence, showing significantly reduced daily drinking.

- Other, additional studies using weight-based dosing found benefits in craving, abstinence, and total drinks.[192]

2013–Addolorato–CNS Drugs
Management of Alcohol Dependence in Patients with Liver Disease

- Addolorate states that ondansetron has a safe profile in alcoholic patients, but that it has not been tested in alcoholic patients with advanced liver disease.[348]

2013–Correa Filho–Addictive Behaviors
A Pilot Study of Full-Dose Ondansetron to Treat Heavy-Drinking Men Withdrawing from Alcohol in Brazil

- Filho suggests that the dose of 16mg/day was ineffective. [349]

2013–Johnson–American Journal of Psychiatry
Determination of Genotype Combinations That Can Predict the Outcome of the Treatment of Alcohol Dependence Using the 5-HT3 Antagonist Ondansetron

- Johnson found that "polymorphisms in the SLC6A4, HTR3A, and HTR3B genes are predictors of reduced drinking in response to ondansetron."[180]

2011–Edwards–Current Pharmaceutical Design
Current and Promising Pharmacotherapies, and Novel Research Target Areas in the Treatment of Alcohol Dependence: A Review

- Edwards states that, in a 304-person study, of patients receiving ondansetron, "those with the LL genotype significantly reduced their drinking compared to the LS and SS individuals."

- He found this consistent with another pilot lab study in humans where "individuals taking .25mg twice a day of ondansetron with the LL genotype reported a significant reduction in drinking."

- In the same study, researchers found no correlation in a reduction in drinking with ondansetron in individuals with the LS or SS genotype.[264]

2011–Lynch–Psychopharmacology
Severity of Drinking as a Predictor of Efficacy of the Combination of Ondansetron and Topiramate in Rat Models of Ethanol Consumption and Relapse

---

- Lynch found that "the combination of ondansetron and topiramate may be a promising treatment for preventing relapse and for treating alcohol dependence in heavy, but not lighter drinkers."[265]

2010–Johnson–The American Journal of Psychiatry
Medication Treatment of Different Types of Alcoholism

- In an analysis describing the treatment for alcoholism that he would recommend based on a patients' presentation, Johnson states, "given that the patient has a moderate severity of alcohol dependence, is still drinking, and had an early onset of problem drinking with a strong family history, the optimal treatment option would be ondansetron." He also states that adverse events are mild.[178]

2008–Myrick–Archives of General Psychiatry
Effect of Naltrexone and Ondansetron on Alcohol Cue-Induced Activation of the Ventral Striatum in Alcohol-Dependent People

---

- In a comparison between the effectiveness of naltrexone and ondansetron, Myrick notes, "Ondansetron by itself was similar to naltrexone and the combination in the overall analysis."

- He found evidence that naltrexone and ondansetron, alone or in combination, "could decrease alcohol cue–induced activation of the ventral striatum."[293]

2006–Heilig–Pharmacology & Therapeutics
Pharmacological Treatment of Alcohol Dependence: Target Symptoms and Target Mechanisms

- Heilig found "ondansetron reduced subjective craving in early onset, but not in late onset subjects, in whom the lowest ondansetron dose in fact increased craving somewhat."

- He notes that "ondansetron has a reasonably well-documented efficacy for early onset alcoholism," and that it appears safe and well tolerated.

- Regarding the difference in its effect depending upon whether alcoholism is early or late onset, Heilig points out that careful clinical assessment beyond a DSM-IV diagnosis of alcohol dependence is important in choosing optimal treatment.

- He hypothesizes that the "optimal patient population for ondansetron likely overlaps with or is the same as" that for naltrexone.[1]

2002—Johnson—Psychopharmacology
Ondansetron Reduces the Craving of Biologically Predisposed Alcoholics

- In pivotal research, Johnson found that "compared with placebo, ondansetron (4 microg/kg b.i.d.) was associated with significant reductions in overall craving in EOA [early onset Type B alcoholics] but not LOA [late onset Type A alcoholics].

- "Ondansetron (4 microg/kg b.i.d) reduced overall craving significantly among EOA. In contrast, ondansetron (1 microg/kg b.i.d.) increased craving significantly in LOA."[350]

1996–Overstreet–Alcoholism: Clinical and Experimental Research
Alternatives to Naltrexone in Animal Models

- Overstreet found that ondansetron "was effective and there was an increase in effectiveness with time."[351]

1993–Johnson–Psychopharmacology
Attenuation of Some Alcohol-Induced Mood Changes and the Desire to Drink by
5-HT3 Receptor Blockade: A Preliminary Study in Healthy Male Volunteers

- In early research, Johnson discovered that "pretreatment with ondansetron significantly attenuated several of the subjective pleasurable effects of alcohol, and also decreased the subjective desire to drink."[352]

Personal Experiences with Ondansetron

Five weeks in on the ondansetron and showing some promise. I have occasionally added naltrexone on days I am drinking as research shows they work well together.

Side effects so far (from ondansetron) have been mild–moderate constipation, lack of energy and noticed my BP has gone up! However worth the results so far....seen a 25% reduction so far. Mixing with the naltrexone has caused me to feel shaky and very hungover the next day but seems to work well together in regards to consumption. I was on Naltrexone (Sinclair method) for 8 months in 2010 and had a 40% reduction. I was drinking 120+ UK units prior to starting on TSM. I can now add another 25% off this amount but still early days.

•••

I came off ondansetron after about 10 weeks as didn't seem too helpful. My drinking went up. I had constipation but that was expected!

Varenicline

Introduction to Varenicline

Varenicline (known by the brand names Chantix or Champix) has recently received approval in several countries as a smoking cessation aid and now is widely available for prescription on this basis.

Since 2007, there has been a small, but growing collection of research indicating that varenicline may also be helpful to people with alcohol dependence who are trying to reduce drinking and minimize craving for alcohol.

However, because the drug has been studied for such a short time in relation to alcohol dependence, there is not a lot known about its overall effectiveness, nor has there been any research on the relationship between specific genetic variations and their impact on effectiveness of varenicline in people with alcohol dependence.

Because both nicotine and alcohol increase dopamine release in the reward pathway, they may play a synergistic role when taken together. In addition, some of the effects of alcohol in the brain seem to be mediated by the area of the brain which are also responsive to nicotine.

Varenicline has been given a black box warning in the USA related to "changes in behavior, hostility, agitation, depressed mood, suicidal thoughts," so mental health should be carefully monitored for anyone who is taking varenicline. However, since the black box ruling, other studies have refuted any link between varenicline and suicidal behavior.

VARENICLINE MEDICATION FAQ

MEDICATION OVERVIEW

What is the medication called?
Varenicline or Varenicline Tartrate

What are common brand names and generic names for this medication?
Chantix (USA), Champix (Elsewhere), varenicline tartrate

What 'type' of medication is this?
Anti-smoking medication

What is it usually prescribed for?
Nicotinic Agonists / Benzazepines

How is it described?

- Varenicline is an anti-smoking medication which cuts nicotine craving in smokers and appears to reduce alcohol craving in some drinkers as well.

- Varenicline is a nicotinic receptor partial agonist—it stimulates nicotine receptors more weakly than nicotine itself does. This medication is the first approved nicotinic receptor partial agonist.

AVAILABILITY & FDA APPROVAL STATUS

A prescription for alcoholism is usually:
Off-Label

Is it FDA approved in the USA? When?
Yes—FDA Approved in 2006—fast-tracked through approval process

Is it HC approved in Canada? When?
Yes—HC Approved in 2008

Is it EMA approved in Europe? When?

Yes—EMA Approved in 2006

How is it available?

By prescription in USA, Canada and parts of Europe

STRENGTH AND CREDIBILITY OF RESEARCH FOR ITS USE IN ALCOHOLISM

How many years has this medication been researched specifically for the treatment of alcoholism?

8 years (Since 2007)

What is the strength of the supporting research?

A literature review by Erwin and Slaton in 2014 of all (8) trials to date stated, "evidence supports the use of varenicline for the reduction in alcohol craving as well as the reduction of overall alcohol consumption in patients with alcohol use disorders."[353]

What credentials does the researcher making the statements above have?

Dr. RM Slaton Pharm.D., BCPS: Associate Professor of Pharmacy at the McWhorter School of Pharmacy

RESEARCH FINDINGS ABOUT EFFECTIVENESS IN TREATMENT FOR ALCOHOLISM

How many patients need to be treated to see one true medication responder? (Known as the 'Number Needed to Treat–NNT)

The NNT Number for varenicline is unknown. (The NNT number is the number that is treated before it is effective in one individual)

How effective is this medication for the treatment of alcoholism?

- In a study of 200 alcohol-dependent adults, taking varenicline cut heavy drinking days a week by 22%.

- "Varenicline significantly reduced alcohol consumption and craving, making it a potentially viable option for the treatment of alcohol use disorders."[354]

In research, how did this medication compare to other medications for the treatment of alcoholism?

Little comparison has taken place between varenicline and other medications.

TREATMENT CANDIDATES FOR THIS MEDICATION

Note: this section highlights study findings that have identified some characteristics that may increase odds of effectiveness. This does not mean it won't help individuals without these characteristics.

What treatment goals might this medication help achieve?

Reduced alcohol consumption; reduced craving.[354]

What are some typical feelings and motivators of people this medication tends to help?

Research has not yet provided insight on this answer.

Has this medication been shown to be more successful in early-onset or late-onset alcoholics?

Research has not yet provided insight on this answer.

Is this medication typically more effective in people with a strong family history of alcoholism?

Research has not yet provided insight on this answer.

Are there specific genetic markers that have been found to be relevant in treatment with this medication?

Research has not yet provided insight on this answer.

Do Alcoholics Have Difficulty Taking this Medication as Prescribed? (i.e. Are there "Compliance" Issues?)

Inability to tolerate the side effects may lead to discontinuation.

Are there other characteristics (gender, taste sensitivity, alcoholism type, co-morbid disorders, smoker status) that may be related to success with this medication?

May be helpful in heavy-drinking smokers.

DIRECTIONS FOR USE & HOW IT WORKS

At what dose and for how long does research suggest the medication should be taken?

The usually recommended regimen is to start with 0.5 mg once daily and increase to a maintenance dose of 1 mg twice daily, continuing therapy for at least 12 weeks after smoking cessation.

Has this medication been tested with other medications for the treatment of alcoholism and found to be complimentary?

Varenicline and naltrexone have been tested together and found to be complimentary for heavy drinkers trying to quit smoking.[355356]

What is known about how this medication actually works in alcoholics? What is the 'Mechanism of Action'?

Researchers indicate: The alpha-4 beta-2 form of the nicotinic acetylcholine receptor (nAChR) modulates the rewarding effects of alcohol. Varenicline is therefore able to modulate alcohol consumption.[357]

SAFETY CONCERNS

Is this medication addictive? Does it have abuse potential?

Varenicline is non-addictive.

How safe is this medication?

- Studies have shown that varenicline is safe in humans who are using alcohol.[357]

- The research also noted a recent FDA ruling that varenicline carry a black box label for "suicidal ideation and suicidal behavior."[357] (Though since this ruling, other studies have reported that there is no strong evidence linking Varenicline with a higher risk of suicidal behavior[358]).

Can this medication be taken while drinking?

While it is not recommended to take this medication while drinking, it can be taken while the alcohol-dependent individual is still drinking though side-effects if taken while alcohol is in one's system may be enhanced.

What are the expected side effects of this medication?

These include nausea, headache, difficulty sleeping, abnormal dreams.

Where can I find a complete list of all side effects, precautions, and instructions in case of emergency or overdose?

A full listing can be found at the nlm.nih.gov site at:

http://bit.ly/nihvarenicline

What does the National Institute of Health (NIH) say about liver impact and where can I find further information on liver impact of this medication?

- Varenicline undergoes minimal hepatic metabolism and is excreted largely unchanged in the urine. The rare reports of hepatotoxicity attributed to varenicline therapy have been mild and self-limiting. Varenicline has not been linked to cases of acute liver failure, chronic hepatitis or vanishing bile duct syndrome.

- Also see the livertox.nlm.nih.gov link at:

http://bit.ly/livertoxvarenicline

What known drug interactions should I watch for and where can I find more information on drug interactions?

- Not known to interact with other drugs in the alcohol treatment medications database. Known to interact with at least 7 other drugs.

- Also see the drugs.com interaction checker at:

http://bit.ly/interactvaren

Where can I find alerts and Black Box Warnings? (Black Box Warnings are cautions affixed to medications by the government)

Visit the nlm.nih.gov site at:

http://bit.ly/nihvarenicline

Were there any known black box warnings at the time this book was written?

Yes. Relates to changes in behavior, hostility, agitation, depressed mood, suicidal thoughts. Relates to mental illness.

OTHER USEFUL INFORMATION

Note: Links to all recommended information sources can be found on the book's website at APrescriptionForAlcoholics.com

Recent Research:

- 2014: Varenicline in the Treatment of Alcohol Use Disorders[353]

- 2014: Varenicline Effects on Drinking, Craving and Neural Reward Processing among non-treatment-seeking alcohol-dependent individuals[359]

- 2013: A Double-Blind, Placebo-Controlled Trial Assessing the Efficacy of Varenicline Tartrate for Alcohol Dependence[354]

CONNECTING WITH OTHERS

Online Forum(s):

- The 'MyWayOut' community started out focused on topiramate but is now a good place to read about and connect with others regarding a variety of medications for the treatment of alcoholism.

- Visit MyWayOut at:

http://bit.ly/mywayoutforum

- A link to Google search results for a search within the MyWayOut forum for this specific medication:

http://bit.ly/mywayvaren

Reviews from others on Drugs.com:

- Not Specifically for Alcoholism:

http://bit.ly/drugcomvaren

Reviews from others on WebMD:

- Generic reviews (not specifically for alcoholism–for smoking cessation):

http://bit.ly/webmdvaren

- Brand name reviews (not specifically for alcoholism–for smoking cessation):

http://bit.ly/webmdvarenbrand

Generic Wikipedia Link:

http://bit.ly/wikivarenicline

DrugBank.ca Link (Detailed Drug Data Including Pricing):

http://bit.ly/drugbankvaren

SIGNIFICANT VARENICLINE RESEARCH & FINDINGS

2015–Vatsalya–International Journal of Neuropsychopharmacology
Effects of Varenicline on Neural Correlates of Alcohol Salience in Heavy Drinkers

---

- Research using MRI scans show that varenicline decreases blood oxygen level-dependent activation in parts of the brain associated with motivation and craving for alcohol in heavy drinkers.[360]

2014–Ray–The American Journal of Drug and Alcohol Abuse
Varenicline, naltrexone, and their combination for heavy-drinking smokers:
Preliminary neuroimaging findings.

- This study tested varenicline alone and with naltrexone on heavy drinking smokers.

- It found that "neuroimaging findings indicate that clinical studies of the combination of varenicline and naltrexone for heavy drinkers trying to quit smoking may be warranted."[355356]

2014–B. L. Erwin–Annals of Pharmacotherapy
Varenicline in the Treatment of Alcohol Use Disorders

- In a literature search looking at 7 randomized, placebo-controlled clinical trials and 1 open-label study the report concluded that "evidence supports the use of varenicline for the reduction of alcohol craving as well as for the reduction of overall alcohol consumption in patients with alcohol use disorders."

- In regards to the goal of complete abstinence the search concluded that varenicline was unlikely to improve abstinence rates.[353]

> **2014–Schacht–Psychopharmacology**
> **Varenicline Effects on Drinking, Craving and Neural Reward Processing among Non-Treatment-Seeking Alcohol-Dependent Individuals**

- In a pilot study testing varenicline's effects on drinking, alcohol craving, and alcohol cue-elicited activation, data indicated that varenicline reduces alcohol craving, increasing self-reported control over alcohol-related thoughts and reducing cue-elicited activation in some areas of the brain.[359]

> **2014–Wackernah–Substance abuse and rehabilitation**
> **Alcohol Use Disorder: Pathophysiology, Effects, and Pharmacologic Options for Treatment**

- "Varenicline is a nicotine agonist used for smoking cessation. Varenicline reduced number of drinks consumed, abstinence, and craving after a priming drink in a 2-hour session in smokers with AUD (Alcohol Use Disorder)."[192]

- "It also reduced number of drinks per week and craving in a 16-week trial, but did not have an effect on total days abstinent."[192]

> **2014–Haass-Koffler–CNS Drugs**
> **Pharmacological Approaches to Reducing Craving in Patients with Alcohol Use Disorders**

- A research review found that "varenicline has been shown to have beneficial effects in preclinical craving models in reducing cue-induced ethanol relapses."

- It cited several studies that showed that following the effect of a priming dose of alcohol, "varenicline attenuated alcohol craving and reduced subjective reinforcing alcohol effects."

- In another study patients, "reported less craving than the placebo group."

- In a third study of alcohol-dependent patients, those taking varenicline reported a significantly lower alcohol craving."[47]

2013–Litten–Journal of addiction medicine
A Double-Blind, Placebo-Controlled Trial Assessing the Efficacy of Varenicline Tartrate for Alcohol Dependence

---

- In a study of 200 alcohol-dependent adults, taking varenicline cut heavy drinking days a week by 22%.

- "Varenicline significantly reduced alcohol consumption and craving, making it a potentially viable option for the treatment of alcohol use disorders."[354]

2012–Mitchell–Psychopharmacology
Varenicline Decreases Alcohol Consumption in Heavy-Drinking Smokers

---

- Mitchell's research found that varenicline significantly decreased alcohol consumption in smokers.[357]

- Mitchell also cited previous studies showing that varenicline is safe in humans who are using alcohol.[357]

- The research also noted a recent FDA ruling that varenicline carry a black box label for "suicidal ideation and suicidal behavior."[357] (Though since this ruling, other studies have reported that there is no strong evidence linking Varenicline with a higher risk of suicidal behavior[358]).

2011–Fucito–Psychopharmacology
A Preliminary Investigation of Varenicline for Heavy Drinking Smokers

---

- Fucito's study found that "varenicline may be a promising strategy for concurrently reducing heavy drinking and promoting smoking changes in heavy drinker."[361]

2009–McKee–Biological Psychiatry
Varenicline Reduces Alcohol Self-Administration in Heavy-Drinking Smokers

---

- The study found that "varenicline significantly reduced alcohol self-administration and was well tolerated, alone and in combination with alcohol in heavy-drinking smokers."[362]

> ### 2007–Steensland–PNAS
> #### Varenicline, an alpha4beta2 Nicotinic Acetylcholine Receptor Partial Agonist, Selectively Decreases Ethanol Consumption and Seeking

- Varenicline reduces both nicotine reward and ethanol seeking and consumption in rodent models.[363]

PERSONAL EXPERIENCES WITH VARENICLINE

I just have to share my experience taking varenicline. I have read some horror stories so I wanted to make sure people know that there are some amazing benefits (at least in my experience).

The results from taking the Rx for 3 weeks has had a life-changing impact on virtually every aspect of my life. Admittedly, I had a serious smoking problem 20 years pack and a half and 2-3 packs when heavily drinking. I have also struggled with alcoholism for many years. It was only in the last few years that I would admit that. I tried to moderate without any success. I would be ?good? For a few days and just have a couple, then it would be back to the same drunk/hung-over cycle.

Anyway, after losing my job I now have the time to work on reinventing myself without the cigs and the booze.

Here is my experience- After a week I cut down to less than 10 cigs a day and strangely enough did not crave any alcohol. Out of habit, I would pour myself a glass of wine or make a cocktail, only to find that I had much less interest. I would have a maximum of 2 glasses if any wine at all. After the second and third week, I started to feel completely in control of the alcohol thing. I would stop after 2 not because I had to, but because I felt I had enough (like normal people). Anyway, I am just blown away that someone as dedicated to drinking 1-2 bottles of wine is now a successful moderator ... There have been other areas that varenicline has helped improve- Slight weight loss (always helps), more energy (maybe from not smoking 2 packs a day- but who cares), a resounding positivity for life (despite losing my job and all my other worries, it has acted as an antidepressant even though it is not classified as one!). Anyway- God bless and I am anxious to hear if anyone else has had similar experiences!

•••

Varenicline has helped me stop smoking and moderate my drinking as well. I've been on varenicline for about 6 weeks now and quit smoking Jan 1st. I have only had one night of going out and drinking too much. I've had about half a dozen days this month where I've had one or two drinks(yep, one or two, that's it). The majority of the month has been AF.

I have had an open bottle of wine in my fridge for 2 weeks now. I don't think that has ever happened before!

I never had any side effects from the drug except some pretty vivid dreams the first couple weeks. I'm very very happy with the results.

•••

I was up at the crack of dawn and doing doing doing. By 11am every morning I was knackered and had already done all the things it would normally take me a week to do and worst of all as I was doing it I was singing with joy. I didn't have any desire to smoke or drink so it wasn't difficult for me and I had never managed to go AF or NF before for more than 3 days so I wasn't complaining. It definitely strongly interferes with the brain and I was only on the lowest dose so I came off it after a month but only once I knew I could go cold turkey on the evil twins Alco and Nico. Hope it works for you too but do be careful if you go up to the next dose and make sure someone knows about it just in case of any downward mood swings.

Disulfiram

Introduction to Disulfiram

Disulfiram gained FDA approval in 1951.[7] For many years disulfiram was the only medication available to aid sobriety[41], and for many doctors, this may be the only drug they have ever heard of or prescribed for this purpose.

However, just because disulfiram is FDA-approved and was the first drug available for this purpose, does not mean it is an appropriate drug for many individuals with alcohol dependence.

On the contrary, disulfiram is very limited in its application and can have some extremely dangerous effects, including death.

Disulfiram is different than all of the other medications in this book because it acts solely as an alcohol deterrent (it does not counter any of the neural drivers of alcohol dependence such as craving or imbalances in systems in the brain).

If disulfiram is in your system and you drink, you will experience debilitating and potentially life-threatening symptoms such as flushing, shortness of breath, tachycardia, headache, nausea, and vomiting. This is the deterrent effect.

I debated whether to include disulfiram in this book because the idea of a medication inflicting punishment is not an approach that I personally like. And while disulfiram was FDA-approved many years ago, more recent research indicates that the drug has lost favor.

In fact, while it is currently widely thought that the medication is still approved in Canada by clinicians that know of it and prescribe it, at some point (as confirmed by a 2012 BC Medical Journal piece), it was removed from health Canada's list of approved medications—possibly as long ago as 2001.[364]

Some researchers have come to the conclusion that it is an outmoded treatment.

Heilig states for example that, "Disulfiram reduces alcohol drinking by severely punishing drinking bouts. For optimal efficacy, punishment must be applied severely and consistently. Taking this to a logical, but undesirable extreme, it could be more effective and safe to use a biosensor and an electric shock generator."[1]

And researcher Michael Soyka simply states that "at present, this treatment cannot be recommended.[41]

Based on this research evidence and disulfiram's seemingly inhuman approach, I developed a negative opinion about disulfiram.

However, once I began to read the comments of individuals who find disulfiram helpful, I realized that even disulfiram has a place in treatment for some people, and perhaps one of those people is you.

Because one of the intentions of this book is not to make a treatment decision for you but to provide you with the tools and information needed around medications so that you can make your own informed decisions, disulfiram was included in the book.

Disulfiram blocks the enzyme aldehyde dehydrogenase, leading to an accumulation of acetaldehyde following intake of alcohol. This, in turn, is what causes the adverse symptoms someone who is trying to 'drink through the disulfiram' will feel. The idea is that the anticipation of these symptoms will help patients choose not to drink.

Disulfiram also inhibits the brain dopamine beta-hydroxylase (DBH), augmenting dopamine. And as with many other medications, there are genetic relationships between disulfiram's effectiveness in specific individuals.

In the case of disulfiram, a 2012 study found that a specific polymorphism of the beta-hydroxylase gene increases the risk of adverse effects in alcohol-dependent patients taking disulfiram.[365]

Results with disulfiram are very patient-specific. For example, for some patients who are extremely committed, welcome supervision, retain some control over their drinking and fear a future temptation (such as attending a social event where they which will trigger a strong desire to drink), disulfiram can be a helpful tool.

Other individuals who are unable to abstain despite taking the medication might be strongly tempted to begin drinking before the medication leaves their system, risking serious medical consequences including death.

Alcoholism is, after all, a disease defined by the alcoholic's continued drinking in the face of severely negative consequences. And alcoholism damages circuits in the brain needed to make seemingly rational decisions. So it is not surprising that these same mechanisms emerge even when an alcoholic has a potentially lethal drug like disulfiram in their system.

Because of the risks of disulfiram, it is sometimes difficult to obtain even in places where it is approved for use. This is a medication that can be obtained via prescription by pharmacies, but sometimes the only place it is available is from a compounding pharmacy (a pharmacy that mixes individual ingredients together to personalize a medication).

As of writing, it is possible to obtain a doctor's prescription for disulfiram in Canada and also for compounding Canadian pharmacies to provide the medication to its customers.

There have been quite a number of research reports on disulfiram over the last twenty decades that cast considerable doubt upon its effectiveness.

According to Markus Heilig: Hester & Miller (2003) concluded that evidence for disulfiram's effectiveness was lacking and Berglund et al. (2003) also found that evidence for efficacy of disulfiram is lacking overall.[1]

Chick et all (1992), Huges and Cook (1997) and Garbutt et al. (1999) all found that data was mixed. In fact, Garbutt et al. found that not only was evidence for disulfiram's effectiveness inconsistent but that there is often significant negative evidence on measures such as relapse.[1]

Heilig also notes that in the largest placebo-controlled study of disulfiram, the study was unable to show that disulfiram had any effect on the likelihood of abstinence over a 1-year treatment period.

It's possible that one of the reasons that research outcomes for disulfiram is so dismal is because it is being measured against the potential of long-term abstinence.

Maybe that is the wrong goal for users of disulfiram because when measured against this bar, disulfiram does not fare well.

However, it is possible that if disulfiram was measured against a different goal, its usefulness would be more clear.

For example, if disulfiram was measured as a medication that was intended for occasional use by highly motivated, non-severe alcoholics on an 'as needed to abstain' basis, perhaps results would be successful.

Adherence and Supervision

Not surprisingly, poor adherence is a major problem with disulfiram treatment and it has been shown that most patients stop treatment within a few months.[41]

Some individuals and their caregivers are able to put systems in place that address the adherence issues—mainly a system that involves supervision.

An extensive review of 13 controlled and five uncontrolled studies of the medication concluded that "supervised disulfiram reduced drinking and improved the rate of retention in treatment compared with unsupervised disulfiram or a no-disulfiram control group."[41]

However, as soon as supervision ends there is little evidence that behavior modification remains.

To 'supervise' adherence to disulfiram, the tablets should be crushed and well mixed with water or another liquid.

There are reports that some individuals who have taken disulfiram this way will throw up to try to remove some of the substance from their system so where a supervised system is in place, one may need to be carefully monitored even after ingesting the medication.

One way to test compliance is the use of a hand-held breath analyzer. Zenics Medical developed the 'Zenalyser' which analyzes breath samples for the concentration of carbon disulphide and acetone produced from metabolism of disulfiram.[366]

To get around the 'supervision' barrier, some long-lasting, implantable formulations of disulfiram have been developed. However there are few studies of this approach and a placebo-controlled trial in 1991 by Johnsen and Morland failed to show its effectiveness.

Who Disulfiram May Help

Those that disulfiram may be helpful for fall within the following criteria and circumstances:

- Those with the motivation and who retain enough control to take a pill either daily or as needed;

- Individuals who opt to use disulfiram without influence or duress from others (if others make a decision that enforces the medication on someone else this can result in negative consequences);

- For someone who recognizes a period of stress or temptation ahead (i.e. attendance at a wedding or business conference; an especially stressful period to get through; or other temptation-laden circumstances where supplementary help is useful);

- For someone who suffers from a lot of mental obsession and debate around drinking (if disulfiram is in one's system it can lessen this internal debate since consequences of drinking once it's in one's system are so negative);

- For someone who welcomes supervision and has a strong third party to supervise (such as a family member or outpatient clinic that is committed to supervision. Though this can be a heavy burden for family to take on.)

- In combination with other strong supports (from friends, community, employer, family, physician, psychological counseling methods, or other non-conflicting medications for the treatment of alcohol dependence).

Who Disulfiram May NOT Help

Disulfiram may NOT be a useful tool for individuals in the following circumstances:

- Not for someone who may seek to 'game' disulfiram (i.e. experiment with drinking alcohol while it's still in ones' system, or not waiting the full recommended amount of time before it has left one's system before drinking);

- Not for someone who does not choose to take it themselves (i.e. someone who is mandated or 'forced' to take it);

- May not be as safe for very severe alcoholics who have already been seen to drink despite very negative consequences (including health threats);

- May not be safe for individuals with existing health concerns (e.g. heart disease, existing liver concerns or taking conflicting medications);

- Never give it to someone unknowingly or who already has alcohol in their system (could lead to severe consequences including death).

DISULFIRAM MEDICATION FAQ

MEDICATION OVERVIEW

What is the medication called?
Disulfiram

What are common brand names and generic names for this medication?
Antabuse, Antabus (similar to Calcium carbimide, temposil)

What is it usually prescribed for?
Enzyme Inhibitors, Alcohol Deterrents / Thiocarbonyl Compounds

How is it described?

- A carbamate derivative used as an alcohol deterrent. When alcohol is ingested after administration of disulfiram, blood acetaldehyde concentrations are increased, followed by flushing, systemic vasodilation, respiratory difficulties, nausea, hypotension, and other symptoms (acetaldehyde syndrome).

- Disulfiram causes a buildup of acetaldehyde five or 10 times greater than normally occurs when someone drinks alcohol. It causes unpleasant effects if you drink even small amounts of alcohol such as flushing, headache, nausea and vomiting. It begins to affect alcohol metabolism within 1-2 hours and reaches a peak in 12 hours. It is slowly excreted from the body over 2 weeks.

AVAILABILITY & FDA APPROVAL STATUS

A prescription for alcoholism is usually:
On-Label

Is it FDA approved in the USA? When?
FDA-Approved in the USA since 1995

Is it HC approved in Canada? When?

Unclear when it was approved; discontinued by Health Canada as of 2001

Is it EMA approved in Europe? When?

Yes—EMA Approved, date unknown

How is it available?

By prescription in the USA, parts of Europe, and Canada (despite the loss of Health Canada approval); may be available in Canada via compounding pharmacies.

TREATMENT CANDIDATES FOR THIS MEDICATION

Note: this section highlights study findings that have identified some characteristics that may increase odds of effectiveness. This does not mean it won't help individuals without these characteristics.

What treatment goals might this medication help achieve?

Short-term complete abstinence on a situation by situation basis

What are some typical feelings and motivators of people this medication tends to help?

Those with high motivation to stop drinking who welcome a deterrent approach.

Has this medication been shown to be more successful in early-onset or late-onset alcoholics?

Effectiveness not related to early or late onset of alcoholism

Is this medication typically more effective in people with a strong family history of alcoholism?

Effectiveness not related to genetic linkage.

Are there specific genetic markers that have been found to be relevant in treatment with this medication?

It has been found that a specific polymorphism of the beta-hydroxylase gene increases the risk of adverse effects in alcohol-dependent patients taking disulfiram.

Do Alcoholics Have Difficulty Taking this Medication as Prescribed? (i.e. Are there "Compliance" Issues?)

- Yes–there are considerable compliance issues with this medication, as taking disulfiram has no impact on any of the elements of the disease that lead to drinking such as craving.

- There may be fewer compliance issues with less severe alcoholics that retain some control over relapse, especially with other strong supports (such as family, friends, community, other medications, active supervision).

DIRECTIONS FOR USE & HOW IT WORKS

At what dose and for how long does research suggest the medication should be taken?

The recommended starting dose is 500 mg once daily for 1-2 weeks, followed by a maintenance dose of 125 to 500 mg daily.

Has this medication been tested with other medications for the treatment of alcoholism and found to be complimentary?

- There has been interest in combining disulfiram with naltrexone, acamprosate, and sodium oxybate as decreasing craving might allow for better adherence to treatment.[367]

- Landabaso found that treatment with a combination of disulfiram and naltrexone (daily dose) resulted in superior abstinence rates after 1 and 2 years compared to disulfiram alone.[367]

- Petrakis found there was no advantage in combining disulfiram with naltrexone.[367]

- Besson combined disulfiram with acamprosate and found the combination to be superior to either medication alone in respect to the duration of abstinence and relapse rate. [367]

- A trial that combined disulfiram with sodium oxybate resulted in reduced relapse rates and increased days of abstinence and treatment adherence. [367]

SAFETY CONCERNS

Is this medication addictive? Does it have abuse potential?

Disulfiram is completely non-addictive.s

How safe is this medication?

- Serious safety concerns exist around disulfiram, particularly where there is a risk of drinking with disulfiram. Disulfiram has caused death when combined with alcohol.

- Similar to a potentially lethal food allergy, individuals close to the alcoholic (for example, family or anyone administering medication or providing food, beverages to the alcohol) should be informed that the alcoholic is taking disulfiram and of the consequences of combining alcohol with disulfiram.

Can this medication be taken while drinking?

Warning: NEVER take disulfiram while drinking or if there is potential for alcohol to still be in ones' system.

What are other common side effects?

Skin rash, headache, drowsiness, weakness, upset stomach, tiredness.

Where can I find a complete list of all side effects, precautions, and instructions in case of emergency or overdose?

You can find this on the US National Library of Medicine website. Search google for 'disulfiram and National Library of Medicine' or visit:

http://bit.ly/disulfiram

What does the National Institute of Health (NIH) say about liver impact and where can I find further information on liver impact of this medication?

- Disulfiram has been associated with a low rate of with serum aminotransferase elevations during chronic therapy and has been linked to clinical apparent acute liver injury which can be severe and result in fatality.

- The severity of liver injury associated with disulfiram can range from asymptomatic elevations in serum aminotransferase levels, to symptomatic liver injury with jaundice, to acute liver failure and death.

- Also see the livertox.nlm.nih.gov website:

    http://bit.ly/livertoxdisulfiram

What known drug interactions should I watch for and where can I find more information on drug interactions?

- There are moderate interaction between disulfiram and naltrexone. Major interaction between disulfiram and alcohol. Known to interact with at least 228 other drugs.

- Also see the drugs.com interaction checker at:

    http://bit.ly/interactiondisulf

Where can I find alerts and Black Box Warnings? (Black Box Warnings are cautions affixed to medications by the government)
Visit:

    http://bit.ly/disulfiram

Were there any known black box warnings at the time this book was written?
Yes. Disulfiram should never be administered to a patient who is in a state of alcohol intoxication or without the patient's full knowledge. The physician should instruct relatives accordingly.

CONNECTING WITH OTHERS

Online Forum(s):

- The 'MyWayOut' community started out focused on topiramate but is now a good place to read about and connect with others regarding a variety of medications for the treatment of alcoholism.

- Visit MyWayOut at:

  http://bit.ly/mywayoutforum

- A link to Google search results for a search within the MyWayOut forum for this specific medication:

  http://bit.ly/mywaydisulfiram

Reviews from others on Drugs.com:

Reviews for generic:

http://bit.ly/drugsdisulfiram

Reviews for branded version:

http://bit.ly/drugsantabuse

Reviews from others on WebMD:

Reviews for generic:

http://bit.ly/webmddisulf

Reviews for branded version:

http://bit.ly/webmdantabuse

Generic Wikipedia Link:

http://bit.ly/wikidisulfiram

DrugBank.ca Link (Detailed Drug Data Including Pricing):

http://bit.ly/drugbankdisulf

PERSONAL EXPERIENCES WITH DISULFIRAM

I don't know of too many people on disulfiram that didn't drink on it. When I was on it I could drink one beer before I started feeling the ill effects and they were enough to keep me from drinking the second beer. Sometimes! The ill effects only lasted about an hour and were limited to hot flashes. I do mean hot too. I felt like my face was going to spontaneously combust at any minute. They recommend 4 days off before you can drink again but I tried sooner. Days one and two weren't enough but I could bear it at three days.

That's just my personal story but I would not recommend drinking on it...

I personally can't believe the stuff is available on the market because any alcoholic will try drinking on it with almost no exceptions.

•••

I would wait out the four/five days, but I always knew where the nearest ER was. What a way to live—counting the moments. I am against this drug as it can be lethal. This is truly when the cure is worse than the sickness. At any rate, it might work for some, but the risks are very real.

•••

I take disulfiram now. Other than an occasional headache(which may not be related to the drug at all) I've experienced no side effects. I have to watch the foods that I eat and avoid caffeine(it can heighten the effects of caffeine). Basically, I eat a lot healthier in the result. I was never a morning drinker so it's been very easy for me just to take the pill with my a.m. vitamins and remove the drinking option from the day. Odd thing that I have the discipline to take a pill every day but not the discipline to drink in moderation. I don't really have cravings but I do get the occasional inner thought "Wouldn't it be nice to have a....wait I can't ...so, I won't."

I use my formerly bar time to exercise, read, focus more on my business, etc. I did a lot if research on it before asking my doctor to prescribe it for me. I know the risks if drinking on it and have no intentions on experimenting. I want to quit ..why would I experiment? Any relapse is premeditated and it can stay in your system for up to two weeks, so it gives you ample time to rethink your relapse I'm certain that had I been forced to take against my will then I would have been consumed with figuring out how to work around the pill. That wasn't my case, I talked it over with my doctor in great depth before we reached the agreement for my prescription. Committed to blood work every few weeks and to monitor my BP. So far, it's working for me.

•••

My brother died as a result of taking Disulfiram and drinking a couple of weeks ago. He was an alcoholic and I'm sure his liver had some damage, but he was physically healthy otherwise—exercised daily and watched what he ate. He went to AA daily and was really trying to overcome his alcoholism. Giving a drug that will kill a person if he drinks to an alcoholic seems to me to be unbelievably irresponsible—why would any doctor ever prescribe this.

•••

Well, I love disulfiram, but I have to take a high dose for it to work, which makes me lethargic. its another tool in my toolbox that helps keep me sober. It stops the mental obsession, because I know I can't drink. There is no "will I or won't I". I won't. I had a client who died drinking on it. I find it helpful. I'm surprised it has such a bad rap... But each to their own. If I took a daily standard dose I can drink on it and not get sick. However, for people who repetitively do that you can get toxicity which damages body organs. If I don't have the mental obsession, I can deal with any physical cravings.

•••

It is true that if someone is hellbent on drinking no matter what, they'll still try to do it on disulfiram and possibly risk their life. I take it precisely because I know I want to quit forever and would not even risk a single sip of alcohol while taking it. Not a chance! Even if all it did was make me puke, that would be enough to keep me away from booze. For me, it works as an excellent insurance policy.

PRAZOSIN & DOXAZOSIN

INTRODUCTION TO PRAZOSIN & DOXAZOSIN

Prazosin is an alpha 1-receptor adrenergic blocker that is used for the treatment of hypertension and noncancerous enlargement of the prostate gland.

It causes blood vessels and muscles to relax.

It is also used to treat anxiety, post-traumatic stress disorder (PTSD) and panic disorder.

It is marketed under the name Minipress by Pfizer and has been FDA-approved since 1976.

Doxazosin (marketed as Cardura and FDA-approved in 1990) is also an alpha adrenergic receptor blocker.

The key difference in these medications is related to their bioavailability—or basically, how long they take to begin working and how long their effects last in ones' system.

For example, prazosin lasts for 4-6 hours, so it is taken twice a day; whereas doxazosin lasts over 36 hours so it can be taken less frequently. Both medications are commonly prescribed by physicians.

The brain's norepinephrine system has been identified as a system involved in alcohol dependence, contributing to withdrawal-induced negative emotional states which contribute to withdrawal-related relapse.[368]

As Prazosin and Doxazosin impact the norepinephrine system, recently there has been some promising research testing their treatment on subjects with alcoholism and additional clinical testing is underway.

As with sertraline, recent research for doxazosin illustrated that doxazosin (and possibly prazosin) may have extremely different effects on people with alcohol dependence based on their family history of alcoholism.

In a double-blind placebo-controlled randomized clinical trial of 41 individuals, FDA-approved Doxazosin was shown to result in "significantly reduced alcohol drinking" in alcohol-dependent patients with a high family history of alcoholism (Type B).[183]

This contrasted with the results from alcoholics with only minimal family history of alcoholism (Type A)–who saw an increase in drinking with doxazosin treatment.[183] For this reason, doxazosin and prazosin also appear on the D-List in the book.

In regards to drug combinations, one study found that combining both prazosin and naltrexone in treatment with rats was more effective than either medication independently.[280]

Another rat study found that combining prazosin and propranolol suppressed alcohol drinking during withdrawal and prolonged abstinence more than either individually.[369]

Phase 2 trials NCT02492334 and NCT02500602 (which have not yet begun recruitment) will test doxazosin's ability to reduce PTSD symptomatology and alcohol use severity.

Several other trials are currently recruiting or underway for doxazosin's impact on other substance use disorders.

Significant Prazosin & Doxazosin
Research & Findings

2015–Kenna–Addiction Biology
Role of the alpha-1 Blocker Doxazosin in Alcoholism: A Proof-of-Concept Randomized Controlled Trial

- Kenna identified that doxazosin has greater bioavailability than prazosin, but had not been studied previously for alcohol dependence.

- Patients with alcohol dependence who took a dose of 16 mg/day (or a maximum tolerable dose) saw a significant reduction in drinking if they had a strong family history of alcoholism; in contrast, those without a family history experienced increased drinking levels.

- As with other recent studies illustrating substantial differences in responses to medication based on genetic markers, Kenna concluded that personalized approaches to medication (i.e. Based on genetic markers and traits for example) were highly significant to treatment outcome.[183]

2015–Simpson–Alcoholism, clinical and experimental research
A Pilot Trial of Prazosin, an Alpha-1 Adrenergic Antagonist, for Comorbid Alcohol Dependence and Posttraumatic Stress Disorder

- In individuals with both PTSD and alcohol dependence, it was shown that "Participants randomized to prazosin had a greater reduction in percent days drinking per week and percent days heavy drinking per week between baseline and week 6 than did placebo participants…"[370]

2015–Verplaetse–Psychopharmacology
Low-Dose Prazosin Alone and in Combination with Propranolol or Naltrexone: Effects on Ethanol and Sucrose Seeking and Self-Administration in the P Rat

- In rats, it was found that "prazosin in combination with propranolol or naltrexone was more effective than either drug alone."[280]

> **2014–Meinhardt–Addiction Biology**
> The Postdependent State in Rats as a Model for Medication Development in Alcoholism

- Meinhardt found that "prazosin can reduce the number of drinking days in alcoholic patients."[371]

> **2014–Rasmussen–Alcohol Clinical Exp**
> Combining the alpha-1 adrenergic receptor antagonist, prazosin, with the β adrenergic receptor antagonist, propranolol, reduces alcohol drinking more effectively than either drug alone

- In rats, "alcohol drinking following propranolol treatment was variable, but the combination of propranolol + prazosin consistently suppressed alcohol drinking during both alcohol withdrawal and following prolonged imposed abstinence, and the combination of these 2 drugs was more effective than was treatment with either drug alone."[369]

> **2014–Wackernah–Substance Abuse and Rehabilitation**
> Alcohol Use Disorder: Pathophysiology, Effects, and Pharmacologic Options for Treatment

- Wackernah summarized: "Prazosin is an alpha 1-receptor adrenergic blocker that is used for the treatment of hypertension. At a titrated target dose of 16 mg daily, prazosin has been shown to reduce stress-induced craving, drinks per weeks, and drinking days. Simpson et al. did not see a reduction in craving, though craving was not stress elicited."[192]

> **2013–Froehlich–Alcoholism, Clinical and Experimental Research**
> Prazosin Reduces Alcohol Drinking throughout Prolonged Treatment and Blocks the Initiation of Drinking in Rats Selectively Bred for High Alcohol Intake

- In rats, Froehlich found that prazosin reduced alcohol drinking and that following termination of prazosin treatment, alcohol drinking slowly returned to baseline. Also, "prazosin retained the ability to reduce alcohol intake with repeated treatments."

- Froehlich concluded that "prazosin may also be useful for deterring the initiation of drinking in individuals with a family history of alcoholism."[372]

**2009–Rasmussen–Alcoholism: Clinical and Experimental Research
The alpha-1-Adrenergic Receptor Antagonist, Prazosin, Reduces Alcohol Drinking in Alcohol-Preferring (P) Rats**

Rasmussen's early findings showed that "the noradrenergic system plays a role in mediating alcohol drinking in rats of the P line and suggest that prazosin-a safe, well-characterized, and well-tolerated drug may be an effective pharmacotherapeutic agent for the treatment of alcohol use disorders."[373]

ZONISAMIDE

INTRODUCTION TO ZONISAMIDE

Zonisamide, like topiramate, is a carbonic anhydrase inhibitor (anti-convulsant), often prescribed for the treatment of seizures. It first became available in Japan in 1989 and then achieved FDA approval in the USA in 2000.

Dr. Clifford M. Knapp of Carnegie Mellon University first reported in 2007 that zonisamide was able to reduce alcohol consumption in mice and rats.[374]

As it is a relatively new drug it has not yet been robustly studied, though initial research in humans looks promising.

Most recent research by Dr. Knapp showed that in a double-blind placebo-controlled clinical trial with 85 participants, "both zonisamide and topiramate produced significant reductions in drinks consumed per day, percent days drinking, and percent days heavy drinking …. These findings indicate that zonisamide may have efficacy in the treatment of alcohol dependence with effect sizes similar to topiramate."[255]

Side effects of zonisamide include kidney stones, drowsiness, ataxia (uncoordinated movements), loss of appetite and gastrointestinal upset.

SIGNIFICANT ZONISAMIDE RESEARCH &

FINDINGS

2015–Knapp–Journal of Clinical Psychopharmacology
Zonisamide, Topiramate, and Levetiracetam

- Knapp reported that in a double-blind placebo-controlled clinical trial with 85 participants, "both zonisamide and topiramate produced significant reductions in drinks consumed per day, percent days drinking, and percent days heavy drinking …. These findings indicate that zonisamide may have efficacy in the treatment of alcohol dependence with effect sizes similar to topiramate."[255]

2014–Wackernah–Substance abuse and rehabilitation
Alcohol Use Disorder: Pathophysiology, Effects, and Pharmacologic Options for Treatment.

- Wackernah states, "Zonisamide was significantly better than placebo in reducing number of heavy drinking days, reduction in number of drinks per week, and urge to drink".[192]

2010–Knapp–American Journal of Drug and Alcohol Abuse
Open Label Trial of the Tolerability and Efficacy of Zonisamide in the Treatment of Alcohol Dependence

---

- In a study assessing the tolerability and efficacy of zonisamide, Knapp found that zonisamide may not impair verbal fluency (as topiramate can) and may reduce alcohol intake.[375]

2010–Arias–Journal of Clinical Psychopharmacology
Placebo-Controlled Trial of Zonisamide for the Treatment of Alcohol Dependence

---

- In a placebo-controlled double-blind trial with 40 subjects assessing zonisamide for safety, tolerability and efficacy for the treatment of alcohol dependence, Arias concluded that there were no adverse events reported and that zonisamide treatment was well tolerated. Zonisamide reduced heavy drinking days, drinks per week and alcohol urge scores. It did not impact the number or rate of days of abstinence.[376]

2010–Rubio–Clinical Neuropharmacology
Effects of Zonisamide in the Treatment of Alcohol Dependence

- In 22 outpatients with alcohol dependence, zonisamide was started at a dose of 50 mg/d and titrated to the maximum dose of 30 mg/day. Rubio found "significant improvement was observed in visual analog scale for craving severity scores, weekly drink consumption, and y-glutamyltransferase." Zonisamide was well tolerated and safe.[377]

2009–Sarid-Segal–American Journal of Drug and Alcohol Abuse
The Anticonvulsant Zonisamide Reduces Ethanol Self-Administration by Risky Drinkers

---

- A double-blind, placebo-controlled study of the effects of 100mg of zonisamide on risky drinkers found that in the second hour of a 2-hour self-administration session alcohol consumption was 50% lower in the zonisamide group compared to the placebo group. Urge to drink was significantly lowered even under a single dose.[378]

2007–Knapp–Pharmacology, Biochemistry, and Behavior
Zonisamide Decreases Ethanol Intake in Rats and Mice

Zonisamide was found to reduce alcohol consumption in mice and rats.[374]

OLANZAPINE

INTRODUCTION TO OLANZAPINE

Olanzapine (marketed as Zyprexa) is an atypical antipsychotic used to treat certain mental illnesses and conditions such as schizophrenia and bipolar disorder.

It may be used in combination with other medication to treat depression.

Olanzapine is FDA-approved, but not for the treatment of alcohol use disorder.

There are some studies which indicate effectiveness in some individuals with alcohol dependence. Hutchinson's work has shown a strong connection with specific genetic markers and effectiveness for the treatment of alcoholism with olanzapine.

Alkermes is currently testing a combination of olanzapine with samidorphan (also reported to decrease drinking) for the treatment of schizophrenia and has reported good results in Phase 2 clinical trials.[379]

Alkermes reports that "ALKS 3831 is designed to offer the efficacy benefits of olanzapine while attenuating the significant weight gain frequently associated with its use."[379]

SIGNIFICANT OLANZAPINE RESEARCH FINDINGS

2014–Littlewood–Psychopharmacology
Dose-Specific Effects of Olanzapine in the Treatment of Alcohol Dependence

- Littlewood's study looked at 129 treatment-seeking alcohol-dependent adults over a 12-week period.

- Results showed that, in comparison to placebo, "participants in the 5 mg group experienced reduced craving for alcohol and participants in the 2.5 mg group decreased in the proportion of drinking days to total days in treatment (PDD) and increased in their control over alcohol use."

- The study found that, "Better control over alcohol use remained significant 6 months post-treatment for the 2.5 mg group. Subjective experiences of the medication suggest that 2.5 and 5 mg were equally well tolerated…"[380]

2014–Wackernah–Substance abuse and rehabilitation
Alcohol Use Disorder: Pathophysiology, Effects, and Pharmacologic Options for Treatment

- Wackernah found that "Olanzapine reduced alcohol cravings in young adult subjects (23 years average age) and reduced the number of drinks per day in AUD [Alcohol Use Disorder or alcoholic] patients with higher baseline drinking habits, but only in individuals with the long version of the D4 dopamine receptor gene (DRD4)."

- The study concluded that "When studied in patients with no DRD4 allele stratification, 5–15 mg daily for 12 weeks was not different from placebo in reducing drinking measures. Given the minimal use of genetic information in AUD patient assessment, olanzapine may be considered on a trial-and-error basis in AUD."[192]

2013–Aubin–Drug and Alcohol Dependence
Emerging Pharmacotherapies for Alcohol Dependence: A Systematic Review
Focusing on Reduction in Consumption

• Aubin reported, "Relapse rates were 37.9% with olanzapine and 29% with placebo."[381]

2012–Gianoli–Experimental and Clinical Psychopharmacology
Treatment for Comorbid Borderline Personality Disorder and Alcohol Use
Disorders: A Review of the Evidence and Future Recommendations
---

• Gianoli summarizes that olanzapine's ability to impact alcohol consumption and craving was identified by Hutchinson et al. (2001).

• He then sites Hutchinson's study where it was found that olanzapine was "differentially effective at reducing cue-elicited cravings based on individual differences in the variable number of tandem repeats (VNTR) in the D4 dopamine receptor gene (DRD4)."

• He summarizes that olanzapine "reduced cravings for all individuals, but only reduced cravings after exposure to alcohol cues AND after a priming dose of alcohol for individuals who were homozygous or heterozygous for the 7 (or longer) repeat allele of the DRD4 VNTR".[382]

2006–Hutchinson–Neuropsychopharmacology
The Effect of Olanzapine on Craving and Alcohol Consumption

• Hutchison summarizes key previous studies indicating that: olanzapine decreases craving after a priming dose of alcohol; craving after a priming dose of alcohol is higher in people with the seven-repeat allele of the DRD4 VNTR polymorphism; that olanzapine is more effective for cue-elicited craving and reduction in alcohol consumption for individuals with specific genetic markers; and non-favourable for individuals without those same markers.

• In this study, Hutchinson finds that "participants who were homozygous or heterozygous for the seven (or longer)-repeat allele of the DRD4 VNTR responded to olanzapine with reductions in cue-elicited craving as well as reductions in alcohol consumption over the course of the 12-week trial, whereas individuals with the shorter alleles did not respond favorably to olanzapine."[383]

2003–Hutchinson–Neuropsychopharmacology
Olanzapine Reduces Craving for Alcohol: A DRD4 VNTR Polymorphism by Pharmacotherapy Interaction

- Hutchinson identified participants who were homozygous or heterozygous for the 7 (or longer) repeat allele of the DRD4 VNTR (classified as DRD4 L), while the other participants were classified as DRD4 S."

- The findings indicated that olanzapine reduces craving for alcohol at baseline for both DRD4 S and DRD4 L individuals, but only reduces craving after exposure to alcohol cues and after a priming dose of alcohol for DRD4 L individuals."[384]

2001–Hutchinson–Psychopharmacology
Olanzapine Reduces Urge to Drink after Drinking Cues and a Priming Dose of Alcohol

- First study to show that olanzapine attenuated the effects of alcohol cues and an alcohol challenge on urge to drink.[385]

1998–Conley–Schizophr Res.
Olanzapine Response in Treatment-Refractory Schizophrenic Patients with a History of Substance Abuse

In a study of schizophrenic patients (38% of which had a history of substance abuse), 69% of those with substance abuse history responded well to olanzapine.[386]

SERTRALINE

INTRODUCTION TO SERTRALINE

Sertraline (brand name Zoloft, marketed by Pfizer) is the only antidepressant to date which has accumulated significant research showing some effectiveness in reducing drinking behaviors in alcoholics with Type A alcoholism.[192]

Type A is the lower risk, later onset type of alcoholism. The alcoholic with this type of alcoholism often does not have a family history of alcoholism.

Type B alcoholics tend to start drinking early in life—before the age of 25, they tend to be more severe in their illness, and often have a strong family history of alcoholism linked to heredity.

Findings seem to point to sertraline as helpful for the less severe type A alcoholics. However, for type B alcoholics, drinking may actually increase on sertraline.

Sertraline's efficacy in less severe alcohol dependence was replicated in late-onset/low-vulnerability alcoholics who were homozygous for the long allele of the 5-HT transporter.[192]

In significant 2011 research by Kranzler, he found that impact on drinking (increase or decrease) in alcoholics taking the antidepressant sertraline relied heavily upon age of onset and genetic markers.

Kranzler found that those with specific genetic marketers reported fewer drinking and heavy drinking days when treated with sertraline whereas individuals without these markers had fewer drinking and heavy drinking days when treated with placebo (and greater number of drinking days with Sertraline).

Sertraline (also known as sertraline hydrochloride) is one of the most popular SSRIs available today, having made over $30 billion for Pfizer since it launched in 1991. There are over 200 million prescriptions for Zoloft and generic sertraline filled annually.[387]

Depression and anxiety are extremely common in people with alcohol dependence—it could be said that they go hand in hand: Depression and anxiety can contribute heavily to the development of alcoholism.

And of course, alcoholism—its imbalancing impact not only on both brain function but also in every area of the alcoholic's life—can contribute to depression.

However, if you are taking, or considering taking an antidepressant or antipsychotic medication it's important to know that some anti-depressants and anti-psychotic medications have actually been shown to cause *increased* drinking. [There is a separate section devoted to this within this book].

There is not yet enough research to draw extremely strong conclusions about who Sertraline will or will not be helpful for in regards to alcohol dependence.

However, some of the main conclusions seem to point to the following:

- There appears to be a strong linkage between Sertraline's effectiveness in alcoholics and specific genetic markers. As has been shown in other medications (acamprosate, topiramate, naltrexone, ondansetron and disulfiram), sertraline is more effective in the treatment of individuals with specific genetic markers. (The genetic variants 5-HTTLPR triallelic SLC6A4 impacts goals including the percentage of heavy drinking days and the % of drinking days.)

- For those experiencing positive effects on drinking, sertraline may help reduce the number of drinking days, increase the time to relapse and increase abstinence rate.

- Sertraline may be a complimentary medication with naltrexone.

- While early research reported that while sertraline seemed to provide an advantage in reducing drinking in alcohol-dependent patients without lifetime depression, it was no better than placebo at reducing drinking in alcoholics with depression.

The D-List contains more information about sertraline and alcoholism.

SIGNIFICANT SERTRALINE RESEARCH

2014–Kenna–Alcohol
Ondansetron and Sertraline May Interact with 5-HTTLPR and DRD4 Polymorphisms to Reduce Drinking in Non-Treatment Seeking Alcohol-Dependent Women: Exploratory Findings

---

- Women taking sertraline who also had specific genetic markers (DRD4 < 7 repeats) drank significantly fewer drinks per drinking day.[347]

2014–Wackernah–Substance Abuse and Rehabilitation
Alcohol Use Disorder: Pathophysiology, Effects, and Pharmacologic Options for Treatment

---

- Wackernah summarized that sertraline (200 mg daily) was found to reduce drinking behaviors in type A alcoholic men; but not in type B alcoholic men or women. "Sertraline's efficacy in less severe alcohol dependence was again replicated in late-onset/low-vulnerability alcoholics who were homozygous for the long allele of the 5-HT transporter."[192]

2014–Aubin–Drug and Alcohol Dependence
Emerging Pharmacotherapies for Alcohol Dependence: A Systematic Review Focusing on Reduction in Consumption

---

- Aubin found that percentage of drinking days was 17.6% with sertraline versus 25.4% with placebo; time to relapse was longer with sertraline than placebo (11 weeks vs. 7.2 weeks), and the percentage of patients remaining abstinent was 50% (sertraline) vs. 21.7% (placebo).[381]

2013–Hashimoto–The world journal of biological psychiatry
Consensus Paper of the WFSBP Task Force on Biological Markers: Biological Markers for Alcoholism

---

- Hashimoto noted that "a polymorphism in the serotonin transporter gene SLC6A4 promoter region has been related to differential treatment response to sertraline."[388]

> ### 2011–Kranzler–Journal of Clinical Psychopharmacology
> ### A Double-Blind, Randomized Trial of Sertraline for Alcohol Dependence: Moderation by Age and 5-Hydroxytryptamine Transporter-Linked Promoter Region Genotype

- Kranzler showed that the effect of age of onset and response to sertraline were conditional on genotype. Those with specific genetic marketers reported fewer drinking and heavy drinking days when treated with sertraline whereas individuals without these markers had fewer drinking and heavy drinking days when treated with placebo.

- Kranzler concluded, "Because AD (Alcohol Dependence) is common, particularly in medical settings, and selective serotonin reuptake inhibitors are widely prescribed by practitioners, these findings have potential public health significance and warrant further evaluation."[179]

> ### 2010–Pettinati–American Journal of Psychiatry
> ### A Double-Blind, Placebo-Controlled Trial Combining Sertraline and Naltrexone for Treating Co-Occurring Depression and Alcohol Dependence

- In a study looking at sertraline and naltrexone, it was found that in patients combining both medications there was a complimentary effect.

- It found, "the sertraline plus naltrexone combination produced a higher alcohol abstinence rate (53.7%) and demonstrated a longer delay before relapse to heavy drinking (median delay=98 days) than the naltrexone (abstinence rate: 21.3%; delay= 29 days), sertraline (abstinence rate: 27.5%; delay=23 days), and placebo (abstinence rate: 23.1%; delay=26 days) groups."

- The study concluded that more patients with depression and alcoholism receiving the sertraline plus naltrexone combination improved abstinence rates, delayed relapse to heavy drinking, had serious adverse events, and tended to not be depressed by the end of treatment.[289]

2004–Dundon–Alcoholism, Clinical and Experimental Research
Dependence 6 Months After Serotonergic Pharmacotherapy

- Dundon found that Type A alcoholics treated with sertraline maintained good outcomes for at least 6 months following pharmacotherapy.

- In contrast, Type B alcoholics (early drinking/genetic linkage) treated with sertraline increased measures of heavy drinking over the 6 months after treatment.[182]

2001–Pettinati–Journal of Clinical Psychopharmacology
Double-Blind Clinical Trial of Sertraline Treatment for Alcohol Dependence

- In an early study of examining sertraline for the treatment of alcohol dependence in 100 alcoholics with and without lifetime depressive disorder, sertraline "seemed to provide an advantage in reducing drinking in alcohol-dependent patients without lifetime depression, illustrated best with a measure of drinking frequency."

- Sertraline was no better than placebo at reducing drinking in alcoholics with depression. Pettinati concluded that subtyping alcoholics on the basis of absence/presence of lifetime depression could help resolve conflicting findings in literature on the treatment of alcoholics with serotonergic medications.[389]

SODIUM OXYBATE (SO)

INTRODUCTION TO SODIUM OXYBATE (SO)

Sodium Oxybate has extensive research supporting its effectiveness in alcoholics. However, it should only be considered a 'Medication Worth Consideration Today', if you live in (or can access healthcare in) Italy.

This is because it has two Achilles heels–its cost and addictive quality. Despite these weaknesses, the drug has gained acceptance and been very successful in Italy.

(Please also see the section–'Are These Drugs Addictive'–for more information and rationale for including SO on the B-List here).

Italian pharmaceutical companies are in development of new formulations which may help to overcome SO's addictive nature.

If this work is fruitful, then SO may be a viable alternative in North America in 10-15 years.

Sodium Oxybate ('SO' or 'SMO') (a drug prescribed for narcolepsy in the United States) is an effective medication for the treatment of alcohol dependence that has been shown to be more effective in several trials, "than naltrexone and disulfiram in maintaining abstinence and preventing craving."[390]

One study in Italy reported that "In the prevention of relapses and maintenance of alcohol abstinence maintenance, 75% to 80% of patients remained abstinent 12 months after the initiation of alcohol treatment."[391]

In 2013, D&A Pharma, manufacturer of the drug in Europe, presented the results of several clinical studies for its Sodium Oxybate formulation 'Alcover', describing it as "a breakthrough treatment of alcohol dependence."[391]

Treatment of alcohol dependence with Sodium Oxybate was in introduced in Italy (1992) and Austria (1999) more than 20 years ago, and according to D&A Pharma, it has been employed to successfully treat "350,000 patients who are 100% refunded at 100% by public healthcare organizations."[391]

It's unfortunately that SO's weaknesses are such a steep hurdle to overcome.

First—this medication can be misused, is addictive, and has become a controlled substance in many countries. (And its short half-life which requires frequent dosing makes the logistics of a supervised dosing approach outside a residential program challenging.)

And second—the drug is expensive—a 10-day supply of Xyrem is reportedly over $4000 USD.[392]

Sodium Oxybate has two names—one which it is known in prescription format, and a second used to describe it in its illicit, street-form.

When used with a prescription, legally, this substance is called 'Sodium Oxybate' (SO) and marketed under the names Xyrem (for narcolepsy) or Alcover (for alcohol dependence and withdrawal).

When used illicitly, the same substance is called Gamma Hydroxybutyric Acid (GHB), and is sometimes called Liquid X, Liquid and Liquid Ecstasy.

Its potential for abuse has led the illicit version—GHB—to become a regulated drug in the United States, (except when in the form of the prescription drug Xyrem or Alcover). The non-prescription version is illegal to manufacture, buy, possess or distribute without a Drug Enforcement Administration license.[393]

When taken as a drug it can induce euphoria and reduce inhibitions. It can also cause suppression of breathing, blackouts, and coma.

In a review of 194 deaths attributed or related to GHB over a 10-year period, it was found that most were from respiratory depression caused by interaction with alcohol or other drugs.[394]

One study also stated that "a major concern in the area of illicit GHB misuse and abuse has been its use for incapacitating victims for the purpose of sexual assault or "date rape."[395]

Unsurprisingly, GHB is illegal to possess without a prescription and heavily regulated in many countries around the world.

Under regulation, the US manufacturer put an extensive risk management program called the 'Xyrem Success Program' in place to prevent the diversion and misuse of sodium oxybate by limiting distribution of the drug and by educating physicians and patients on proper use of the drug.

Under this program, reportedly, the manufacturer has successfully been able to limit the medication from becoming part of the illicit market.[395]

To maintain safety and deter addiction, in the European studies of SO (conducted in Germany, Austria, Italy and Poland), careful management and control of the medication was put in place so that the medication could only be taken at "therapeutic dose intervals" (which means only a certain amount at certain time intervals was taken by patients, safeguarding against addiction development).[391]

Under these conditions, the Director of the Italian Scientific Committee on Addiction Medicine concluded that SO was both effective and very safe.[391]

Control and management of Sodium Oxybate as a treatment for alcohol addiction could be likened to the use of methadone (also an addictive and dangerous substance if abused) which is used (in a controlled and monitored way) to help heroin addicts reduce or eliminate heroin use.

Unfortunately, no matter how effective an alcohol dependence drug may be, if it has the potential for abuse it is highly unlikely that even the most inspired pharmaceutical marketing campaign will overcome this barrier to convince North American doctors to prescribe an addictive medication to a patient population that has a proven susceptibility to addiction.

However, there may be a silver lining to this cloud, which means that perhaps in the next decade Sodium Oxybate could be revisited as a viable and non-addictive option for alcohol dependence.

A great deal of research has been done in the last decade to try to build safeguards into medications to stop them from being consumed in an abusive manner, or to try to prevent them from becoming addictive in the first place.

An abuse-proof painkiller, for example, has the potential to create a new billion dollar market for drug manufacturers.

Extended-release (also known as 'slow release' or 'controlled release') formulations of medications slow down the absorption, reducing peak concentrations after administration, a property that reduces the addictive potential of medication.

Researchers are able to make further modifications to drug formulations which make it difficult for drugs to be tampered with—for example, infusing drugs with polymers, so that when a drug is crushed, instead of turning to inhalable powder, it turns to putty.

Sodium oxybate is one such medication where a new formulation has been developed to impede its potential for abuse.

D&A Pharma has announced the development of two new formulations.

The first is a solid/pill form of Sodium Oxybate, code-named 'SMO.IR' (which has only been available in a liquid format in the past); and the second is an extended-release version of the Sodium Oxybate pill form. Research was published in 2015 showing that 'no deleterious interaction was observed' between SMO.IR and alcohol.[396]

Another Italian company, Laboratorio Farmaceutico CT Srl is also involved in development of the second version and reports that it has been authorized for a phase 2 clinical study in the USA.[397]

SIGNIFICANT SODIUM OXYBATE RESEARCH FINDINGS

2015–Mirijello–European Review for Medical and Pharmacological Sciences
Novel Strategies to Treat Alcohol Dependence with Sodium Oxybate according to Clinical Practice

- Results of a 2009 survey of 50 addiction medical professionals concluded that there was "some concern has been raised about the risk of developing addiction to, misuse or abuse of SMO, especially in patients with AD and poly-drug addiction and psychiatric co-morbidity (borderline personality disorder)." However, it also pointed to the fact that trials have shown that "episodes of craving for and abuse of SMO in alcoholics are a very limited phenomenon (~10%)".

- Dosing recommendations recommended that "following simple rules of administration (i.e. not to exceeding 50-100 mg/kg/day, adequately fractioned), SMO can be considered a safe and efficient drug for the treatment of alcohol dependence."[398]

- The study also found that that combining Sodium Oxybate and naltrexone was superior to either drug alone in inducing and maintaining abstinence, "which was achieved in almost 70% of alcoholics after 3 months of treatment"[398]

- Regarding dosing, there was a strong consensus that "the craving for alcohol is likely suppressed by increasing the dosages of SMO. However, due to the very short half-life (25-30 minutes) of the drug, before prescribing > 100 mg/kg/day of SMO (the maximum approved daily dose), fractioning of the drug from three to six daily administrations could be considered a safer approach. On the other hand, due to their lack of efficacy, doses of SMO < 50 mg/kg/day are not suggested."[398]

536 · MEDICATIONS FOR ALCOHOLISM

2015–Patat–British Journal of clinical pharmacology
Pharmacodynamic Interactions of a Solid Formulation of Sodium Oxybate and Ethanol in Healthy Volunteers

---

- "SMO.IR, a solid immediate-release formulation of sodium oxybate, is being developed to reduce the risk of criminal or accidental misuse of the drug and to obtain worldwide approval for the treatment of alcohol dependence."[396]

2014–Caputo–Journal of psychopharmacology (Oxford, England)
Sodium Oxybate in Maintaining Alcohol Abstinence in Alcoholic Patients according to Lesch Typologies: A Pilot Study

---

- Caputo reported, "all patients significantly reduced their alcohol intake… cases of SO abuse were very limited…"[399]

2014–Keating–Clinical Drug Investigation
Sodium Oxybate: A Review of Its Use in Alcohol Withdrawal Syndrome and in the Maintenance of Abstinence in Alcohol Dependence

---

- Keating reported that sodium oxybate was "at least as effective as naltrexone or disulfiram in the maintenance of abstinence in alcohol-dependent patients …sodium oxybate was generally well tolerated."[390]

2014–Skala–Expert opinion on pharmacotherapy
Sodium Oxybate in the Treatment of Alcohol Dependence: From the Alcohol Withdrawal Syndrome to the Alcohol Relapse Prevention

---

- Skala commented that "SMO has proved safe and effective in the treatment of alcohol withdrawal syndrome and in the prevention of relapses. Craving for and abuse of SMO have been reported, in particular in some subtypes of alcoholic patients, e.g., those affected by coaddiction and/or psychiatric comorbidity."[400]

2011–Leone–The Cochrane database of systematic reviews
Gamma-Hydroxybutyrate (GHB) for Treatment of Alcohol Withdrawal and Prevention of Relapses

---

- In a Cochrane review, Leone wrote, "GHB did appear to be better than Naltrexone and Disulfiram in maintaining abstinence and preventing craving, based on two trials and one trial respectively for these comparisons." Leone noted that the most reported side effects were dizziness and vertigo and that GHB should be used "only under strict medical surveillance."[401]

2009–Griffiths–Drug Alcohol Dependence
Illicit Gamma-Hydroxybutyrate (GHB) and Pharmaceutical Sodium Oxybate
(Xyrem®): Differences in Characteristics and Misuse

- Regarding the terminology used to describe this substance, Griffiths wrote, "it is important, however, to recognize that illicit GHB and sodium oxybate have different risks or liabilities of abuse and using "GHB" to refer to both illicit GHB and sodium oxybate has blurred this distinction in the scientific literature and in the popular press"[395]

16 | D-List Drugs – Drugs That Can Increase Drinking

"SSRIs can trigger an increase (rather than a decrease) in alcohol consumption."[178]

Dr. Bankole Johnson

One area of research I felt it was critical to share—for every person with alcohol dependence to know about, whether they wish to treat their illness with medication or not—is around anti-depressants and antipsychotics and their impact on drinking.

If medications exist that will help you drink less, then it is also feasible that there are medications that may have the opposite effect—increasing drinking.[402]

And that is the case with several different medications—some of which are likely to be prescribed to alcoholics.

Depressive symptoms can be observed in approximately 80% of alcoholics, with 30% meeting criteria for major depression. Many alcoholics have grappled with suicide and the rate of suicide amongst the alcoholic population is very high.

The potential for people with schizophrenia to experience alcoholism or another substance use disorder is also very high—47 percent of schizophrenics were found to have met the criteria for substance use disorder (excluding smoking) in their lives in one 1990 study.[403]

Thus, a large number of alcoholic patients are prescribed anti-depressants and anti-psychotics. (Don't let the term 'anti-psychotic' make you think that this category of drug may never be prescribed to you. Many of the top medications prescribed for depression and anxiety are actually called anti-psychotic medications).

And unlike medications for the treatment of alcoholism, it has become somewhat acceptable in 12-step programs for alcoholics to take anti-depressants. So, even 12-steppers are at risk here.

It's truly another one of the ugly paradoxes in the world of alcohol dependence treatment: some of the only medications that are ever prescribed to help alcoholics with their treatment, can make them worse.

And they are prescribed despite the lack of research into their effects in this group.[404]

COMMON ANTIDEPRESSANTS–SSRIS

Several leading addiction scientists have raised a red warning flag in this area–particularly with the common category of antidepressants–SSRIs.

Dr. Henry Kranzler is one scientist who has conducted research on alcoholics taking the medication sertraline (marketed as Zoloft). You can read about the study results later in this chapter in the section on Sertraline.

He concluded the following:

> *"Alcoholism subtypes may moderate the response to treatment with medications that affect serotonergic tone, which differs as a function of age of alcoholism onset."*[179]

Kranzler's significant findings showed that in the first week of his study, sertraline reduced drinking in alcoholics, whether they were Type A or Type B.

But by week 12, whereas in Type A alcoholics (late onset), sertraline continued to reduce drinking levels, those with Type B alcoholism taking sertraline were drinking more than those on placebo.[179]

And of the findings Kranzler says:

> *"Because alcohol dependence is common, particularly in medical settings, and selective serotonin reuptake inhibitors are widely prescribed by practitioners, these findings have potential public health significance and warrant further evaluation."*[179]

Another well-respected scientist, Dr. Johnson Bankole has also seen issues in regards to alcoholism and SSRIs.

Bankole has found that (unlike Kranzler's findings, where Type B alcoholics were seen to increase drinking)[179], SSRI's can increase drinking in Type B alcoholics.

In one journal he writes, "SSRIs can trigger an increase (rather than a decrease) in alcohol consumption among late-onset alcoholics."[178]

Other researchers, such as Dr. Alen Francisco have seen increases in drinking related to SSRIs. In 2014 research, Francisco reported that SSRIs produced long-lasting increases in alcohol consumption after alcohol deprivation in rats.[404]

These findings hold important implications for a large segment of those suffering with alcoholism.

For example, Kranzler found that the most negative affect of sertraline was in Type B alcoholics with a specific genetic variation–'L'L'.

This is not an uncommon variant, with a prevalence of approximately 25%, making Kranzler's findings extremely significant.

Type B alcoholics make up approximately 65% of all alcoholics.

If 25% of these Type B alcoholics have the 'L'L' variation, it means that 16.25% of *all* alcoholics might react with some level of increased drinking to SSRIs like sertraline.

Conversely, of the 25% of Type A alcoholics (making up 35% of the population of alcoholics) who carry this variation, 8.75% of all alcoholics could be treated with some level of success with SSRI's like sertraline.

He states that "In view of the findings reported here, the prevalence of the L' allele in the general population could determine the impact of SSRI treatment on outcomes among alcoholics."

•••

Please use caution here.

This is an emerging area–and one which requires a great deal more research before it's understood.

If you have been prescribed an anti-depressant or anti-psychotic—don't stop taking it.

But if you have been on one of these medications and experienced this yourself, rest assured that it's likely a biological response brought on by your genetics. (Not a reflection of a 'bad attitude' or any of that nonsense).

Anti-depressants and anti-psychotics can literally save the lives of people who suffer from debilitating psychological pain. People discontinuing these medications too quickly or without a doctor's supervision can expose themselves to enormous harm. As it says in the legal print at the start of this book—do not stop taking medication or change dosage without consulting a physician.

However, if you are an alcoholic and you take these medications, or your physician wishes to prescribe them to you, this is an area you need to be aware of. Bring this information to your doctor.

Scientists don't know exactly why this occurs, but there are some theories.

We do know that the serotonin and noradrenaline systems are heavily involved in the loss of control over drinking. And these are the same systems targeted by antidepressants and antipsychotics.

And given that neither alcoholism nor depression's impact and exact mechanisms or causes of actions in these complicated systems are well understood, it is perhaps not surprising that adverse reactions and their mechanisms are not well understood either.

•••

OTHER MEDICATIONS

SSRIs are not the only type of medication to be aware of.

Some of the research findings in this area show a wide range of medications that have been shown to increase drinking in either humans or in animal models.

We'll start here with more information about sertraline, but will continue on to cover many other different medications you need to be aware of.

SERTRALINE

Sertraline is a popular antidepressant that is marketed under the brand name Zoloft.

You may have noticed that Sertraline appears on two lists in this book— it's on the B-List, with other medications that are well worth consideration, and here on the F-List—as a medication that may increase drinking.

That's because research has shown that whether you increase or decrease your drinking with sertraline is very much to do with your genes and the type of alcoholism you have.

While it seems to decrease drinking in Type A alcoholics (late onset alcoholism, with less of a family background), research has shown that sertraline can increase drinking in Type B (early onset) alcoholics.[192]

Kranzler found that in the first week of treatment with sertraline, all patients in the study showed a substantial decrease in drinking.

But, while in the twelfth week of treatment, Type A alcoholics (late onset alcoholism) had a reduction in drinking days, Type B alcoholics (early onset alcoholism), experienced more drinking days, and more heavy drinking days than those taking placebo.[179]

In week 12:

- Type As taking sertraline had fewer drinking days than Type As on placebo

- Type Bs taking sertraline had more drinking days than Type Bs on placebo

In week 12, for individuals with the L'/L' genetic variation (but not the S' variation)[179]:

- Type As taking sertraline had fewer heavy drinking days than Type As on placebo

- Type Bs taking sertraline had "significantly more" heavy drinking days than those on placebo

Looking at the entire period, for individuals with the L'/L' genetic variation (but not the S' variation)[179]:

- Type A's taking sertraline were marginally less likely than Type A's taking placebo to drink on any given day

- Type B's taking sertraline were "significantly more likely" to drink on any given day than Type B's on placebo.

Kranzler also used a test called the 'Short Index of Problems' (SIP) that measures alcohol-related problems.

Among L'/L' carriers (but not S' carriers), he found[179]:

- Type B's taking sertraline scored a mean of 24, whereas Type Bs on placebo scored a mean 6.5. (The higher the score, the more alcohol-related problems you are experiencing).

And finally he measured GGTP, a liver enzyme that reflects recent drinking.

For L'L' carriers he found[179]:

- Type B patients taking sertraline had a mean of 165.8, while those on placebo scored 35.2. (The lower the score, the greater the drinking)

- Type A patients taking sertraline had a mean of 49.3, while those on placebo scored 92.

DOXAZOSIN

Doxazosin is an alpha-1-blocker that was studied in a double-blind placebo-controlled randomized clinical trial for its usefulness in treatment-seeking alcohol dependent individuals. It also appears on the B-list for it's effectiveness in Type B (early onset) alcoholics.

By contrast, individuals without a strong family history of alcoholism (Type A) were seen to increase their drinking when taking doxazosin.[183]

Because both doxazosin and prazosin are both alpha adrenergic receptor blockers (though they effect bioavailability differently). While tests have only shown that doxazosin could be problematic for Type A individuals, given their commonalities, it is possible that prazosin may be problematic for Type A alcoholics too.

ONDANSETRON

As with sertraline and doxazosin, the drug, ondansetron, also appears both on the B-List and here on the D-List.

This is because response to this medication is highly dependent on the type of alcoholism you manifest.

Ondansetron is a serotonin (5HT3) receptor agonist typically used for postoperative nausea and vomiting. While it has shown significant reductions in craving and drinking levels in individuals with Type B early onset alcoholism, it may not be useful for those with Type A alcoholism.

Instead, studies such as Dr. Bankole Johnson's pivotal 2002 work have found that in Type A alcoholics, ondanseron (even at low doses) could increase craving and negatively affect abstinence.[350]

ATOMOXETINE

Atomoxetine (brand name Strattera) is an SNRI, or 'selective noradrenaline reuptake inhibitor' originally developed to treat depression but approved as a medication for attention-deficit hyperactivity disorder.

It was found to increase alcohol consumption in rats after relapse.[404]

FLUOXETINE & VENLAFAXINE

Scientists have found that both the SSRI fluoxetine (brand names Prozac and Sarafem) and the popular SNRI venlafaxine (brand names Effexor and Trevilor) enhanced the alcohol deprivation effect (ADE) and led to an increase in drinking lasting at least 5 weeks in research animals.[404]

FLUPENTHIXOL DECANOATE, AMISULPRIDE, TIAPRIDE

In a review of 13 placebo-controlled trials, with the exception of one isolated outcome, none of the following antipsychotics improved abstinence, or reduced drinking or craving in patients with primary alcohol dependence: amisulpride (atypical antipsychotic), aripiprazole (antipsychotic), flupenthixol decanoate (antipsychotic), quetiapine (atypical antipsychotic), tiapride (selective dopamine antagonist).[405]

The extensive review found that "relapse prevention and abstinence/drinking days were significantly worse in patients treated with flupenthixol decanoate compared to placebo."[405][381]

Flupenthixol decanoate is an antipsychotic marketed under brand names Fluanxol, Navane, Taractan, and others.

Even after what the study called the "damning result" from the flupenthixol decanoate study was removed, placebo performed better than the remaining antipsychotics as a group in several measurements including percentage of abstinent days.[405]

Additional research reported that flupenthixol decanoate, amisulpride, and tiapride all performed poorly in placebo-controlled studies on measures of alcohol intake, craving, and abstinence.[192]

Amisulpride is marketed as Amazeo, Amipride, Amival, Solian, Soltus, Sulitac and Sulprix.

Tiapride is marketed as Hipokin, Tiager, Tiaprid, Boinlil, Cuckool, Delpral, and numerous other names.

LISURIDE

Lisuride (a dopamine agonist and partial agonist for several serotonin receptors) was found to shorten the duration of abstinence: "relapse rates at 6 and 12 months were significantly higher; time to first drink was significantly shorter with lisuride."[381]

Lisuride is marketed under the names Dopergin, Dopergine, and Arolac.

RITANSERIN

Ritanserin is a serotonin receptor antagonist developed for schizophrenia and migraine. The atypical antipsychotic risperidone (used to treat schizophrenia and bipolar disorder) was developed from ritanserin and is marketed under the brand names Risperdal, Risdon, and Sizodon.

Research showed that "multiple large clinical trials revealed poor results with ritanserin when compared to placebo when measuring daily drinks, craving in heavy drinkers, and relapse rates."[192]

TIAGABINE

Tiagabine is an anti-convulsive medication that is also used in the treatment of panic disorder. It is marketed under the name Gabitril.

In one trial looking at its usefulness in alcohol dependence, "abstinence rates were 7% for Tiagabine and 14.3% for placebo."[381]

17 | THE FUTURES LIST – 60+ DRUGS TO WATCH

PROMISING MEDICATIONS

The biggest discoveries often start with one small discovery—sometimes so small it seems unimportant and insignificant at the time, until years later when we understand its value.

The substances in this chapter are on the cusp of our understanding in regards to their potential for treatment of alcohol dependence.

Perhaps a medication in this chapter will one day become the next super drug to help people with alcohol addiction.

As this list shows, there are numerous drugs that have shown that they might have potential to become effective treatments (or part of a treatment cocktail) for alcohol dependence.

Unfortunately, the vast majority will never see the light of day when it comes to FDA approval of treatments for alcoholism.

Some of them are already generic, so they do not have pharmaceutical industry backing; some have been approved for other purposes and, therefore, will never be marketed by the pharmaceutical company that owns it for the treatment of alcohol dependence; others were abandoned at an early stage in clinical research before further development was taken because the cost or risk was too high.

For a drug to become an FDA-approved, pharmaceutical-company-marketed, on-label medication for the treatment of alcohol dependence, many variables have to fall into place.

The most promising drugs need this combination of factors to achieve this:

- Show both effectiveness and safety and no sign of addictive qualities

- Are not yet generic

- Have not yet achieved FDA-approval for other purposes

- Are not far more likely to achieve FDA-approval for another, more profitable purpose

- Are patent protected (and will maintain this patent for at least another decade)

- Have not been abandoned by the pharmaceutical company due to risk or other business issues

If a medication has all of these characteristics then it has the possibility of both becoming approved by the government AND being marketed by a pharmaceutical company.

To be clear–just because a drug has been shown to be effective means very little. Too many other factors are involved for a drug to gain your doctor's attention.

Of all of the drugs below, there are only a handful that seem to hold promise based on the criteria above. They are:

- Adial Pharmaceuticals' ADO4

- Invidior's Arbaclofen Placarbil (STX209)

- Laboratorio Farmaceutico CT Srl's GET73

- Alkermes Samidorphan and ALKS-3831

- Cerecor's LY2456302 (CERC-501) (though Eli Lilly's sale to Cerecor casts some doubt on the drug's future)

- Eli Lilly's LY2940094 (though little research available on efficacy for alcohol dependence)

- Eolas Therapeutics/AstraZeneca's EORA101 (though still in very early research stages)

CLINICAL TRIAL PARTICIPATION

Quite a few of the medications written about in this section are currently recruiting for clinical trials.

If you would like to find out more about participating in a clinical trial, you can visit the US National Institute of Health website where clinical trials are listed and search for the trial using the trial's registration number.

The NIH website is:

http://www.ClinicalTrials.gov

Where possible, I've included the trial registration number in the description below. They usually begin with the letters 'NCT'. You can find a study on the ClinicalTrials website by searching using the registration number.

For example, the study for arbaclofen placarbil has the trial number 'NCT02511886'. Search for this in the search box and information about the study will come up.

The Status Field will indicate if a trial has begun to recruit participants, and by clicking on the study you can find out more about what is being tested, and who to contact for more information.

You can find other studies without knowing the trial number by searching for a drug's generic name and the term 'alcoholism' or 'AUD' or 'Alcohol Use Disorder'.

The keywords you use can impact your search results. For example, I searched for 'alcohol use disorder and fluoxetine' and 11 studies appeared. I searched for 'alcoholism and fluoxetine' and only 4 study results appeared.

DRUG NAMING

Some of the medications in the C-List do not have names yet and are named with a cryptic code–for example: 'GSK1144814'.

The first letters of these codes often signify the drug company behind the medication. For example:

- ADX = Addex Therapeutics
- AD = Adial Pharma
- STX = Seaside Therapeutics
- GSK = GlaxoSmithKline
- LY = Eli Lilly and Company
- PXT = Pharnext
- ABT = AbbVie
- TKM = Tekmira
- MN = MediciNova
- CM = Curemark

THE DRUG LIST

AD04

AD04 is a serotonin-3 (5HT3) antagonist containing ondansetron which interrupts the reinforcing effects of alcohol, reducing the urge to drink and helping alcoholics drink at safer levels. It is not a new molecular entity, but a unique combination of substances already known about. It is likely that AD04 will be for Type B early onset alcoholism (not Type A, where ondansetron does not perform well).

It is believed that the reinforcing effects of alcohol are exaggerated in patients that have certain mutations in genes that control serotonin function in the brain.

AD04 was developed by Adial Pharmaceuticals (a privately held company). Prolific researcher Dr. Bankole Johnson is the founder and Chairman of Adial, and AD04 is the brainchild of Johnson's work. It is designed to be used in individuals with specific genetic mutations that are identifiable through DNA testing of patient blood samples. AD04 contains a very low dose of ondansetron, which is currently used as an anti-emetic for post-operative and post-chemotherapy nausea. Research suggests that higher doses may be less effective in treating individuals with alcoholism than lower doses.

At this time, AD04 is in phase 3 trials for alcohol dependence. It has not yet received FDA-approval but company CEO William Stilley anticipates a commercial launch in 2017.[40697]

AMITIFADINE (EB-1010)

In testing with laboratory rats, amitifadine (an antidepressant drug in development by Euthymics Bioscience) was effective in attenuating alcohol binge drinking and two measures of negative affect (depression) induced by abstinence.

The study concluded, "Given the safety profile of amitifadine, low risk for weight gain, lack of sexual side effects, and low abuse liability, we propose amitifadine would be effective in treating the co-occurrence of alcoholism and depression, and at doses that are safe and well tolerated in humans."[407]

AMPEROZIDE

Amperozide is a 5-HT2 receptor antagonist that has been shown to reduce alcohol intake in laboratory rats.[351] It is an atypical antipsychotic which inhibits dopamine release and was originally investigated for schizophrenia in humans. It is not FDA-approved and its main use is in veterinary medicine to decrease aggression and stress in pigs.

Brian A McMillen of East Carolina University provides a little background on this medication:

> "We (the late Bob Myers and myself) demonstrated that amperozide would reduce alcohol consumption in rats bred to drink large quantities and reduce consumption and reward effects of cocaine.
>
> Winger had an abstract that it reduced morphine self-administration by monkeys. We all but had a contract finalized to test the drug in alcoholic-clients as they were discharged from a local state in-patient facility, but Kabi Pharmacia abandoned the drug and then Pharmacia merged with Upjohn and then they were bought by Pfizer and the patent is long gone now.
>
> It is used by the Swedish pig farmers to reduce aggression amongst their piglets and prevent a wasting syndrome when the piglets are weaned and separated from their sows—together about a 25% loss if not managed (what I know about pig farming you can put in a thimble).
>
> The Kabi scientists at Malmo were visited by a few police chiefs trying to find out what the drug was because the addicts were using it to get clean."[408]

ARBACLOFEN PLACARBIL (STX209)

In 2014 Reckitt Benckiser Group spun its pharmaceuticals division off into a company named Individior. Its primary product is Suboxone, a heroin addiction drug,[409] and Individior continues to look for opportunities to expand in the addiction arena.[92]

XenoPort is a biopharmaceutical company that has developed a drug called Arbaclofen Placarbil. Arbaclofen Placarbil is a GABA-B agonist that was originally codenamed STX209 and has not yet received FDA approval.

Individior was granted exclusive worldwide rights for the development and commercialization of Arbaclofen Placarbil in 2013.

Arbaclofen Placarbil is a "patent protected new chemical entity,"[93] with applications in autism and fragile X syndrome. The company hopes to launch it commercially in 2020. It has already been tested in over 1300 human subjects.[93] It is reported to be able to "suppress alcohol cravings, reduce alcohol intake and potentially help maintain abstinence in alcohol-dependent people."[92]

At the time of writing, Reckitt Benckiser had registered a phase 2 trial to test this medication in people with alcohol dependence– clinicaltrials.gov.org identifier NCT02511886, which has not yet started recruiting.

XenoPort also has the restless leg medication Horizant in its stable of drugs. Horizant, is gabapentin enacarbil, the extended release version of gabapentin discussed in the chapter on A-List drugs.[410]

ARIPIPRAZOLE

An atypical antipsychotic (marketed as Abilify or Aripiprex) is a partial agonist of both the dopamine and serotonin receptors. It was first proposed in 2003 for use in alcoholism and then "subsequently tested in a multisite RCT but failed to meet its primary outcomes…in another double-blind, comparison trial was shown to reduce craving, but to a lesser extent than with naltrexone."[47]

A 2012 summary of studies with aripiprazole and alcohol dependence[411] concluded that the existing studies, (while promising), were not statistically impactful to demonstrate significantly that aripiprazole effectively combated alcohol dependence. Of the 2010 summary, however, there were individual trial findings that showed aripiprazole's promise in possibly reducing number of drinks per day and reducing urges after follow-up drinks.[192]

One study found for example that "Despite objective evidence that ventral striatum activation is blunted with aripiprazole, and that aripiprazole may be as efficacious as naltrexone in reducing craving and increasing the time to relapse in patients with a goal of abstinence, its precise usefulness in alcohol-dependent patients is not clear."[192]

Respected researcher Dr. Raymond Anton is currently recruiting participants for a Phase 3 trial with aripiprazole (NCT01292057).

BRUCINE

Brucine is a poisonous alkaloid related to strychnine. Brucine was found to significantly suppress voluntary alcohol intake and reduced preference for alcohol in laboratory rats. The effect was found to be dose-related and apparent across the 10 days of treatment.[412] Brucine is not FDA-approved.

BENFOTIAMINE

Benfotiamine—a high dose Vitamin B1—completed Phase 4 trials in chronic long-term alcoholics where it was found to be beneficial—particularly for women. Severe alcoholism can be associated with significant nutritional and vitamin deficiency, especially vitamin B1 (thiamine) which is related to neurological deficits impacting mood and cognition.

The study found that "alcohol consumption decreased from baseline levels for 9 of 10 BF treated women after 1 month of treatment compared with 2 of 11 on PL. Reductions in total alcohol consumption over 6 months were significantly greater for BF treated women."[413]

Further research into the subset of men that were studied also found that it appeared to "reduce psychiatric distress and may facilitate recovery in severely affected males with a lifetime alcohol use disorder and should be considered for adjuvant therapy in alcohol rehabilitation."[414]

CARBAMAZEPINE

Carbamazepine is a prototypical anti-epileptic medication used as an anticonvulsant and analgesic and first FDA-approved in 1962 and now available in generic form. It has been seen to protect against some symptoms of alcohol withdrawn, but may also reduce relapse rates,[1] and has been shown to outperform placebo in longer time to relapse to heavy drinking.[192]

CHLORZOXAZONE

Chlorzoxazone is an FDA-approved centrally acting muscle relaxant used to treat muscle spasms. Research studying Chlorzoxazone for its effect on reduction in consumption is in the planning phase.[381]

In 2014 Cui et al. reported that chlorzoxazone had decreased alcohol consumption in laboratory rats but that in a clinical trial of 20 social alcohol users it had failed to reduce the number of drinks consumed per week.[415]

CLOZAPINE

Clozapine is an atypical antipsychotic medication used to treat schizophrenia. It is FDA-approved but carries at least five black box warnings for adverse effects. One report stated that while "the atypical antipsychotic clozapine has been shown to reduce alcohol use in patients with schizophrenia, its toxicity severely limits its use in patients."[416]

Some reports indicate that clozapine augmented by lamotrigine may have positive outcomes.[417]

CITALOPRAM

Citalopram is a generic antidepressant drug in the SSRI class. It received FDA-approval to treat major depression in 1998. While citalopram has been found to reduce alcohol consumption in moderate drinkers (particularly men), this effect has not been seen in heavy drinkers.[192]

When researchers combined naltrexone and citalopram together and treated patients with co-occurring alcohol dependence and depression both medications were reasonably well tolerated and well-adhered to resulting in improvements in mood and drinking. However, no synergistic effect was found between the two (no interaction effect was found beyond what was expected for each individual medication alone).[418]

Clinical trial CT01657760 is currently recruiting for a trial to test the effect of citalopram on craving.

D-PENICILLAMINE

D-Penicillamine is an amino acid metabolite of penicillin though it has no antibiotic properties. It has been used to treat rheumatoid arthritis since the 1960s.

In testing, animals treated with a combination of naltrexone and D-Penicillamine did not demonstrate the characteristic drinking spike seen after abstinence (called the Alcohol Deprivation Effect), indicating that this combination may prevent the appearance of this effect.[285]

D-SERINE; D-CYCLOSERINE

D-serine is an amino acid that acts as a signaling molecule in the brain. It is being studied for the treatment of ALS.

One report states that "NMDAR modulators can reduce aversion-resistant alcohol drinking, and support testing of D-serine and D-cycloserine as immediately accessible, FDA-approved drugs to treat AUDs"[419]

One 2015 study, which combined d-cycloserine with cue-exposure-based extinction training (which means experiencing an alcohol trigger or cue and practicing not responding to it by drinking in order to weaken the response over time) found positive results, "Following treatment with CET plus DCS, cue-induced brain activation in the ventral and dorsal striatum was decreased compared to treatment with CET plus placebo.[420]

DIHYDROMYRICETIN

Dihydromyricetin is a flavonoid compound that counteracts acute alcohol intoxication.

It has been reported to reduce alcohol consumption in laboratory rats. In his 2012 work published in the Journal of Neuroscience, Dr. Yi Shen argues that "dihydromyricetin could be a novel candidate for medication development in alcohol use disorders."[371421]

DIVALPROEX SODIUM (VPA)

Divalproex Sodium is an FDA-approved treatment for seizures caused by epilepsy.

The anti-convulsant "significantly decreased relapse to heavy drinking in a blinded study against placebo and also decreased amount of drinking and craving compared to baseline. A small non-blinded study found VPA treatment increased abstinence at 6 weeks post-detoxification, though this was not statistically significant."[192]

Another study (NCT01760785) is underway.

DIZOCILPINE (MK-801) & PHENCYCLIDINE

Research by Holter et al. (1996), Hundt et al. (1998), Vengeliene et al. (2005) found that "drugs non-competitively antagonizing NMDA receptors, such as dizocilpine and phencyclidine... can also reduce voluntary alcohol drinking and alcohol deprivation effect reflecting relapse."[422]

Both dizocilpine and phencyclidine (PCP) have the potential for abuse.

DULOXETINE

Duloxetine is a serotonin-norepinephrine reuptake inhibitor which is FDA-approved and prescribed for depression.

There is at least one trial of duloxetine where planning is underway to examine its ability to reduce alcohol consumption in dependent individuals[381][423]

Another clinical trial (NCT00929344) is underway comparing duloxetine to pregabalin for alcohol dependence.

DUTASTERIDE

The FDA-approved Dutasteride inhibits the conversion of testosterone to dihydrotestosterone (DHT), making it useful in the treatment of enlarged prostate (and used off-label by some to fight hair loss).

Dutasteride reduces alcohol's sedative effects and may reduce drinking[424].

Researchers found, "Heavy drinkers had fewer heavy drinking days during the 2 weeks following the dutasteride sessions and fewer total drinks in the first week after dutasteride."[424]

Recruitment is underway for a Phase 4 reduction in consumption trial (NCT01758523) for dutasteride.[381]

ESCITALOPRAM

Research found that depression and anxiety drug escitalopram was "not effective for preventing relapse when administered as a monotherapy, however, combination therapy did appear to be effective."[381]

A Phase 1 trial (NCT01657760) is underway to look at the effects of escitalopram on craving and dopamine response.

ETICLOPRIDE

Eticlopride is a selective dopamine antagonist that acts on dopamine receptor D2. Eticlopride was seen to decrease alcohol seeking behavior triggered by alcohol cues in laboratory rats.[371]

FENOFIBRATE & PPARs

Fenofibrate belongs to a category of drugs called PPARs (peroxisome proliferator-activated receptors).

It is FDA-approved and commonly used to treat high cholesterol and high triglyceride levels.

Some PPARs have been shown to reduce voluntary alcohol intake in animals. Fenofibrate was shown to do this in two recent studies, by Karahanian et al. in 2014 and Blednov et al. in 2015.

Clinical trials currently being led by respected addiction researcher Barbara Mason of the Scripps Research Institute are designed to test the hypothesis that alcohol-dependent individuals treated with fenofibrate will report decreased craving for alcohol following alcohol cues, as well as decreased drinking.[425]

Trial NCT02158273 to study fenofibrate's impact on craving is currently recruiting.

Other PPAR's are Pioglitazone (PPAR gamma agonist) & Tesaglitazar (Dual PPAR alpha and PPAR gamma agonist).

Pioglitazone (a common FDA-approved diabetes drug that decreases inflammation[426]) and tesaglitazar (a drug originally proposed for type 2 diabetes but discontinued) have been shown to significantly decrease alcohol intake in mice.

Pioglitazone was effective only for 6 hours after administration of the drug though tesaglitazar showed a long-lasting effect."[425]

As with fenofibrate, gemfibrozil is a PPAR used to treat high cholesterol and triglyceride levels. It has shown reduced alcohol drinking in rats.[425]

FLUOXETINE

Fluoxetine is used to treat depression or obsessive-compulsive disorder.

In alcohol-dependent rats, a combination of desipramine and fluoxetine did lower alcohol self-administration in early withdrawal and recovery was delayed in dependent animals, "indicating a potent effect."[427]

Unfortunately, in human testing, fluoxetine lacked consistent evidence in regards to alcohol dependence. Research on alcohol dependent patients indicated little impact on levels of alcohol dependence or was sporadic.[192]

GABAB PAMS

One of baclofen's 'problems', is that it is a generic drug. As such, despite its effectiveness, pharmaceutical companies do not stand to make much profit from it and are therefore unmotivated to lobby or market it.

But GABAB PAMs (including ADX71441, CGP7930, GS39783, BHF177, rac-BHFF, KK-92A) represent a new area of research that potentially brings with it the beneficial effects of baclofen with some additional advantages.

GABAB PAMs are 'positive allosteric modulators' of GABAB receptors. They have a similar pharmacological profile to the GABAB receptor agonist baclofen (reviewed extensively earlier in the book).[428]

It is theorized that positive allosteric modulators of the GABAB receptor reproduce several of the positive anti-alcohol effects of baclofen while minimizing the adverse effects (such as sedation and motor incoordination).

Addex Pharmaceuticals announced recently that they had entered into a collaboration with the National Institute on Alcohol Abuse and Alcoholism (NIAAA) to evaluate a GABAB PAM called ADX71441. It was shown by Addex in laboratory animal testing that animals responded positively on several different measures of alcohol dependent behavior when given ADX71441.[429]

Other GABAB PAMs (CGP7930, GS39783, BHF177, rac-BHFF) have been shown to reduce daily alcohol intake in rats. One of these– GS39783–showed the complete suppression of binge-like drinking after treatment.[43] KK-92A is another GABAB PAM which has been shown to attenuate the effects of nicotine in rats.[430]

This class of drugs has been called, "a major step forward… demonstrating the ability to reproduce the suppressive effects of baclofen on several alcohol-related behaviors."[43] Testing of GABAB PAMS is still at the preclinical stage.

NEUROKININS

Neurokinins (NK1Rs) such as GSK1144814, GSK1521498, GSK598809, GSK618334, Tradipitant (VLY-686, LY686017 represent a category of new compounds in drug pipeline for which scientists hold great promise. They are a family of peptide transmitters involved in the reward pathway for drugs of abuse, including alcohol.[431]

Tradipitant (also known as VLY-686 or LY686017 and licensed worldwide by Vanda Pharmaceuticals after Eli Lilly developed it) is one such drug.

George et al.'s 2008 study of LY686017, published in Science, showed that this Neurokinin 1 receptor antagonist altered challenge-induced craving and robustly altered cortisol response to challenge.

Magnetic resonance imagery showed that responses to negative affective stimuli were dampened and responses to positive affective stimuli were up-regulated in the same study.[432]

An article on the research stated that the drug "reduces responses to stress in some recovering alcoholics, and eases their cravings to have a drink." The study was conducted on 50 recovering alcoholics, all of whom reported high levels of anxiety at the start of the study.

"The 25 randomly selected to be given the drug reported fewer cravings than those assigned to receive a placebo, and they had a lessened response to stressful situations. ...This might be an approach that could be used for people who drink to relieve stress in their lives, or have anxiety disorders."[433]

Glaxo Smith Kline also has a neurokinin that is being studied in schizophrenia. GSK1144814 is a dual Neurokinin-1 and neurokinin-3 receptor antagonist. [381]

GSK1144814 was also studied in relation to alcoholism in clinical trial NCT01181908 which showed the (tolerable) effects of the combination of GSK1144814 and alcohol in healthy volunteers.

NICOTINIC RECEPTOR LIGANDS (CYTISINE, LOBELINE)

Varenicline is a nicotinic receptor ligand which is helpful for alcohol-dependent smokers (and appears in the B-List).

The nicotinic receptor ligands cytisine and lobeline have also showed promise in reducing alcohol consumption and nicotine-induced alcohol drinking in several trials.[434]

GET73

In 2013, Italian researchers showed evidence that that a new compound with a huge name–((N-[(4-trifluoromethyl)benzyl]4-methoxybutyramide)) reduces alcohol intake in laboratory animals.[104] The short form for the compound is GET73.

A 2015 report showed evidence that GET73 can play a neuroprotective role against alcohol-induced neurotoxicity in the brains of rats, "thus lending further support to the significance of developing GET73 as a therapeutic tool for use in the treatment of alcohol use disorders."[435]

GET73 is the brainchild of Italy's Labratorio Farmaceutico, which also brought Alcover (GHB) to the world.

GET73's discovery is significant given that it was designed as a GHB derivative, thought to possess a more favorable pharmacodynamic and pharmacokinetic profile.

GHB (Gamma-Hydroxybutyric Acid) has been shown to be very effective for individuals with alcohol dependence though its use in practice is extremely hampered by its high price and the potential for addiction and abuse.

Researchers hope that GET73 will contain all of GHB's anti-alcohol effects while overcoming the negative aspects of the medication.[436]

Phase 1 and 2 trials for the study of GET73 in alcoholism (NCT01842503), is currently recruiting.

GSK1521498

So far, research into mu-opioid antagonist GSK1521498 looks promising. In research with naltrexone, in alcohol-preferring rats, "GSK1521498 showed significantly greater effectiveness than naltrexone, supporting its potential use for promoting abstinence and preventing relapse in alcohol addiction."[437]

And in humans, "GSK1521498 has been shown generally to be well tolerated compared with placebo, with no detectable deleterious effects on anxiety, mood or other aspects of hedonic function, or on liver or other blood safety parameters. Importantly, its coadministration with ethanol did not affect its tolerability."[437]

Researcher Dr. Hisham Ziauddeen concluded, "these findings… support continued development of GSK1521498 for the treatment of alcohol addiction."

GSK598809 AND GSK618334

GSK598809 and GSK618334 are dopamine d3 receptor antagonists.[381]

At least 12 studies have been completed for GSK598809 on alcoholism, substance abuse and other compulsion-related illnesses.

Three studies have been completed on GSK618334 for alcohol dependence and substance abuse (NCT01036061, NCT00814957, NCT00513279).

GUANFACINE

Guanfacine is an FDA-approved medication utilized in the treatment of attention deficit hyperactivity disorder and hypertension.

Researchers hypothesize that "noradrenergic medications that are promising for comorbid PTSD and substance use disorders include prazosin, guanfacine, and atomoxetine."[438]

Two trials to look at guanfacine and alcohol are currently recruiting (NCT00585754 and NCT02164422)

IBUDILAST (AV-411 OR MN-166)

Ibudilast is an anti-inflammatory drug used in Japan.

This non-selective phosphodiesterase inhibitor was tested in alcohol-dependent rats in 2015. It was found that when administered "twice daily, ibudilast reduced alcohol drinking in rats by approximately 50% and reduced drinking by alcohol-dependent mice at doses which had no effect in non-dependent mice. These findings support the viability of ibudilast as a possible treatment for alcohol dependence."[439]

Ibudilast has reached Phase 2 of clinical trials. Highly respected researcher Dr. Lara Ray recently completed the latest US-based clinical trial, NCT02025998.

IDAZOXAN + DESIPRAMINE + HALOPERIDOL

Researchers stated that "although the atypical antipsychotic clozapine has been shown to reduce alcohol use in patients with schizophrenia, its toxicity severely limits its use in patients." So they "recreated a clozapine-like drug to reduce alcohol drinking" in laboratory animals.

The 'clozapine-like' drug, which mimicked aspects of clozapine's pharmacology, was created by combining low dose haloperidol with a norepinephrine α-2 receptor antagonist, idazoxan, and a norepinephrine reuptake inhibitor, desipramine.[416]

The drug combination reduced alcohol drinking and alcohol preference significantly in laboratory animals.[416]

Desipramine and naltrexone are currently being tested in trial NCT00338962 at Yale University.

IVERMECTIN

Ivermectin (IVM) is an FDA-approved medication used to treat rosacea. In laboratory rat testing researchers found that "The IVM group drank significantly less ethanol over the 30-day period compared to the placebo."

A study of human subjects with alcoholism was completed in March 2015, with results yet to be released.[440]

JMV 2959

JMV 2959 is a ghrelin receptor antagonist (GHS-R1A) that reduces alcohol preference. It is in the pre-clinical study phase for obesity.[381]

JNJ-39220675

There has been little research done with Histamine H3 receptor antagonists, despite the fact that the histamine system has been implicated in addiction and a mutation of the HNMT gene was found in abundance in alcoholics from two different populations.

Some researchers speculate that carriers of the mutation may have low levels of histamine in the amygdaloid nuclei, a structure associated with anxiety.[441]

Very early research into one histamine H3 receptor antagonist, JNJ-39220675, found that "After 3 days of deprivation, rats were exposed to alcohol again 15 min after receiving a subcutaneous injection of JNJ-39220675. The animals displayed reduced intake of alcohol after a period of abstinence, just when the urge for drinking is enhanced."[441]

KUDZU (PUERARIN)

A substance called kudzu (which contains the isoflavone puerarin, a phytoestrogen extract) has long been reported to be helpful to alcoholics.

It is the only eastern medication mentioned by the NIAAA.[421] The mechanism is not entirely understood, but it is proposed that the extracts of the kudzu root may alter alcohol dehydrogenase or monoamine oxidase–acetaldehyde pathways,129,130 leading to reduced alcohol consumption."[192]

In limited research, it has been shown to reduce alcohol consumption and increase a number of abstinent days.[192] Some research has reported that a single dose of kudzu "quickly reduces alcohol consumption in a binge drinking paradigm."[442]

Recent research was also conducted by Dr. Scott E. Lukas of Harvard's McLean Hospital.

LY2456302 (CERC-501)

Eli Lilly research found that "LY2456302 reduced ethanol self-administration in alcohol-preferring (P) rats and, unlike naltrexone, did not exhibit significant tolerance upon 4 days of repeated dosing.

LY2456302 is a centrally-penetrant, potent, kappa-selective antagonist with pharmacokinetic properties favorable for clinical development and activity in animal models predictive of efficacy in mood and addictive disorders."

Eli Lilly sold Phase 2-ready Kappa Opioid Receptor Antagonist LY2456302 to Cerecor pharmaceuticals in February 2015.[443] A phase 2 trial (NCT02218736) is currently in the recruitment phase for the use of LY2456302 in people with anxiety disorders.

LY2940094

LY2940094 is a Nociceptin receptor antagonist and considered to be Eli Lilly's most advanced anti-depressant in development. The nociceptin receptor is related to stress response.

In December 2014, a Phase 2 clinical trial (NCT01798303) for the treatment of alcohol dependency was concluded. Results have not yet been released for this trial.

LY379268

In laboratory animal studies, scientists found that "LY379268 treatment attenuated alcohol self-administration, cue-induced and stress-induced reinstatement of alcohol seeking in both non-dependent and post dependent animals."[371]

LAMOTRIGINE

Lamotrigine is GlaxoSmithKline's FDA-approved anticonvulsant drug used in the treatment of epilepsy and bipolar disorder and off-label to treat depression.

Several studies have looked at lamotrigine and shown its ability to reduce alcohol craving. Kalyoncu et al. first reported its effects in a series of case reports in 2005. In 2006 Rubio, Lopez-Munoz and Alamo studied lamotrigine in a 12-week open-label study of patients with the dual diagnoses of bipolar disorder and alcohol dependence, and reported that lamotrigine "improved mood symptoms, decreased both alcohol craving and consumption."

One other study conducted in 2007 by Vengeliene, Heidbreder and Spanagel showed that lamotrigine reduced alcohol seeking and relapse-like drinking behavior in laboratory animals.[382]

LEVETIRACETAM

Levetiracetam is an FDA-approved generic anti-convulsant from UCB Pharmaceuticals Inc., which has shown mixed results. One open-label trial found positive results though other double-blind, placebo-controlled trials failed to show any benefits on alcohol dependence from levetiracetam. And one study found that "moderate-to-heavy drinkers taking levetiracetam increased their drinking during the study period."[192]

Respected researcher Dr. Clifford M. Knapp's 2015 research found that levetiracetam was able to "significantly reduce the percent days heavy drinking."[255]

MT-7716

MT-7716 is a nociception (NOP) receptor agonist that regulates alcohol intake and anxiety-like behavior in rats.[444] Mitsubishi Tanabe Pharma Corporation discontinued US trials in 2013 though research has continued with the help of US government grants.

CRF1 RECEPTOR AGONISTS

There has been a great deal of interest in CRF1 Receptor Agonists—as the corticotropin-releasing Hormone (CRH) System plays a key role in the extreme sensitivity to stress experienced by detoxified alcoholics, it would seem that these substances might hold promise for addiction treatment. CRF1 Receptor agonists include MTIP, MPZP, Antalarmin, MJL-1-109-2, R121919, Pexacerfont (BMS-562086).

Hansson et al.'s 2006 research and Gehlert et al.'s 2007 research showed that CRH1 antagonism suppressed alcohol self-administration in recently detoxified alcohol-dependent laboratory animals[432], effectively attenuating the levels of alcohol consumption during acute withdrawal in rats.[371]

But unfortunately in a 2015 report for the CRH1 Antagonist Pexacerfont, researchers stated that "the extensive preclinical data on CRH1 antagonism as a mechanism to suppress alcohol seeking may not translate to humans."[445]

Other CRF1 receptor agonists include MTIP, Antalarmin, R121919, emicerfont (GW876008), verucerfont (GSK561679), CP316311, SSR125543A, R121919/NBI30775, 19567470/CRA5626, and ONO-2333Ms"[157]

Eli Lilly discontinued Phase 1 trials of MTIP for alcoholism in 2013.

MECAMYLAMINE

Mecamylamine is a generic nicotinic acetylcholine receptor (similar to varenicline), originally marketed by Merck, Sharp, and Dohme, which has been proposed as smoking cessation aids.

Two trials have been completed with Mecamylamine in alcoholic individuals: NCT00342563 and NCT00563797.

The second trial found that "Mecamylamine was more effective than placebo in reducing drinking in nonsmokers."[446]

MEMANTINE

Memantine is an FDA-approved medication for Alzheimer's disease that acts on the glutamatergic system by blocking NMDA receptors. Recruitment is underway for a Phase 2 study of memantine combined with naltrexone by Yale University (NCT01519063).

METADOXINE

Alcobra's Metadoxine is used to treat chronic and acute alcohol intoxication as well as alcoholic liver disease.

2006 research by Guerrini et al. on 160 alcoholics in a treatment unit at the University of Pisa (Italy) found that metadoxine was associated with significantly higher abstinence rates than placebo at 6 months (44.8% for metadoxine vs. 21.6% for placebo)."[381][447]

2011 research by Leggio et al. showed that metadoxine resulted in a significant decrease in drinks per week, as well as a decrease in craving.[448]

In September 2015 metadoxine received fast track designation (medications on fast track can receive FDA approval more quickly) for Fragile X syndrome.

MIFEPRISTONE

Mifepristone is used with another medication called misoprostol to end early pregnancy.

A 2012 study by Vendruscolo found that mifepristone blocked the development of compulsive alcohol self-administration in alcohol-dependent laboratory rats.

Dr. Barbara Mason's 2012 study in humans also indicated that mifepristone suppressed alcohol cravings and relapse.[449]

Two studies by highly respected researchers at different institutions (Dr. Mason at Scripps Institute, and Dr. Carolina Haass-Koffler at Brown University) are currently recruiting participants: NCT02179749 and NCT02243709.

MILNACIPRAN

Milnacipran is an SNRI (serotonin-norepinephrine reuptake inhibitor) that is FDA-approved to treat fibromyalgia.

In laboratory rat tests, "a robust, dose-dependent suppression" of alcohol self-administration was seen. It was also shown that milnacipran reduced excessive ethanol consumption and prevented relapse after protracted abstinence in alcohol-dependent rats.[427]

MIRTAZAPINE

Mirtazapine is an FDA-approved antidepressant marketed as Remeron. It is a noradrenergic and specific serotonergic antidepressant (NaSSA).

Individual case reports indicate that the widely used and well-tolerated antidepressant may reduce alcohol consumption.

Limited research show that the use of mirtazapine for patients with alcohol dependence and depression may experience an improvement in mood and alcohol craving.[450]

A double-blind, randomized, placebo-controlled, 2-armed clinical trial was conducted with 59 males. Results suggested that "high consumers of alcohol with a heredity for AUD benefit from treatment with mirtazapine.[451]

One trial for alcohol use and depression (NCT02185131) is currently recruiting subjects.

MODAFINIL

Modafinil is an FDA-approved wakefulness-promoting agent used to treat disorders such as narcolepsy.

In the first randomized double-blind placebo-controlled trial of modafinil in a sample of alcohol-dependent individuals, results were mixed. Modafinil was well tolerated with no abuse potential reported.

However, "no significant main effects of modafinil were found for the primary alcohol outcome variables compared to placebo," though "overall abstinence rates were higher in the modafinil compared to the placebo."

Response to modafinil seemed to vary depending upon inhibition levels: it was beneficial to those with poor levels of inhibition, and detrimental to alcohol use for individuals with strong initial inhibition."[452]

ORG 25935 (SCH 900435)

ORG 25935 is a selective inhibitor of the glycine transporter developed by N.V. Organon that in 2007 showed a reduction in alcohol consumption in animal testing. Merck Sharp & Dohme Corp terminated phase 1 trial NCT00764660 for unknown reasons.

One Yale-led study is currently underway for its impact in healthy adults on cognition (NCT00700076).

OSU6162

Recent human studies of monoamine stabilizer OSU6162 showed that the medication was safe and tolerable in humans, but was not large enough to draw conclusions regarding its effectiveness for alcohol dependence.

Scientists identified OSU6162 as a potential medication for alcohol dependence after 2012 research by Steensland et al., 2015 research by Tolboom et al., and 2015 research by Feltmann et al. showed its relevance in animal testing.[453]

ODELEPRAN (LY2196044, OPRA II)

LY2196044 is an opioid antagonist that resulted in reductions in heavy drinking days, increased percent days abstinent, and reduced drinks per day when tested in individuals with specific genetic mutations related to the dopamine system.

Eli Lilly discontinued further research in April 2013.[454]

OREXIN RECEPTOR ANTAGONISTS (SB334867, LSN2424100)

The orexin system also has been implicated in the motivational properties of alcohol. Research done in 2014 looked at several orexin receptor antagonists and found that one of them, GlaxoSmithKline's SB334867, significantly reduced alcohol intake in alcohol-dependent laboratory rats. Other orexin receptor antagonists in preclinical study were found to have implications for alcohol intake in rats.[455]

Ely Lilly has been researching their orexin receptor antagonist, LSN2424100.

Suvorexant, Merck's dual orexin receptor antagonist for the treatment of insomnia has been shown to be completely safe in large-scale Phase III human trials for a different indication, demonstrating the safety of orexin receptor antagonists.[456]

In 2015 Euolas Therapeutics Inc Eolas Therapeutics, Inc entered into a worldwide license and partnership agreement with AstraZeneca for an orexin-1 receptor antagonist (EORA101) which is still in preclinical trials for the treatment of addictions, including alcoholism.[101]

PXT 3003

Combinations of naltrexone and baclofen have been shown to be effective in rats for alcoholism, but its safety and effectiveness has not been tested in combination in humans.[242]

However, Pharnext's PXT 3003, a unique combination of naltrexone and baclofen was given EMA and FDA Orphan Drug approval for the treatment of Charcot-Marie-Tooth Disease after successful clinical trials in humans showed the safety (and efficacy) of the drug combination.

Planning for a Phase 3 trial is underway for Charcot-Marie-Tooth Disease.

Orphan Drug Approval allows PXT 3003 to have marketing exclusivity for 10 years in Europe and seven years in the US if it is finally approved.[220]

Unfortunately, no trials for PXT 3003 in relation to alcohol dependence are planned.

PROPRANOLOL

Propranolol is a common generic medication used to treat high blood pressure and irregular heart rhythms.

In rats, alcohol drinking followed by treatment with propranolol showed variable results, but the combination of propranolol and prazosin "consistently suppressed alcohol drinking during both alcohol withdrawal and following prolonged imposed abstinence, and the combination of these two drugs was more effective than was treatment with either drug alone."[369]

In addition, in laboratory rats, combining propranolol with naltrexone was more effective in reducing the impact of alcohol than either drug alone.[280]

A phase 2 trial (NCT01634347) is currently recruiting for propranolol's effects on drug or alcohol craving.

QUETIAPINE

The anti-psychotic drug quetiapine (marketed as Seroquel) has shown mixed results.

In one study, it showed drink reduction and reduced impulsivity in early-onset, light-drinking alcoholics.[192]

But in other trials "quetiapine significantly reduced depressive symptoms and improved sleep but had no effect on other nondrinking outcomes"[457]; and did not reduce alcohol consumption in patients with BPD and alcohol dependence."[458]

One study (NCT01662297) which will look at insomnia in dually diagnosed (addiction and mental health issues) veterans is currently recruiting to test trazodone versus quetiapine.

RISPERIDONE

Risperidone is an FDA-approved drug used to treat schizophrenia and bipolar disorder.

In hamsters, risperidone only transiently decreased alcohol drinking. However, when desipramine was paired with risperidone, the combination produced a more "substantial and relatively sustained effect than risperidone alone." Data from this study may help in the "development of new treatments for patients with schizophrenia and alcoholism, and also for those with alcoholism alone."[459]

ROLIPRAM

Rolipram is a selective PDE4 inhibitor thought to represent a new treatment option for alcoholism due to its effects on the cAMP cascade (a messenger important in biological processes).

One preclinical study found that rolipram acutely reduced ethanol self-administration in a dose-dependent fashion and also, after chronic dosing, reduced ethanol preference and consumption.

This was consistent with a previous study showing that rolipram could reduce ethanol consumption in mice."[460]

RETIGABINE (EZOGABINE)

Retigabine was FDA-approved in 2010 as an anticonvulsant. Research in rats shows that the administration of retigabine may produce a decrease in alcohol consumption.[461]

SAMIDORPHAN (ALKS33 / RDC-0313), ALKS 5461, ALKS-3831

Alkerme's Samidorphan (3-carboxamido-4-hydroxy naltrexone) is a novel opioid receptor antagonist that is currently in Phase 2 clinical development for the treatment of alcoholism.

At least two clinical studies have been completed in relation to alcohol dependence (NCT00981617 and NCT00800319).

Safety and tolerability were tested in healthy adults with results published in February 2015.[95]

Results from the study indicated "samidorphan was generally well tolerated, with somnolence reported as the most common adverse event."[95]

Samidorphan has been reported to have "similar efficacy to naltrexone but possibly with reduced side effects."

A Phase 2 trial (NCT02161718) is currently recruiting for individuals to test ALKS-3831, which is a combination of olanzapine and samidorphan in patients with schizophrenia and alcohol use disorders. Recent results in a second clinical trial (NCT01903837) have shown that ALKS 3831 provides the same effectiveness as olanzapine without the significant weight gain frequently associated with its use."

Alkermes anti-depressant ALKS-5461 is a combination of buprenorphine and samidorphan.

ALKS-5461 has had good results in phase 3 trials for major depressive disorder and is in phase 1 for cocaine abuse and kidney disorders. Additional trials are progressing (NCT02158546, NCT02521857, NCT02545439).

SCH23390

SCH23390 is a dopamine D1-like receptor antagonist.

Recent research showed that cue-induced conditioning for alcohol-seeking was reduced by SCH23390.[462]

In other tests SCH23390, "dose-dependently decreased the seeking behavior in the cue-induced reinstatement test in non-dependent and dependent Wistar rats."[371]

SoRI-9409

The delta opioid receptor antagonist SoRI-9409 is in preclinical study.[381]

It previously was shown to produce a selective and long-lasting decrease in alcohol consumption in heavy-drinking rats.[367]

TKMALDH2

TKMALDH2 from Tekmira Pharmaceuticals Corp is in "early development to treat alcohol use disorder."[334]

It is a once-a-month treatment designed for 'alcohol avoidance'.

Previously the only other medication in this category was disulfiram.[463]

PART

5

PART 5: RANDY'S STORY & RESOURCES

18 | BEARING WITNESS

RANDY'S STORY

Some people believe there are no coincidences or accidents. That things unfold as they always were meant to unfold.

Logic tells me that's nonsense. But there's another little voice that tells me otherwise.

The little voice says that I was meant to meet Randy, meant to watch him struggle, be his friend, research all this stuff, write this book, lose him.

The little voice says maybe *you* were meant to read this book.

Maybe this book was intended *just* for you—someone I have never met. And maybe what you do next is one more link in a chain of events that are unfolding just as they were intended to.

•••

When we bear witness, we tell the stories that are too big, too profound to keep inside anymore.

Sometimes, by telling someone's story, we are saying, "This is what happened. It shouldn't have been this way. Let's not do this to anyone *ever again.'*

I think this whole book is my way of sharing that sentiment. So here's Randy's story.

•••

I'm going to tell you some stories about Randy. But before I do, I hope you can keep this picture of him in your mind:

Randy was a guy who once had a beautiful wife (his high school sweetheart), a young son, a lovely house, a hockey team he played on, a boat on his driveway, a group of good friends, a close family, vacations in the Caribbean, and a white- collar job he excelled at.

He was good natured, funny and good looking. He was gifted with anything mechanical, could excel at any sport, and was a born entertainer. He was the life of the campfire, singing songs and entertaining with his guitar.

Growing up, he was a good kid. He stayed out of trouble. He followed rules, went to college, didn't pick fights. He spent summer weekends on the beach with his family looking for someone to take him waterskiing.

He was an extremely *normal* guy. And in so many things he was blessed.

If there was a picture next to the phrase 'wasted potential' in the dictionary, it would be his. And he knew it. He told me that once.

It was like a cruel twist of fate gave him all these gifts, and then gave him a disease that wasted all of them.

Randy was on a train. People joined him and sat with him on the journey sometimes. Some for longer than others. Eventually the train went faster and faster. We all got off one by one and then watched him as the train went out of control, crashed and burned. Nobody could stop it, not even him.

I've heard people explain his alcoholism by saying, "He had 'deep seated' issues," or 'demons'. I think I probably knew him better than anyone did, in his last few years anyway. And I don't think that demons or issues were behind his alcoholism.

When sober, which he was the majority of the time, he was happier and more mentally balanced than just about anyone I knew.

I believe he simply had a disease in his brain, deeply rooted in his DNA, passed to him from his father, called alcoholism.

I hope that as you read, you'll remember how I just described him. Because you won't see the happy, healthy, blessed Randy in my stories.

And if you find yourself starting to judge, please remember that what happened to him could happen to anyone–you or I.

•••

One of the stories that I remember vividly is this one. It's not the worst story, but for some reason it stays with me, it symbolizes something–maybe powerlessness.

Once, after being sober for a few months, Randy saved up his money and purchased a used bike.

It was a big expense for him–he rarely spent money on himself when sober.

When Randy loved something (whether it was a cup of coffee, or a cat), he loved it enthusiastically and emphatically.

And he loved this bike like that. Probably in the same way that a kid on a bike feels freedom for the first time, Randy felt free when he rode that bike.

A few weeks after he bought it, he relapsed.

When Randy was drinking it was very common for him to drink and drive, but he had seen police in his area, so instead of driving, he rode the bike to the liquor store instead.

He was a week or two into the binge when this happened, so he probably looked like a mess—with stained clothes and a scruffy face.

Leaving the liquor store, he had two bags full of bottles—one on each arm. But between the effect of intoxication and the weight and awkwardness of the bags, he was having trouble riding his bike, wobbling around, zigzagging.

Over 6 feet tall, he lost control, flew off the bike, hit the ground hard and just missed landing on his own smashed bottles.

As he said to me later, he just picked himself up, turned around and rode back to the store.

He was afraid the store would close and he'd have no alcohol all night. That was a scary thought, and so he bought more to replace the smashed bottles, and once again rode off on his bike.

He soon realized that he was having just as much trouble as the first time. He fell off again.

This time, he gave up on the bike and dropped it on the lawn of a house he had been passing by.

He didn't lock the bike and didn't go back to get it. He had to get home to drink.

By the time he had sobered up again, a week or two later, of course the bike was long gone.

We cruised slowly past the spot at the side of the busy road where he had abandoned it, and it was such a sad, puzzled look he gave to the patch of lawn where he'd left it.

That was life for Randy though.

It was just one more regret piled on hundreds of others that were part of living with alcoholism.

And the lost bike was really just one of the little ones.

The ones that weighed most heavily on him were the regrets he felt about losing precious time and connection with his son, disappointing his family, and hurting people he loved.

•••

A few months after I met him, I found out he was a binge drinker.

He would follow his urge to drink at any cost.

He would start drinking and then be unable to stop. He would drink eighteen hours a day, non-stop for weeks at a time. If you have ever seen someone drink like this, you'll know without a shadow of a doubt, that there is something wrong with them.

I never had a single doubt in my mind that alcoholism was a biological disease—a major malfunction of some system in the body—after I saw this.

He didn't enjoy this. It made him sad, lonely, depressed and sick. He couldn't really explain why he did it, but it was like he was a prisoner to it.

When I first came across him during one of these binges, I had never seen anything like it.

He sat in a dark basement surrounded by hundreds of cans and bottles, piles of partially eaten take-out food, wrappers and garbage. It was unfathomable that one person could drink so much. When alcoholism took hold of Randy, he was obsessed with and driven by alcohol over all else.

The room stank and he stank. It was disgusting. He looked at me, ashamed. Spills and carpet stains dried around him. He wore stained clothes he hadn't changed in days, he had grown a beard, his face was puffy and bloated. He reeked of vomit and alcohol.

It's not a pretty picture and I guess I could keep it to myself. But there is too much secretiveness and shame in alcoholism already. This is what the disease looks like behind the closed doors of many homes—maybe yours.

I came to learn that he had destroyed his very successful sales career, most of his family refused any contact with him, he had few friends, he had been bankrupt, and he owned nothing but his Ford F10. Eventually, during the time I knew him, he was evicted four times and became a regular visitor to the food bank.

He'd been in and out of rehab programs, treatment programs and Alcoholics Anonymous for years.

On a scale of 1-10, where 10 is a seriously ill alcoholic, I would give him a 12.

•••

On several occasions I tried to help Randy access medical services he needed.

We met very kind people in the healthcare system from time to time. People who seemed to understand, saw him as a human, and truly seemed to care.

But every now and then during these times I observed the failure of a few others in the helping professions to treat him with respect and dignity.

The sudden discontinuation of alcohol in one's system can send your brain into a state of anxiety that most of us have only ever felt momentarily if we've lost a child at the fair, or discover we've left our wedding ring in a public bathroom.

And it was during times when his brain was going into anxiety overdrive, as alcohol left his system—that Randy would sometimes experience this disregard from the healthcare profession.

Sadly, there is a different set of care standards for people with addictions.

Once, I spent a day with him when he wanted to stop a binge and was seeking help from a public detox facility.

Some detox facilities seem to want people visiting them to feel like naughty children. They sometimes seem like detention centers, not places where sick people seek help. Even if people seeking help checked themselves in freely (as Randy did), no cell phones or computers were allowed at any time. If they left they weren't allowed back. They were grouped together in rooms on cots just feet away from one another.

When people die of alcohol withdrawal syndrome (AWS), one of the main reasons is because of the complications of seizures they can experience.[141]

Any alcoholic experiencing AWS, who has had a seizure during detoxification (as Randy had), needs medication to protect them from the further possibility of a deadly seizure.

The detox place we went to, despite being associated with a hospital, and despite being full of people who needed medical help, had no medical staff. And they wouldn't let him in without the seizure medication he needed.

As he had stopped drinking before our drive there, by the time we tried to register at the center, he started experiencing alcohol withdrawal syndrome.

It was Sunday, and so we headed to a hospital emergency room to get the needed prescription. As he vomited and shook, we were sent to the back of the line. People who were 'really sick' came in, waited their turn, were checked out and left while we sat there waiting.

Five hours later we gave up, and taking the letter the detox facility had given us (on their hospital letterhead, specifying the necessary medication), we drove to a walk-in clinic.

After waiting another hour to see him, the doctor dismissively said no to the prescription.

I pointed the letter out to him once more.

He said no.

I told him I would escort Randy straight back to the facility where the staff would store the medication. I asked him to call the detox facility to verify the letter.

He said no.

I told him I wouldn't leave his office until he called the facility.

He finally called them.

He was terse with them on the phone, hung up on them, and then said no. I had no patience left. It took everything I had not to whack a row of clinic brochures off the counter as we left.

Randy was quiet and placid through the whole exchange. I was new to this treatment, but he was used to this. It had been drilled into him that he was to blame; that he'd brought it on himself.

We drove back to the emergency room and four hours of shaking and vomiting later finally met a very kind doctor who gave us the prescription. He seemed to be one of the rare few that understood.

I puzzled later over this experience. Had I not been there with my car to drive him from facility to facility, and with money to pay for the prescription, he would not have been able to access the detox facility himself.

I started to understand why, even when alcoholics reach out for help (something which can be difficult to begin with), it seems so difficult to obtain it.

Of course (as I knew would happen), later AA friends scolded me for enabling him. They said "Randy is a big boy" and that I should not have helped in the first place. "He's taking advantage of you," they said.

Maybe you agree with them. A lot of people would.

But perhaps try re-reading those paragraphs again, and this time remove Randy from the picture.

Replace him with your beloved (non-alcoholic) spouse, or child or friend.

Imagine you are trying to access medical care so that they do not have a seizure and die while trying to access further care.

In that scenario, would that experience—the delays and refusal of treatment for your loved one—someone who is ill and at serious risk of a seizure that could result in permanent brain damage—would that be okay with you? Or would it infuriate you?

Does it represent a good standard of care in a first world country?

Did your perception of whether the experience was okay or not change when you took the alcoholic out of the picture?

If it did, then that may be a measure of your own stigma. We all start off with it. We are all a product of the same societal influences.

•••

When Randy relapsed, his family and friends were always angry, disappointed, worried, and afraid for him. He knew his mother woke up in the middle of the night with her heart racing, terrified for his safety. His father was furious at him for what he 'did to his mother', and wouldn't talk to him for months afterward.

He didn't want to hurt anyone—didn't want to do this to them. But each time he relapsed, he did it again.

He said to me, sobbing, frustrated, feeling the weight of letting his family down, "my god, I try, please, tell them how hard I have tried."

And I agree with him—Randy tried *so hard* not to be an alcoholic.

I truly never saw anyone try so hard to change in my life.

I think some around him would disagree with me. Friends told me angrily, that before I knew him, he would always leave any kind of treatment program early.

And now that I know what I know about 12-step programs and treatment centers, and how they don't really help at all, I don't blame him for leaving early.

He was genetically hard-wired for alcoholism.

I'm sure he was well aware that treatment was doing nothing for him.

•••

When Randy relapsed, as he consistently did, this is what it was like.

He would drink until he had spent every dollar he had. His credit card would be maxed out and his bank account emptied.

Then he'd pawn anything he owned to buy alcohol. His apartment would be bare—left with no possessions—no TV, no laptop, no cellphone.

When he came out of the 2-3 week binge, he would have to pick up the pieces of his life.

Two hours after his last drink, he would start to go through physical withdrawal.

He would experience severe anxiety, shakiness, weakness, be hot one minute and freezing cold the next.

His throat would be raw and swollen from so much alcohol, but through it he would vomit and dry heave.

A few times during withdrawal he had a seizure.

He'd be weak, exhausted, with stomach problems, insomnia and wasted muscles. He never complained about this though. He always felt he deserved it.

But emotionally, things would be much worse.

He would have to deal with the embarrassment of his drunken behavior (lies, missed fathers' days, missed visits with his son, missed work, missed payments) and the relationship carnage that he had created during the binge—angry friends, angry family, angry customers, angry everyone.

Deeply ashamed, he'd face all these people, including his AA sponsor, who was inevitably frustrated and disappointed in him and threatening to no longer sponsor him.

As is AA's practice, he would face his actions and make amends to everyone.

Eventually it was too much for most people. Most of his family shunned him and no longer invited him to family gatherings, little occasions—like Christmas.

Friends gave up on him. It's hard to continue to help and support someone who seems to be hurting themselves over and over again. Few friendships can endure that forever.

The truck would have to be rescued from impoundment. There would be overdue bills to pay, and later, tickets for leaving his vehicle too long somewhere would arrive in the mail.

He was often put out immediately by whoever his landlord or roommate was.

Penniless and homeless, he would go to the few remaining people in his life that would still talk to him and shame-faced, beg ten dollars here, fifty dollars there, enough to find a place to stay—a shelter, a couch or a cockroach-infested motel room. There was no dignity.

With stress, anxiety and shame weighing him down, he would put his life back together, go to daily AA meetings, find work as a contractor, repay each penny, try to put shaky relationships back together, get through isolation and loneliness and enormous guilt, work out to rebuild his physical strength, buy back a few belongings from the pawn shop.

He would continue to try to seek help, setting up an appointment with a psychiatrist that specialized in addiction or turning to a local center for mental health.

And then, in two to three months, he would do it all over again.

French-American cardiologist and former alcoholic, the late Dr. Olivier Ameisen was truly on the mark when he wrote, "Addiction is a living nightmare in which you wake up *to* the horror, not *from* it.[22]

You know those people you walk past downtown? The ones lying on a hot air vent, covered in a piece of cardboard on a downtown street? I always wondered, 'what goes on in someone's life for them to end up there?'

But now I have a better idea of the answer to that. I always thought Randy was one binge away from becoming one of those people.

•••

I was told at Alanon meetings and by others not to help him.

They said, "He has to hit rock bottom before he will change. Practice 'tough love.'" I'd feel guilty for the $50 I'd lend him or for giving him a drive somewhere. I thought they were right, so for a long time I did nothing to help him—I wouldn't lift a finger—and I'd get angry at anyone who did.

But every time I saw this cycle, I'd wonder, if he hasn't hit this so-called 'rock bottom' yet, what can rock bottom *possibly* look like?

Because every three months I saw him go through a hell that would knock most human beings off their feet and put them in a psychiatric ward for a month.

It was unbelievable to see what he endured. It was unbelievable to see him get back on his feet again and again.

•••

He might have been an addict, but he had a big heart, and he never stopped being a human being who hurt—a lot.

I never saw Randy cry about his own material losses. But I did see this big guy bawl his eyes out like a child in pain over the hurt he had caused people he cared for over and over again.

He would say, "I am such a F—ing idiot! I'm such a stupid F-up!"

And he always defended to me the people who treated him badly. He knew how much his alcoholism had hurt them too and was somehow able to forgive them.

As the alcohol left his system after a binge sometimes I'd help him write a 'to do' list.

He was so overwhelmed by the enormity and anxiety of everything he had to fix that the list usually had no more than four tasks on it.

I found an old one the other day while I was cleaning up. It had tasks like, 'eat soup', and 'find truck' written on it.

As anyone would be, he would be overwhelmed by the enormity and anxiety of everything he had to fix.

•••

In between binges, my friend was a different person. At first he was relieved and happy to be sober and in control again. It was like he had gotten something out of his system and could think straight again.

He rebuilt his life each and every time.

When he was sober he was a dedicated and popular member of AA. Shamefaced, after a binge he'd walk back into a meeting and get his first chip all over again. After he died I found lots of those chips. They were a little reminder of something that had offered so much hope.

He read the AA big book, wrote in a journal, practiced the steps, worked with a sponsor, prayed, made amends, and attended meetings nearly every day.

AA was comforting to him. And he loved a lot of the people there (and they loved him). Without the community he had in AA maybe he would not have lasted as long as he did.

But it had no effect whatsoever when it came to helping him control alcoholism.

And inevitably, after a few months, that straight thinking would disintegrate.

•••

I'd been doing some research, so one day Randy and I watched Claudia Christian's amazing documentary 'One Little Pill'.

It was utterly enthralling.

This pill, naltrexone—why hadn't we heard about it? Where could we get some? Would it work? We were so hopeful.

There are some very vivid scenes of drinking in that documentary, and I believe Randy was very strongly triggered by the alcohol cues in those scenes.

The next morning he went to his family doctor and convinced his reticent doctor to give him a prescription for naltrexone. Then he went to the liquor store. He didn't bother to stop at the pharmacy in between.

I picked him up at his apartment and despite the fact that he was already drunk, I marched him off to the pharmacy where we handed in the prescription. I was used to double-takes when I was with him—the sober girl, and the drunk guy.

They didn't have naltrexone—barely knew of it. We waited in the drugstore as they called around to other pharmacies for us and finally located 30 pills at one of them.

Thirty pills was the entire supply of naltrexone in a city of several hundred thousand people. Either there was a huge, unprecedented run on naltrexone or not too many doctors were prescribing it. I hope nobody else needed them. Another car ride, and three hundred uninsured dollars later, we had the pills and he took one.

Naltrexone stopped the binge in its tracks.

He went to work the next day.

That was unheard of.

The next night he came over with a bottle of wine.

He took a pill, and took a drink of wine.

The rest of the bottle sat there on the counter, untouched for the rest of the evening. I still have a photograph of it. It was unbelievable.

The naltrexone seemed to work.

There is research that shows that those with the most severe alcoholism (as Randy clearly had) are also the ones who may have the most difficulty in compliance with naltrexone—or in other words, they are likely to stop taking it when they are supposed to.

And that's what happened with Randy—he stopped taking it.

In a way it was devastating. Here was something that worked for him, but also didn't work for him. Hope came and hope went.

Someone asked me—'why did he stop? That was so stupid!'

I said he stopped for the same reason he drank—because there was a very sick brain inside his head making all of the decisions. There was not enough healthy brain left to just keep taking that damn one little pill.

One of my biggest regrets is that I didn't take the next step with him.

I could have driven him across the border to receive the monthly naltrexone injection. Things might have been very different for him.

But I didn't.

•••

Randy could tell his AA sponsor any transgression he had ever made. As is customary in AA, they worked through many of his most painful moments in life together.

But he only once brought medication up with his sponsor, and the reaction he received taught him never to bring it up again.

I brought it up with his sponsor too—someone I thought was intelligent, logical and well-reasoned. The sponsor sent me a link to an article that said medication was a waste of time and a crutch. I also got the very clear message not to bring it up again.

It was my first experience bringing the idea of medication to an AA member, other than Randy, and it taught me that AA and medication didn't mix.

•••

After the naltrexone experience, Randy jumped through a lot of hoops to get into a well-respected public program that indicated they treated alcoholics with, among other things, medication.

I'd read a lot more about other medications and we were hopeful that he'd find something that could help him manage the disease.

We went back and forth, an hour drive each way, several times.

There was an initial interview meeting, then another day spent watching a presentation made by a social worker, and then a few months of waiting for an appointment with the addictions specialist. Again – this experience of reaching out for help and finding that actually getting it was very difficult.

Finally, he drove into the city again for the doctor's appointment.

I talked to him after the appointment. I was hopeful that he had finally met an enlightened doctor–one with experience and knowledge in medical treatment of alcoholics.

But that wasn't the case.

He said the doctor was not very enthusiastic about medication. The 'medical' advice he'd received?

Keep going to AA.

•••

When he binged, Randy almost always drove drunk.

And he wasn't alone in this–attend enough AA meetings and you'll find it's common practice for alcoholics. (And while it seems to me that combatting alcoholism should be high on the radar for organizations that advocate against drunk driving, inquiries to a few of the major ones in North America told me it isn't).

The second last time I saw my friend binge, he had not eaten for at least a week, had been drinking 40 ouncers of vodka day and night for two weeks, had been seen stumbling around half naked in the parking lot of a seedy motel, was still driving around in his truck to pick up liquor, was vomiting up dark liquid and had several severe bruises and gashes on his body from falls.

I found him this way after the police called me to report that he'd been in a car accident and left the scene. (They didn't know he'd been drinking). He was in a motel right next to the accident location.

You don't need to be a doctor to predict that if this is what your life looks like, it won't be long before you are in a drawer at the morgue.

This was bad, but it wasn't unusual. And so, long before this particular binge, I had become convinced that he would be dead within 5 years.

I told a member of his family this and suggested that she should try to enjoy him while he was still around.

He was fun to be around when he was sober, and when he was drinking he was never mean—just the opposite—sometimes he was grumpy and stubborn, but usually he was quite introspective, honest and gentle.

I guess she heard me because after that conversation he was invited to their house for dinner a few times.

•••

Einstein says the definition of insanity is doing the same thing over and over, and expecting different results.

But that's what we did. He'd relapse, we—his friends and family—would get mad at him. He'd grovel. Holier than thou, we'd deign to let him back into our 'good graces' saying, "this is the last time!" Then the whole thing would happen all over again.

If Randy was relapsing on a regular, consistent basis, why were we always so disappointed and angry with him each time? What good did it really do? In retrospect, it was just very harmful. I started to take a new approach.

Later I thought of it as a kind of palliative care.

If a 'palliative care' approach existed for severe addicts, instead of this one where we just wait for rock bottom, and make life no easier for the alcoholic, then maybe Randy's last few years on this earth could have been not so hellish. Maybe he would still be here.

It took me a lot of time—and seeing the cycle over and over again to come to this perspective.

I know many people would call some of my behavior 'enabling'–I would once have done the same. But eventually I came to the conclusion that if 'tough love' was going to save Randy it would have worked already.

When he drank before, I was sometimes unkind. I would stay away from him until he stopped. If he showed up at the house I wouldn't let him in. But given the perspective that things weren't going to change for Randy, I started to behave differently.

For example, when he was in the middle of a binge, I knew he was lonely and trapped in a basement or dingy motel, so I'd take him with me to a dog park.

I got more than a few funny looks from people, but I didn't care. He was not a threat to anyone, and he loved the dogs.

I'd take him to the beach for an hour for fresh air and some company and food. We'd sit on a rock and when he started getting antsy for more alcohol I'd take him back.

If he stopped by the house, instead of keeping him locked out as I would have before, I let him in for a while.

And if he wanted to go to detox, I'd take him.

When I wrote this part of the book, Randy was still alive. I knew he would die, but not so soon.

And during that time when he was alive I wrote this, "I sometimes think forward to the day when I am at his funeral and, as sad as I know it will be, I don't want to have any regrets about making his life worse than it already was. I want to know that he knew I saw him as a good human who deserved dignity, and showed him love and kindness."

The best advice I can give to anyone, when it comes to how you interact with someone you love, whether they are an addict or not, is to think about how you will feel at their funeral.

I'm no saint. I didn't always treat him well—I was angry at him. I did a lot of things wrong. But I'm thankful that mostly I was kind to him, and I was particularly kind after I realized he wasn't going to get better. And I'm so glad of that.

And because of this, while I do feel regret and guilt at his death, I feel far less, I know, than others.

•••

I had not seen him for a while, but I heard later that over the summer of 2015 Randy was doing really well—on the outside anyways.

He had friends over for a barbecue and played guitar out in his garden for them.

He walked his puppy around his townhouse complex and made friends with new neighbors.

He was spending time with his son—the person on this earth he loved the most–who was working with him over the summer.

He was working hard–something he loved to do, making money in his roofing company, paying off debts, working out, dating.

He was spending time with people in his family that would still include him in their lives and as usual, he kept on trying to mend fences, repairing relationships with friends and family that shunned him. He reunited with his childhood best friend. They planned to play hockey together again in the fall. He looked tanned and fit.

But on May 21 he texted me saying he was "struggling hard." We talked but there was not much I could do.

If his life was a train wreck, then this was the start of the final moments of that wreck–when things start happening in slow motion and you can see it happening in front of you, but you can't stop it.

A week later he gave away his dog.

Around June 8 he started to drink again.

A few more weeks of hard drinking, and on June 24 he told me he wanted to kill himself. He said he no longer wanted to hurt the people that loved him. He didn't see how he could move on with his life–be in a relationship with anyone every again–when he could never seem to stay sober. He didn't want to make his mom cry anymore. He was out of hope.

I took him to detox the next day. All the way there he kept asking me to turn around and telling me he just wanted to kill himself and I kept telling him it would be okay, to reconsider. (It wasn't the first time I'd heard this from him during a relapse).

I got him into the detox, but a few hours later he checked himself out.

The detox called the police. They had a duty to do so because he was suicidal. That's another pattern for people with addiction that is very common. Eventually an addict that the medical system has failed enters the criminal justice system—so that system can fail him too.

Over the next few weeks he continued to drink. He texted and called friends and family and said goodbye.

He said he loved them and told them he was going to die soon. Some responded. Others didn't. Some called the police. Others ignored him.

I could have been there more for him, but I'd made a decision to live my own life. That feels bad enough, so I can't imagine how the people who loved him that completely ignored him feel now, in retrospect.

But at the time, I guess they'd already made a decision to get off the train too. Ultimately, we all have one life to live. We have to live it for ourselves. Sometimes being around someone as sick as Randy is so destructive, we just have to let them go.

There was a period of three days in a psych ward where he was forced to stop drinking (nobody visited). I drove him home and he started back up again.

The police were called and visited him several times. He was always drinking when they called on him—he was never taken seriously.

Show me an alcoholic who has ever committed suicide when he or she was sober.

On July 12 Randy was arrested for drunk driving. That was probably the last straw—more than he could bear.

On July 22 Randy went to the police station for finger printing for the drunk driving charge.

I believe that sometime the next day, July 23, 2015 he hung himself.

He got off the train too.

No more smiling, no more laughing, no more guitar playing, no more drinking, no more Randy.

•••

Randy's sponsor talked about Randy's 'allergy to alcohol' at his funeral.

Hearing this stupid notion (which I'd heard many times before from AA members and read in the AA Big Book), made me cringe.

The last thing I wanted Randy's funeral to serve as was a platform to continue to further the antiquated, incorrect notions about this disease.

Alcoholism is no more an allergy than any mental or physical illness is. If it were, I would have just about stabbed him to death with my daughter's EpiPen years ago.

I notified Randy's psychiatrist a few weeks after his death that Randy had taken his life.

It's not a shameful secret that he killed himself, at least, I won't let it be. It's a fact of this untreated disease.

And it was his way—a way I know took enormous courage—the only way he knew—for Randy to stop the devastation his disease left in his wake.

His psychiatrist—an addiction specialist—a doctor with medical training—wrote me, "thank you for letting me know. I had no idea. Addiction is a horrible condition... The use of that stuff destroys the soul."

I know he had cared about Randy. But the words he used stuck with me. His soul? Really?

It's no wonder that in the days before his death Randy wrote to me and told me he felt like a monster.

I replied to the shrink: "It definitely destroyed parts of his brain, but his soul was still beautiful." In retrospect—it was mean-spirited of me. I was lashing out.

But again—these beliefs and phrases—they aren't right. No doctor would say that Alzheimer's had destroyed someone's 'soul', or that schizophrenia had destroyed a 'soul'.

I can't think of anyone—perhaps other than a murderer or pedophile—who would deserve that description.

An 'allergy' to alcohol? An illness that destroys 'the soul'?

It is the subtleties of language and behavior like these that are the shadows of the massive, looming illogic with which we treat this illness.

Despite the wealth of medical knowledge we have that addiction is an illness of the brain, despite the medical treatments that exist, his sponsor thought he had an allergy and his doctor thought he needed to fix his soul.

No wonder Randy never got better. He never really had a chance.

YOUR STORY

But you do have a chance.

Whether you are just starting to realize you are developing dependence, or you already know you have a serious problem with alcoholism, today you have a far better chance than Randy ever had.

He didn't have this book.

You do.

These medications exist. And now all of this information is here, in one place, for you.

It's up to you now.

My hope for you is that you don't become another sad story.

I couldn't save Randy. But my hope is that this book might help save someone else. Maybe you.

I wish you all the best, and I hope you can do what you need to do to live the beautiful and amazing life you were meant to live.

I hope you can find a way to be happy, joyous, and free.

Namaste.

19 | RESOURCES

APRESCRIPTIONFORALCOHOLICS.COM

If you would like additional information on this topic, I encourage you to visit the book website, located at APrescriptionForAlcoholics.com.

There you will find:

- At least one free excerpt from this book that you can share with others.

- A list of recommended reading which includes some of the best and most informative research articles, reports, popular press articles, and books.

You'll also find links to:

- Key research, reports, and publications mentioned in this book

- Forums and support groups

- Links to online pharmacies

The site will be updated and expanded over time, so please join the mailing list for updates.

SPREAD THE WORD

If this book or the medications in it have made a difference to you, please consider helping to spread the word.

You can do this by:

- Sharing the free chapter found on the website with a friend (www.APrescriptionforAlcoholics.com)

- Passing the book on to someone you know.

- Donating a few copies to a library, school, doctor's office or recovery program.

- Posting about the book on social media.

BIBLIOGRAPHY

The bibliography is also available at the book website (APrescriptionforAlcoholics.com). The site will be updated in the future to include a searchable database of links to bibliography publications. Some printable publications are already available on the website.

If you would like to be updated when the full database is available, sign-up for the newsletter at the book website.

1. Heilig M, Egli M. Pharmacological treatment of alcohol dependence: Target symptoms and target mechanisms. *Pharmacol Ther.* 2006;111(3):855-876. doi:10.1016/j.pharmthera.2006.02.001.
2. Batki SL, Pennington DL. Toward personalized medicine in the pharmacotherapy of alcohol use disorder: Targeting patient genes and patient goals. *Am J Psychiatry.* 2014;171(4):391-394. doi:10.1176/appi.ajp.2014.14010061.
3. Addiction Medicine: Closing the Gap Between Science & Practice | CASAColumbia. http://www.casacolumbia.org/addiction-research/reports/addiction-medicine. Accessed November 11, 2015.
4. Heilig M. The Thirteenth Step Addiction in the Age of Brain Science. 2015.
5. Ferri M, Amato L, Davoli M. Alcoholics Anonymous and other 12-step programmes for alcohol dependence. *Cochrane Database Syst Rev.* 2006;3(3):CD005032. doi:10.1002/14651858.CD005032.pub2.
6. White N. Alcoholics Anonymous has a terrible success rate, addiction expert finds. *Tor Star.* 2014:2-5. http://www.thestar.com/life/2014/03/28/alcoholics_anonymous_has_a_terrible_success_rate_addiction_expert_finds.html.
7. Author Unknown. Medication for the Treatment of Alcohol Use Disorder: A Brief Guide. *NIAAA.* 2013. https://www.ncbi.nlm.nih.gov/pubmedhealth/PMH0058549/.
8. Kraft S. WHO Study: Alcohol Is International Number One Killer, AIDS Second. *MedicalNewsToday.com.* 2011.

http://www.medicalnewstoday.com/articles/216328.php. Accessed April 30, 2015.

9. World Health Organisation. Global status report on alcohol and health 2014. 2014:1-392. doi:/entity/substance_abuse/publications/global_alcohol_report /en/index.html.

10. Bradley K, Kivlahan D. Medications for alcohol use disorder--reply. *JAMA*. 2014;312(13):1352. doi:10.1001/jama.2014.10167.

11. Dealing With Addiction: Why The 20th Century Was Wrong: Peter Ferentzy: 9781105004100: Amazon.com: Books. http://www.amazon.com/Dealing-With-Addiction-Century-Wrong/dp/1105004104. Accessed October 27, 2015.

12. Merchant B. Less Than 1% of Oil-Soaked Birds Survive: TreeHugger. *TreeHugger*. 2010. http://www.treehugger.com/natural-sciences/less-than-1-of-oil-soaked-birds-survive.html. Accessed June 8, 2015.

13. A Look At My Book. 2011. http://www.peterferentzy.com/Excerpt--A-Peek-Inside.html. Accessed October 21, 2015.

14. Anahad O. Drugs to Aid Alcoholics See Little Use, Study Finds. *New York Times*. 2014:2014-2016. http://nyti.ms/1sqM915.

15. Glaser G. The Irrationality of Alcoholics Anonymous. *Atl*. 2015. http://www.theatlantic.com/features/archive/2015/03/the-irrationality-of-alcoholics-anonymous/386255/. Accessed April 28, 2015.

16. Batten L. Science and Technology Select Committee Inquiry on alcohol guidelines. Royal College of Physicians' Written Evidence. 2011;(September):1-12. doi:10.1111/j.1750-3841.2007.00606.x.

17. Nutt D. Presentation: Alcohol Dependence: a Treatable Brain Disease with Serious Health Consequences. In: ; 2014. ttp://progressinmind.elsevierresource.com/videos/lectures/burd en-terms-increasing-mortality-rates.

18. Nutt D. Alcohol dependence: a treatable brain disease with serious health consequences. *Present ECNP*. 2014.

19. MADD - Drunk Driving Statistics. http://www.madd.org/drunk-driving/about/drunk-driving-statistics.html. Accessed September 3, 2015.

20. Unknown A. Children of Alcoholics. *Am Acad Child Adolesc Soc*. 2011;17(17):11-13. http://www.aacap.org/AACAP/Families_and_Youth/Facts_for _Families/Facts_for_Families_Pages/Children_Of_Alcoholics_1 7.aspx. Accessed April 30, 2015.

21. Kendall RE. Alcohol and suicide. *Subst Alcohol Actions Misuse*.

1983;4(2-3):121-127. http://www.ncbi.nlm.nih.gov/pubmed/6648755. Accessed April 30, 2015.
22. M.D. OA. The End of My Addiction. http://us.macmillan.com/theendofmyaddiction/olivierameisen. Accessed May 18, 2015.
23. Measuring America's drinking habit is tricky – here's how to do it - The Washington Post. http://www.washingtonpost.com/news/wonkblog/wp/2014/10/03/measuring-americas-drinking-habit-is-tricky-heres-how-to-do-it/. Accessed October 8, 2015.
24. Hazelden Introduces Antiaddiction Medications into Recovery for First Time | TIME.com. http://healthland.time.com/2012/11/05/hazelden-introduces-antiaddiction-medications-in-recovery-for-first-time/. Accessed November 2, 2015.
25. Release P. Lundbeck Introduces Selincro As the First and Only Medicine for the Reduction of Alcohol. *Eur Pharm Rev.* 2013:2-4.
26. Une recommandation temporaire d'utilisation (RTU) est accordée pour le baclofène - Point d'information - ANSM : Agence nationale de sécurité du médicament et des produits de santé. http://www.ansm.sante.fr/S-informer/Points-d-information-Points-d-information/Une-recommandation-temporaire-d-utilisation-RTU-est-accordee-pour-le-baclofene-Point-d-information. Accessed November 11, 2015.
27. Michael Botticelli Sworn in as Deputy Director of the Office of National Drug Control Policy | whitehouse.gov. https://www.whitehouse.gov/ondcp/news-releases-remarks/botticelli-sworn-in-as-deputy-director-of-ondcp. Accessed October 30, 2015.
28. Obama Tells Outdated Opioid Treatment Industry It's Time To Change. http://www.huffingtonpost.com/entry/obama-opioid-addiction-treatment_5627b3d6e4b0bce347034174. Accessed October 29, 2015.
29. Alkermes PLC > Investor Relations > Press Release. http://phx.corporate-ir.net/phoenix.zhtml?c=92211&p=irol-newsArticle&ID=2072722. Accessed October 22, 2015.
30. Video & Transcript: President Obama Speech in Charleston, West Virginia on Prescription Drug Abuse and Heroin Addiction, Oct. 21, 2015 | Shallow Nation. http://www.shallownation.com/2015/10/21/video-president-obama-speech-in-charleston-west-virginia-on-prescription-drug-abuse-and-heroin-addiction-oct-21-2015/. Accessed October 29, 2015.

31. Addiction Resources | The Business of Recovery. http://www.thebusinessofrecovery.com/addiction-resources---the-business-of-recovery.html. Accessed October 9, 2015.

32. Del Re a C, Gordon AJ, Lembke A, Harris AHS. Prescription of topiramate to treat alcohol use disorders in the Veterans Health Administration. *Addict Sci Clin Pract.* 2013;8(1):12. doi:10.1186/1940-0640-8-12.

33. theNNT. http://www.thennt.com/. Accessed November 26, 2015.

34. Kalk NJ, Lingford-Hughes AR. The clinical pharmacology of acamprosate. *Br J Clin Pharmacol.* 2012;77(2):315-323. doi:10.1111/bcp.12070.

35. Addolorato G, Leggio L, Ferrulli A, et al. Effectiveness and safety of baclofen for maintenance of alcohol abstinence in alcohol-dependent patients with liver cirrhosis: randomised, double-blind controlled study. *Lancet.* 2007;370(9603):1915-1922. doi:10.1016/S0140-6736(07)61814-5.

36. Fletcher DK. New Treatments for Alcohol Related Problems. *Presentation.* 2014.

37. Mason BJ, Quello S, Goodell V, Shadan F, Kyle M, Begovic A. Gabapentin treatment for alcohol dependence a randomized clinical trial. *JAMA Intern Med.* 2014;174(1):70-77. doi:10.1001/jamainternmed.2013.11950.

38. Spanagel R, Vengeliene V, Jandeleit B, et al. Acamprosate produces its anti-relapse effects via calcium. *Neuropsychopharmacology.* 2013;39(4):783-791. doi:10.1038/npp.2013.264.

39. Higuchi S. Efficacy of Acamprosate for the Treatment of Alcohol Dependence Long After Recovery From Withdrawal Syndrome. *J Clin Psychiatry.* 2015;(February):181-188. doi:10.4088/JCP.13m08940.

40. Mason BJ, Lehert P. Acamprosate for Alcohol Dependence: A Sex-Specific Meta-Analysis Based on Individual Patient Data. *Alcohol Clin Exp Res.* 2012;36(3):497-508. doi:10.1111/j.1530-0277.2011.01616.x.

41. Soyka M, Kranzler HR, Berglund M, et al. World Federation of Societies of Biological Psychiatry (WFSBP) Guidelines for Biological Treatment of Substance Use and Related Disorders, Part 1: Alcoholism. *world J Biol psychiatry.* 2008;9(1):6-23. doi:10.1080/15622970801896390.

42. Rosack J. Once-Promising Alcoholism Drug Runs Into FDA Roadblock. *Psychiatr News.* 2014. http://psychnews.psychiatryonline.org/doi/full/10.1176/pn.37.17.0024a. Accessed May 7, 2015.

43.   Agabio R, Colombo G. GABAB receptor ligands for the treatment of alcohol use disorder: preclinical and clinical evidence. *Front Neurosci.* 2014;8:140. doi:10.3389/fnins.2014.00140.

44.   De Beaurepaire R. Suppression of alcohol dependence using baclofen: A 2-year observational study of 100 patients. *Front Psychiatry.* 2012;3(DEC):1-7. doi:10.3389/fpsyt.2012.00103.

45.   Johnson B a, Ait-Daoud N. Topiramate in the new generation of drugs: efficacy in the treatment of alcoholic patients. *Curr Pharm Des.* 2010;16(19):2103-2112. doi:10.2174/138161210791516404.

46.   Leavitt SB. Evidence for the Efficacy of Naltrexone in the Treatment of Alcohol Dependence (Alcoholism). *Addict Treat Forum.* 2002.

47.   Haass-Koffler CL, Leggio L, Kenna G a. Pharmacological Approaches to Reducing Craving in Patients with Alcohol Use Disorders. *CNS Drugs.* 2014;28(4):1-18. doi:10.1007/s40263-014-0149-3.

48.   Harris AHS, Bowe T, Del Re AC, et al. Extended Release Naltrexone for Alcohol Use Disorders: Quasi-Experimental Effects on Mortality and Subsequent Detoxification Episodes. *Alcohol Clin Exp Res.* 2015;39(1):79-83. doi:10.1111/acer.12597.

49.   Greutman MD, Gales MA, Gales BJ, Greutman MD, Gales BJ. Gabapentin in Alcohol Dependence. *J Pharm Technol.* 2015:8755122515575543. doi:10.1177/8755122515575543.

50.   Unknown A. Clinical Trial Indicates Gabapentin Is Safe and Effective for Treating Alcohol Dependence. *Scripps.edu.* 2013. http://www.scripps.edu/newsandviews/e_20131111/mason.html. Accessed May 3, 2015.

51.   ADial: Pharmacotherapeutics for dependence-related diseases. http://www.adialpharma.com/products/. Accessed October 22, 2015.

52.   Litten RZ, Bradley AM, Moss HB. Alcohol biomarkers in applied settings: Recent advances and future research opportunities. *Alcohol Clin Exp Res.* 2010;34(6):955-967. doi:10.1111/j.1530-0277.2010.01170.x.

53.   Author Unknown. The Corporate, Political and Scientific History of Naltrexone. *Low Dose Naltrexone.* 2015. http://www.lowdosenaltrexone.org/gazorpa/History.html.

54.   Together J, Field AE. Medication for Alcoholism : An Expanding Field. 2012.

55.   Alcohol dependency: burden in terms of stigmatization - Psychiatry. http://progressinmind.elsevierresource.com/videos/lectures/burden-terms-stigmatization. Accessed October 5, 2015.

56. Clinical relevance of alcohol reduction | Progress in Mind: Focus on Alcohol Use Disorders Resource Centre. http://progressinmind.elsevierresource.com/videos/lectures/clinical-relevance-alcohol-reduction. Accessed October 5, 2015.

57. Fda. Novel New Drugs 2014. *Cent Drug Eval Res.* 2015;(January):0-18. doi:http://www.fda.gov/downloads/Drugs/DevelopmentApprovalProcess/DrugInnovation/UCM430299.pdf.

58. What Addicts Need. http://www.newsweek.com/what-addicts-need-93767. Accessed October 23, 2015.

59. Pink Ribbons Inc. takes a close look at breast cancer fundraising | National Post. http://news.nationalpost.com/arts/the-women-behind-pink-ribbons-inc-hope-to-change-the-discourse-of-breast-cancer. Accessed October 20, 2015.

60. Eddy DM. The Origins of Evidence-Based Medicine. A Personal Perspective. *Virtual Mentor.* 2011;13(1):55-60. doi:10.1001/virtualmentor.2011.13.1.mhst1-1101.

61. Dodes L. The Sober Truth: Debunking the Bad Science Behind 12-Step Programs and the Rehab Industry. *Book.* 2014. http://www.amazon.com/The-Sober-Truth-Debunking-Programs/dp/0807033154. Accessed April 30, 2015.

62. Miller JC. 12-step treatment for alcohol and substance abuse revisted: Best available evidence suggests lack of effectiveness or harm. *Int J Ment Health Addict.* 2008;6(4):568-576. doi:10.1007/s11469-008-9146-4.

63. Letters 30. http://www.orange-papers.org/orange-letters30.html. Accessed October 29, 2015.

64. Dying To Be Free - The Huffington Post. http://projects.huffingtonpost.com/dying-to-be-free-heroin-treatment. Accessed October 30, 2015.

65. Donovan DM, Ingalsbe MH, Benbow J, Daley DC. 12-step interventions and mutual support programs for substance use disorders: an overview. *Soc Work Public Health.* 2013;28(3-4):313-332. doi:10.1080/19371918.2013.774663.

66. DuPont RL, McLellan a. T, White WL, Merlo LJ, Gold MS. Setting the standard for recovery: Physicians' Health Programs. *J Subst Abuse Treat.* 2009;36(2):159-171. doi:10.1016/j.jsat.2008.01.004.

67. Alcoholics Anonymous World Services. Three Talks to Medical Societies by Bill W., Co-Founder of Alcoholics Anonymous. *Alcohol Anon.* 1949:4-32.

68. As Bill Sees It: The A.A. Way of Life-- Selected Writings of A.A.'s Co-Founder: Alcoholics Anonymous World Service, Bill W: 9780916856038: Books - Amazon.ca.

http://www.amazon.ca/As-Bill-Sees-It-Co-Founder/dp/0916856038. Accessed September 28, 2015.

69. Wilson B. A Communication to AAs Physicians - Vitamin B. *Unpublished.* 1965.

70. Goodman C, Ahn R, Harwood R. Case Studies : LAAM , Naltrexone , Clozapine , and Nicorette. *Dep Heal Hum Serv.* 1997. http://aspe.hhs.gov/health/reports/cocaine/FINAL.htm.

71. Ferentzy P, Turner NE. *The History of Problem Gambling: Temperance, Substance Abuse, Medicine, and Metaphors.* Springer Science & Business Media; 2013. https://books.google.com/books?id=gZlAAAAAQBAJ&pgis=1. Accessed September 3, 2015.

72. *The Big Book of Alcoholics Anonymous.*

73. Inside Addiction Treatment With Dr. Marvin Seppala | The Fix. https://www.thefix.com/content/inside-addiction-with-marvin-seppala. Accessed October 30, 2015.

74. Founding Story |. http://www.compassion4addiction.org/about/founding-story/. Accessed October 27, 2015.

75. Larimer ME, Palmer RS, Marlatt GA. Relapse prevention: An overview of Marlatt's Cognitive-Cehavioral Model. *Alcohol Res Heal.* 1999;23(2):151-160. doi:10.1186/1747-597X-6-17.

76. Mignon SI. Physicians' Perceptions of Alcoholics. *Alcohol Treat Q.* 1996;14(4):33-45. doi:10.1300/J020V14N04_02.

77. Ghfoduhg KDG, Dofrkrolvp W, Dq ZD V, Lq L. Disease theory of alcoholism.

78. Nunes E V. Gabapentin: a new addition to the armamentarium for alcohol dependence? *JAMA Intern Med.* 2014;174(1):78-79. doi:10.1001/jamainternmed.2013.11973.

79. Schomerus G, Lucht M, Holzinger A, Matschinger H, Carta MG, Angermeyer MC. The stigma of alcohol dependence compared with other mental disorders: A review of population studies. *Alcohol Alcohol.* 2011;46(2):105-112. doi:10.1093/alcalc/agq089.

80. Juman RM. The Deadly Stigma of Addiction. *Fix.* 2012:1-30.

81. "My hope that women will not be afraid": Classic Actresses who had Breast Cancer | Comet Over Hollywood on WordPress.com. http://cometoverhollywood.com/2015/10/23/my-hope-that-women-will-not-be-afraid-classic-actresses-who-had-breast-cancer/. Accessed October 28, 2015.

82. Pescosolido BA, Martin JK, Long JS, Medina TR, Phelan JC, Link BG. "A disease like any other"? A decade of change in public reactions to schizophrenia, depression, and alcohol dependence. *Am J Psychiatry.* 2010;167(11):1321-1330.

doi:10.1176/appi.ajp.2010.09121743.

83. Inside The $35 Billion Addiction Treatment Industry - Forbes. http://www.forbes.com/sites/danmunro/2015/04/27/inside-the-35-billion-addiction-treatment-industry/. Accessed October 21, 2015.

84. Targeting Addiction | The University of Virginia Magazine. http://uvamagazine.org/articles/targeting_addiction/. Accessed October 23, 2015.

85. Butler D. Translational research: crossing the valley of death. *Nature.* 2008;453(7197):840-842. doi:10.1038/453840a.

86. Uxj DQG, Dqg G, Wkdw F, et al. List of off-label promotion pharmaceutical settlements. 2005.

87. Mason BJ, Quello S, Goodell V, Shadan F, Kyle M, Begovic A. Gabapentin treatment for alcohol dependence a randomized clinical trial. *JAMA Intern Med.* 2014;174(1):70-77. http://www.embase.com/search/results?subaction=viewrecord&from=export&id=L372116393\nhttp://dx.doi.org/10.1001/jamainternmed.2013.11950\nhttp://elvis.ubvu.vu.nl:9003/vulink?sid=EMBASE&issn=21686106&id=doi:10.1001/jamainternmed.2013.11950&atitle=Gabapent.

88. Release C, Markets I. Major restructuring initiative announced and 2015 guidance revised - Lundbeck. 2015;(56759913):1-24.

89. Big pharma pulling back from mental health | CTV News. 2012. http://www.ctvnews.ca/health/health-headlines/big-pharma-pulling-back-from-mental-health-drug-research-studies-1.1015154. Accessed October 22, 2015.

90. The great neuro-pipeline "brain drain" (and why Big Pharma hasn't given up on CNS disorders). http://www.ddw-online.com/therapeutics/p216813-the-great-neuro-pipeline-brain-drain-(and-why-big-pharma-hasn-t-given-up-on-cns-disorders)-fall-13.html. Accessed October 23, 2015.

91. Kaitin KI, Milne CP. A Dearth of New Meds. *Sci Am.* 2011;305(2):16-16. doi:10.1038/scientificamerican0811-16.

92. RB spin-out Indivior says addiction pipeline will deliver - News - pharmaphorum. http://www.pharmaphorum.com/news/rb-spin-out-indivior-says-addiction-pipeline-will-deliver. Accessed June 9, 2015.

93. Unknown A. Reckitt Benckiser Pharmaceuticals and XenoPort Enter Into Global Licensing Agreement for Arbaclofen Placarbil (NASDAQ:XNPT). *Website.* 2013. http://investor.xenoport.com/releasedetail.cfm?ReleaseID=848226. Accessed June 4, 2015.

94. Indivior understands a patient's journey with addiction. http://indivior.com/diseases-of-addiction/the-patient-journey/.

Accessed October 22, 2015.

95. Turncliff R, DiPetrillo L, Silverman B, Ehrich E. Single- and multiple-dose pharmacokinetics of samidorphan, a novel opioid antagonist, in healthy volunteers. *Clin Ther.* 2015;37(2):338-348. doi:10.1016/j.clinthera.2014.10.001.

96. Neuroscience Drug Discovery Research | AstraZeneca. http://openinnovation.astrazeneca.com/az-rd-focus-areas/neuroscience/. Accessed October 22, 2015.

97. ADial Pharmaceuticals Announces Publication of Study on AD04 for the Treatment of Patients With Alcohol Use Disorder | Reuters. http://www.reuters.com/article/2013/08/12/idUSnGNX6Pzsp s+1d0+GNW20130812. Accessed October 16, 2015.

98. Addex Therapeutics : Addex' ADX71441 Demonstrates Robust Efficacy in Multiple Preclinical Models of Alcohol Use Disorder. http://www.addextherapeutics.com/investors/press-releases/news-details/article/addex-adx71441-demonstrates-robust-efficacy-in-multiple-preclinical-models-of-alcohol-use-disorde/. Accessed October 22, 2015.

99. Kroll D. XenoPort And NIAAA To Test Alcoholism Treatment. *Forbes.* 2014. http://www.forbes.com/sites/davidkroll/2014/09/10/xenoport-and-niaaa-to-test-alcoholism-treatment/. Accessed June 9, 2015.

100. Welcome to XenoPort. http://www.xenoport.com/. Accessed October 22, 2015.

101. AstraZeneca Working with Eolas Therapeutics on Anti-Addiction Drug | Xconomy. http://www.xconomy.com/san-diego/2015/06/30/astrazeneca-working-with-eolas-therapeutics-on-anti-addiction-drug/. Accessed October 22, 2015.

102. Heptares - Pipeline. http://www.heptares.com/pipeline/. Accessed October 22, 2015.

103. Unknown A. SMO. *http://www.da-pharma.fr/*. 2015.

104. Ferraro L, Loche A, Beggiato S, et al. The new compound GET73, N-[(4-trifluoromethyl)benzyl]4-methoxybutyramide, Regulates hippocampal Aminoacidergic transmission possibly via an allosteric modulation of mGlu5 receptor. Behavioural evidence of its "anti-alcohol" and anxiolytic properties. *Curr Med Chem.* 2013;20(27):3339-3357. http://www.ncbi.nlm.nih.gov/pubmed/23862615. Accessed July 9, 2015.

105. A Conversation With Michael Botticelli, The New Director Of National Drug Control Policy - The Diane Rehm Show. http://thedianerehmshow.org/shows/2015-06-11/a-conversation-with-michael-botticelli-the-new-white-house-drug-

czar. Accessed October 29, 2015.

106. SAMHSA bans drug court grantees from ordering participants off MAT. http://www.alcoholismdrugabuseweekly.com/m-article-detail/samhsa-bans-drug-court-grantees-from-ordering-participants-off-mat.aspx. Accessed October 29, 2015.

107. Linchpin: Are You Indispensable?: Seth Godin: 8601400965627: Amazon.com: Books. http://www.amazon.com/Linchpin-Are-Indispensable-Seth-Godin/dp/1591844096. Accessed October 27, 2015.

108. Thomas PE. Suppression of alcohol dependence using high-dose baclofen: A self-case report. *Prog Neurol Psychiatry*. 2012;16(1):30-31. doi:10.1002/pnp.226.

109. "John" David Sinclair - Times West Virginian: Obituaries. http://www.timeswv.com/obituaries/john-david-sinclair/article_eb3ee6be-f39c-11e4-8145-4f42ac610bd0.html. Accessed December 7, 2015.

110. Unknown A. Lundbeck Nalmefene Patent Overview. *Eur Pat Off.* 2015.

111. Unknown A. US2014005216A1 - nalmefene lundbeck patent jan 2014.pdf. *Pat Appl*. 2014.

112. Sinclair JD. Method for treating alcoholism with nalmefene - Patent. *United States Pat Database*. 1992:1-7.

113. Sinclair JD. US Patent for Naltrexone. *United States Pat Database*. 1989:1-8.

114. Babylon Confidential: A Memoir of Love, Sex, and Addiction: Claudia Christian, Morgan Grant Buchanan: 9781937856069: Amazon.com: Books. http://www.amazon.com/Babylon-Confidential-Memoir-Love-Addiction/dp/1937856062. Accessed December 7, 2015.

115. Glaser G. Her Best-Kept Secret: Why Women Drink-And How They Can Regain Control. *Book*. 2014. http://www.amazon.com/Her-Best-Kept-Secret-Drink-And-Control/dp/1439184380. Accessed April 30, 2015.

116. Cameron J, Kaplan B, Parfitt D, Roskams AJ, Trimmer P. BrainFacts. 2012:96.

117. Vengeliene V, Bilbao A, Spanagel R. The alcohol deprivation effect model for studying relapse behavior: a comparison between rats and mice. *Alcohol*. 2014;48(3):313-320. doi:10.1016/j.alcohol.2014.03.002.

118. Heinz A, Beck A, Grüsser SM, Grace AA, Wrase J. Identifying the neural circuitry of alcohol craving and relapse vulnerability. *Addict Biol*. 2009;14(1):108-118. doi:10.1111/j.1369-1600.2008.00136.x.

119. Volkow ND, Koob G. Brain disease model of addiction: why is it

so controversial? *The Lancet Psychiatry.* 2015;2(8):677-679. doi:10.1016/S2215-0366(15)00236-9.

120. Dr. Nora Volkow on Addiction: A Disease of Free Will | National Institute on Drug Abuse (NIDA). https://www.drugabuse.gov/videos/dr-nora-volkow-addiction-disease-free-will. Accessed November 4, 2015.

121. Koob GF, Volkow ND. Neurocircuitry of addiction. *Neuropsychopharmacology.* 2010;35(1):217-238. doi:10.1038/npp.2010.4.

122. Anonymous. [Editorial] Animal farm. *Nature.* 2014;343(6168):5. doi:10.1126/science.343.6168.234-a.

123. American S. Seeking Connections: Alcoholism and our Genes. 2007.

124. Gilpin NW, Koob GF. Neurobiology of Alcohol Dependence: Focus on Motivational Mechanisms. *Alcohol Res Health.* 2008;31(3):185-195. http://www.pubmedcentral.nih.gov/articlerender.fcgi?artid=277 0186&tool=pmcentrez&rendertype=abstract.

125. Bierut LJ. Genetic vulnerability and susceptibility to substance dependence. *Neuron.* 2011;69(4):618-627. doi:10.1016/j.neuron.2011.02.015.

126. A Family History of Alcoholism. http://pubs.niaaa.nih.gov/publications/FamilyHistory/famhist.h tm. Accessed June 8, 2015.

127. In the Realm of Hungry Ghosts: Close Encounters with Addiction: Gabor Mate M.D.: 9780676977417: Psychopathology: Amazon Canada. http://www.amazon.ca/gp/product/0676977413/ref=as_li_tf_tl ?ie=UTF8&tag=whenthebodysa-20&linkCode=as2&camp=15121&creative=330641&creativeASI N=0676977413. Accessed September 29, 2015.

128. Dick DM, Kendler KS. The impact of gene-environment interaction on alcohol use disorders. *Alcohol Res.* 2012;34(3):318-324. http://www.pubmedcentral.nih.gov/articlerender.fcgi?artid=360 6909&tool=pmcentrez&rendertype=abstract. Accessed May 29, 2015.

129. Vetreno RP, Crews FT. Current hypotheses on the mechanisms of alcoholism. *Handb Clin Neurol.* 2014;125:477-497. doi:10.1016/B978-0-444-62619-6.00027-6.

130. Begleiter H, Porjesz B. Potential biological markers in individuals at high risk for developing alcoholism. *Alcohol Clin Exp Res.* 1988;12(4):488-493.

131. Porjesz B, Rangaswamy M, Kamarajan C, Jones K a.,

Padmanabhapillai A, Begleiter H. The utility of neurophysiological markers in the study of alcoholism. *Clin Neurophysiol.* 2005;116(5):993-1018. doi:10.1016/j.clinph.2004.12.016.

132. Fromme K, de Wit H, Hutchison KE, et al. Biological and behavioral markers of alcohol sensitivity. *Alcohol Clin Exp Res.* 2004;28(2):247-256. doi:10.1097/01.ALC.0000113420.28472.25.

133. Ray L a, Chin PF, Miotto K. Naltrexone for the treatment of alcoholism: clinical findings, mechanisms of action, and pharmacogenetics. *CNS Neurol Disord Drug Targets.* 2010;9(1):13-22. doi:10.2174/187152710790966704.

134. Ray L, Mackillop J, Monti PM. Subjective responses to alcohol consumption as endophenotypes: advancing behavioral genetics in etiological and treatment models of alcoholism. *Subst Use Misuse.* 2010;45(11):1742-1765. doi:10.3109/10826084.2010.482427.

135. Barr CS, Schwandt M, Lindell SG, et al. Association of a functional polymorphism in the mu-opioid receptor gene with alcohol response and consumption in male rhesus macaques. *Arch Gen Psychiatry.* 2007;64(3):369-376. doi:10.1001/archpsyc.64.3.369.

136. Filbey FM, Ray L, Smolen A, Claus ED, Audette A, Hutchison KE. Differential neural response to alcohol priming and alcohol taste cues is associated with DRD4 VNTR and OPRM1 genotypes. *Alcohol Clin Exp Res.* 2008;32(7):1113-1123. doi:10.1111/j.1530-0277.2008.00692.x.

137. Ramchandani VA, Umhau J, Pavon FJ, et al. A genetic determinant of the striatal dopamine response to alcohol in men. *Mol Psychiatry.* 2011;16(8):809-817. doi:10.1038/mp.2010.56.

138. Ray L a., Bujarski S, Squeglia LM, Ashenhurst JR, Anton RF. Interactive effects of OPRM1 and DAT1 genetic variation on subjective responses to alcohol. *Alcohol Alcohol.* 2014;49(3):261-270. doi:10.1093/alcalc/agt183.

139. Maguire EA, Gadian DG, Johnsrude IS, et al. Navigation-related structural change in the hippocampi of taxi drivers. *Proc Natl Acad Sci U S A.* 2000;97(8):4398-4403. doi:10.1073/pnas.070039597.

140. Kalivas PW, O'Brien C. Drug addiction as a pathology of staged neuroplasticity. *Neuropsychopharmacology.* 2008;33(1):166-180. doi:10.1038/sj.npp.1301564.

141. Article R, Schuckit MA. Recognition and Management of Withdrawal Delirium (Delirium Tremens). *N Engl J Med.* 2014;371(22):2109-2113. doi:10.1056/NEJMra1407298.

142. Amato L, Minozzi S, Davoli M. Efficacy and safety of

pharmacological interventions for the treatment of the Alcohol Withdrawal Syndrome. *Cochrane database Syst Rev.* 2011;(6):CD008537. doi:10.1002/14651858.CD008537.pub2.

143. Alcohol's Effect on the Brain - GRM7 and Alcoholism. http://wagnergen677s09.weebly.com/alcohols-effect-on-the-brain.html. Accessed September 15, 2015.

144. Meyerhoff DJ, Durazzo TC. Proton Magnetic Resonance Spectroscopy in Alcohol Use Disorders: A Potential New Endophenotype? *Alcohol Clin Exp Res.* 2008;32(7):1146-1158. doi:10.1111/j.1530-0277.2008.00695.x.

145. Lukas SE, Lowen SB, Lindsey KP, et al. Extended-release naltrexone (XR-NTX) attenuates brain responses to alcohol cues in alcohol-dependent volunteers: A bold FMRI study. *Neuroimage.* 2013;78:176-185. doi:10.1016/j.neuroimage.2013.03.055.

146. Volkow ND, Fowler JS, Wang GJ, Baler R, Telang F. Imaging dopamine's role in drug abuse and addiction. *Neuropharmacology.* 2009;56 Suppl 1:3-8. doi:10.1016/j.neuropharm.2008.05.022.

147. Heinz A, Siessmeier T, Wrase J, et al. Correlation between dopamine D2 receptors in the ventral striatum and central processing of alcohol cues and craving. *Am J Psychiatry.* 2004;161(10):1783-1789. doi:10.1176/appi.ajp.161.10.1783.

148. Gilman JM, Hommer DW. Modulation of brain response to emotional images by alcohol cues in alcohol-dependent patients. *Addict Biol.* 2008;13(3-4):423-434. doi:10.1111/j.1369-1600.2008.00111.x.

149. Oscar-Berman M, Valmas MM, Sawyer KS, Ruiz SM, Luhar RB, Gravitz ZR. Profiles of impaired, spared, and recovered neuropsychologic processes in alcoholism. *Handb Clin Neurol.* 2014;125:183-210. doi:10.1016/B978-0-444-62619-6.00012-4.

150. Sinclair S. Development of an alcohol-deprivation effect in rats. *Q J Stud Alcohol.* 1968.

151. Oscar-Berman M, Bowirrat A. Genetic influences in emotional dysfunction and alcoholism-related brain damage. *Neuropsychiatr Dis Treat.* 2005;1(3):211-229. doi:18568071.

152. Farris SP, Miles MF. Ethanol modulation of gene networks: implications for alcoholism. *Neurobiol Dis.* 2012;45(1):115-121. doi:10.1016/j.nbd.2011.04.013.

153. Levey DF, Le-Niculescu H, Frank J, et al. Genetic risk prediction and neurobiological understanding of alcoholism. *Transl Psychiatry.* 2014;4:e391. doi:10.1038/tp.2014.29.

154. Gelernter J, Kranzler HR, Sherva R, et al. Genome-wide association study of alcohol dependence:significant findings in African- and European-Americans including novel risk loci. *Mol Psychiatry.* 2014;19(1):41-49. doi:10.1038/mp.2013.145.

155. Edenberg HJ, Foroud T. Genetics of alcoholism. *Handb Clin Neurol.* 2014;125:561-571. doi:10.1016/B978-0-444-62619-6.00032-X.

156. Genetic Strategies to Detect Genes Involved in Alcoholism and Alcohol-Related. http://pubs.niaaa.nih.gov/publications/arh26-3/172-180.htm. Accessed November 16, 2015.

157. Zorrilla EP, Heilig M, de Wit H, Shaham Y. Behavioral, biological, and chemical perspectives on targeting CRF(1) receptor antagonists to treat alcoholism. *Drug Alcohol Depend.* 2013;128(3):175-186. doi:10.1016/j.drugalcdep.2012.12.017.

158. The Scripps Research Institute - News and Views. https://www.scripps.edu/newsandviews/e_20020225/koob2.html. Accessed September 15, 2015.

159. Sulovari A, Kranzler HR, Farrer LA, Gelernter J, Li D. Eye color: A potential indicator of alcohol dependence risk in European Americans. *Am J Med Genet Part B Neuropsychiatr Genet.* 2015;168(5):347-353. doi:10.1002/ajmg.b.32316.

160. Leao RM, Cruz FC, Vendruscolo LF, et al. Chronic Nicotine Activates Stress/Reward-Related Brain Regions and Facilitates the Transition to Compulsive Alcohol Drinking. *J Neurosci.* 2015;35(15):6241-6253. doi:10.1523/JNEUROSCI.3302-14.2015.

161. Laaksonen E, Lahti J, Sinclair JD, Heinälä P, Alho H. Predictors for the efficacy of naltrexone treatment in alcohol dependence: Sweet preference. *Alcohol Alcohol.* 2011;46(3):308-311. doi:10.1093/alcalc/agq101.

162. Kampov-Polevoy AB, Garbutt JC, Janowsky DS. Association between preference for sweets and excessive alcohol intake: A review of animal and human studies. *Alcohol Alcohol.* 1999;34(3):386-395. doi:10.1093/alcalc/34.3.386.

163. Weafer J, Burkhardt A, de Wit H. Sweet taste liking is associated with impulsive behaviors in humans. *Front Behav Neurosci.* 2014;8:228. doi:10.3389/fnbeh.2014.00228.

164. Kampov-Polevoy A, Lange L, Bobashev G, Eggleston B, Root T, Garbutt JC. Sweet-liking is associated with transformation of heavy drinking into alcohol-related problems in young adults with high novelty seeking. *Alcohol Clin Exp Res.* 2014;38(7):2119-2126. doi:10.1111/acer.12458.

165. A KP, Lange L, Bobashev G, Eggleston B, Root T, Jc G. Sweet - liking is associated with transformation of heavy drinking into alcohol- related problems in young adults with high novelty seeking. *Alcohol Clin Exp Res.* 2014;38(7). doi:10.1111/acer.12458.

166. Kareken D a., Dzemidzic M, Oberlin BG, Eiler WJ a. A Preliminary Study of the Human Brain Response to Oral Sucrose and Its Association with Recent Drinking. *Alcohol Clin Exp Res.*

2013;37(12):2058-2065. doi:10.1111/acer.12194.

167. Defining Alcohol-Related Phenotypes in Humans. http://pubs.niaaa.nih.gov/publications/arh26-3/208-213.htm. Accessed May 22, 2015.

168. Spanagel R, Vengeliene V. New pharmacological treatment strategies for relapse prevention. *Curr Top Behav Neurosci*. 2013;13:583-609. doi:10.1007/7854_2012_205.

169. In Clue to Addiction, Brain Injury Halts Smoking - New York Times. http://www.nytimes.com/2007/01/26/science/26brain.html?_r =0. Accessed May 26, 2015.

170. Naqvi NH, Bechara A. The hidden island of addiction: the insula. *Trends Neurosci*. 2009;32(1):56-67. doi:10.1016/j.tins.2008.09.009.

171. Lewandowski CM. SAMHSA - Reasons for Not Receiving Treatment. 2014;1. doi:10.1017/CBO9781107415324.004.

172. Unknown. Lundbeck Shareholder Magazine. 2011.

173. Rehm J. The risks associated with alcohol use and alcoholism. *Alcohol Res Health*. 2011;34(2):135-143. doi:Fea-AR&H-65.

174. L B. [Benefits in reducing alcohol consumption : how nalmefene can help]. PubMed Commons. *Encephale*. 2015;40(6):2014-2015. doi:10.1016/j.encep.2014.10.012.

175. Sinclair J, Chick J, Sørensen P, Kiefer F, Batel P, Gual A. Can Alcohol Dependent Patients Adhere to an "As-Needed" Medication Regimen? *Eur Addict Res*. 2014;20(5):209-217. doi:10.1159/000357865.

176. Soyka M, Rösner S. Opioid antagonists for pharmacological treatment of alcohol dependence - a critical review. *Curr Drug Abuse Rev*. 2008;1(3):280-291.

177. Weerts E, Kaminski BJ. Comparison of baclofen vs. naltrexone treatment during abstinence on reinstatement of alcohol self-administration in baboons. *Drug Alcohol Depend*. 2015;146:e18-e19. doi:10.1016/j.drugalcdep.2014.09.731.

178. Johnson B a. Medication treatment of different types of alcoholism. *Am J Psychiatry*. 2010;167(6):630-639. doi:10.1176/appi.ajp.2010.08101500.

179. Kranzler HR, Armeli S, Tennen H, et al. A double-blind, randomized trial of sertraline for alcohol dependence: moderation by age and 5-hydroxytryptamine transporter-linked promoter region genotype. *J Clin Psychopharmacol*. 2011;31(1):22-30. doi:10.1016/j.ypsy.2011.07.076.

180. Johnson B a., Seneviratne C, Wang XQ, Daoud NA, Li MD. Determination of genotype combinations that can predict the outcome of the treatment of alcohol dependence using the 5-HT3 antagonist ondansetron. *Am J Psychiatry*. 2013;170(9):1020-

1031. doi:10.1176/appi.ajp.2013.12091163.

181. Neergaard L. In a lab that looks like a bar, researchers hunt new ways to curb heavy drinking. *Chicago Trib.* 2015:2-4. http://www.chicagotribune.com/lifestyles/health/sns-bc-us-med--healthbeat-alcohol-treatment-20150101-story.html.

182. Dundon W, Lynch KG, Pettinati HM, Lipkin C, Alcohol B. Dependence 6 Months After Serotonergic. *Alcohol.* 2006;28(7):1065-1073. http://www.pubmedcentral.nih.gov/articlerender.fcgi?artid=143 5448&tool=pmcentrez&rendertype=abstract. Accessed June 15, 2015.

183. Kenna GA, Haass-Koffler CL, Zywiak WH, et al. Role of the α1 blocker doxazosin in alcoholism: a proof-of-concept randomized controlled trial. *Addict Biol.* 2015. doi:10.1111/adb.12275.

184. Lunau K. Off-label drugs are off the charts in Canada - Macleans.ca. *Macleans Mag.* 2012. http://www.macleans.ca/society/health/off-label-is-off-the-charts/. Accessed June 16, 2015.

185. Miller K. Off-Label Drug Use: What You Need to Know Prescription drugs are often prescribed for uses other than what the. *WebMD.* 2015.

186. Kelvin Ogilvie AE. Prescription Pharmaceuticals in Canada - Off-Label Use. *Standing Senat Comm Soc Aff.* 2014.

187. Lee MR, Leggio L. Combined Pharmacotherapies for the Management of Alcoholism: Rationale and Evidence to Date. *CNS Drugs.* 2014;28(2):107-119. doi:10.1007/s40263-013-0137-z.

188. Christian C. One Little Pill Documentary about Naltrexone and TSM. *Vimeo.com.* 2014. https://vimeo.com/ondemand/onelittlepill.

189. Karpyak VM, Biernacka JM, Geske JR, et al. Genetic markers associated with abstinence length in alcohol-dependent subjects treated with acamprosate. *Transl Psychiatry.* 2014;4(10):e453. doi:10.1038/tp.2014.103.

190. Heilig M. Acamprosate: an alcoholism treatment that may not be what we thought. *Neuropsychopharmacology.* 2014;39(4):781-782. doi:10.1038/npp.2013.272.

191. Yahn SL, Watterson LR, Olive MF. Safety and efficacy of acamprosate for the treatment of alcohol dependence. *Subst Abuse.* 2013;6:1-12. doi:10.4137/SART.S9345.

192. Wackernah RC, Minnick MJ, Clapp P. Alcohol use disorder: pathophysiology, effects, and pharmacologic options for treatment. *Subst Abuse Rehabil.* 2014;5:1-12. doi:10.2147/SAR.S37907.

193. Mason BJ. Acamprosate, Alcoholism, and Abstinence. *J Clin*

Psychiatry. 2015;(February):e224-e225. doi:10.4088/JCP.14com09632.

194. Venturella F, Asaro A, Faillace G, et al. The control of abstinence in the treatment of alcohol dependence: the use of acamprosate in relapse prevention. *J Biol Res Italy.* 2014;87(1). doi:10.4081/jbr.2014.2142.

195. Maisel NC, Blodgett JC, Wilbourne PL, Humphreys K, Finney JW. Meta-analysis of naltrexone and acamprosate for treating alcohol use disorders: When are these medications most helpful? *Addiction.* 2013;108(2):275-293. doi:10.1111/j.1360-0443.2012.04054.x.

196. Witkiewitz K, Saville K, Hamreus K. Acamprosate for treatment of alcohol dependence: Mechanisms, efficacy, and clinical utility. *Ther Clin Risk Manag.* 2012;8:45-53. doi:10.2147/TCRM.S23184.

197. Donoghue K, Elzerbi C, Saunders R, Whittington C, Pilling S, Drummond C. The efficacy of acamprosate and naltrexone in the treatment of alcohol dependence, Europe versus the Rest of the World: a meta-analysis. *Addiction.* 2015;(November 2014):n/a - n/a. doi:10.1111/add.12875.

198. O'BRIEN CC. Intensive Calcium Therapy as an initial Approach to the Psychotherapeutic Relationship in the Rehabilitation of the Compulsive Drinker. *J Psychol.* 1964;57:125-129. doi:10.1080/00223980.1964.9916681.

199. Miller PM, Book SW, Stewart SH. Medical Treatment of Alcohol Dependence: A Systematic Review. *Int J Psychiatry Med.* 2012;42(3):227-266. doi:10.2190/PM.42.3.b.

200. Mason BJ, Heyser CJ. Acamprosate: a prototypic neuromodulator in the treatment of alcohol dependence. *CNS Neurol Disord Drug Targets.* 2010;9(1):23-32. doi:10.2174/187152710790966641.

201. Rösner S, Hackl-Herrwerth A, Leucht S, Lehert P, Vecchi S, Soyka M. Acamprosate for alcohol dependence. *Cochrane Rev.* 2010;128(6):379. doi:10.1016/B978-0-12-398338-1.00040-3.

202. Ooteman W, Naassila M, Koeter MWJ, et al. Predicting the effect of naltrexone and acamprosate in alcohol-dependent patients using genetic indicators. *Addict Biol.* 2009;14(3):328-337. doi:10.1111/j.1369-1600.2009.00159.x.

203. Rösner S, Leucht S, Lehert P, Soyka M. Acamprosate supports abstinence, naltrexone prevents excessive drinking: evidence from a meta-analysis with unreported outcomes. *J Psychopharmacol.* 2008;22(1):11-23. doi:10.1177/0269881107078308.

204. Ooteman W, Koeter MWJ, Verheul R, Schippers GM, van den Brink W. The effect of naltrexone and acamprosate on cue-induced craving, autonomic nervous system and neuroendocrine

reactions to alcohol-related cues in alcoholics. *Eur Neuropsychopharmacol.* 2007;17(8):558-566. doi:10.1016/j.euroneuro.2007.02.012.

205. Jung YC, Namkoong K. Pharmacotheraphy for alcohol dependence: Anticraving medications for relapse prevention. *Yonsei Med J.* 2006;47(2):167-178. doi:10.3349/ymj.2006.47.2.167.

206. Verheul R, Lehert P, Geerlings PJ, Koeter MWJ, van den Brink W. Predictors of acamprosate efficacy: results from a pooled analysis of seven European trials including 1485 alcohol-dependent patients. *Psychopharmacology (Berl).* 2005;178(2-3):167-173. doi:10.1007/s00213-004-1991-7.

207. Kim SG, Han BD, Park JM, Kim MJ, Stromberg MF. Effect of the combination of naltrexone and acamprosate on alcohol intake in mice. *Psychiatry Clin Neurosci.* 2004;58(1):30-36. doi:10.1111/j.1440-1819.2004.01189.x.

208. Heyser CJ, Moc K, Koob GF. Effects of naltrexone alone and in combination with acamprosate on the alcohol deprivation effect in rats. *Neuropsychopharmacology.* 2003;28(8):1463-1471. doi:10.1038/sj.npp.1300175.

209. Weinstein A, Feldtkeller B, Feeney A, Lingford-Hughes A, Nutt D. A pilot study on the effects of treatment with acamprosate on craving for alcohol in alcohol-dependent patients. *Addict Biol.* 2003;8(2):229-232. doi:10.1080/1355621031000117464.

210. Garbutt JC, West SL, Carey TS, Lohr KN, Crews FT. Pharmacological Treatment of Alcohol Dependence. *JAMA.* 1999;281(14):1318. doi:10.1001/jama.281.14.1318.

211. Spanagel R, Hölter SM, Allingham K, Landgraf R, Zieglgänsberger W. Acamprosate and alcohol: I. Effects on alcohol intake following alcohol deprivation in the rat. *Eur J Pharmacol.* 1996;305(1-3):39-44. http://www.ncbi.nlm.nih.gov/pubmed/8813529. Accessed June 2, 2015.

212. Lhuintre JP, Moore N, Tran G, et al. Acamprosate appears to decrease alcohol intake in weaned alcoholics. *Alcohol Alcohol.* 1990;25(6):613-622. http://www.ncbi.nlm.nih.gov/pubmed/2085344. Accessed June 2, 2015.

213. Lhuintre JP, Daoust M, Moore ND, et al. Ability of calcium bis acetyl homotaurine, a GABA agonist, to prevent relapse in weaned alcoholics. *Lancet.* 1985;1(8436):1014-1016. http://www.ncbi.nlm.nih.gov/pubmed/2859465. Accessed June 2, 2015.

214. Young K a, Franklin TR, Roberts DCS, et al. Nipping cue reactivity in the bud: baclofen prevents limbic activation elicited

by subliminal drug cues. *J Neurosci.* 2014;34(14):5038-5043. doi:10.1523/JNEUROSCI.4977-13.2014.

215. Gache P, Beaurepaire R De, Jaury P, Joussaume B, Rapp A, Selle PD La. Prescribing Guide for Baclofen in the Treatment of Alcoholism – for Use by Physicians. *Britiish J Med Med Res.* 2014;4(5):1164-1174. doi:10.9734/BJMMR/2014/7069.

216. Ameisen O. Complete and prolonged suppression of symptoms and consequences of alcohol-dependence using high-dose baclofen: A self-case report of a physician. *Alcohol Alcohol.* 2005;40(2):147-150. doi:10.1093/alcalc/agh130.

217. Author Unknown. Baclofen Authorized in France - June 13, 2014 : BaclofenForAlcoholism. *Reddit.* 2014. http://www.reddit.com/r/BaclofenForAlcoholism/comments/2 ifiqx/baclofen_authorized_in_france_june_13_2014/. Accessed April 3, 2015.

218. Addolorato G, Leggio L, Ferrulli A, et al. Dose-response effect of baclofen in reducing daily alcohol intake in alcohol dependence: Secondary analysis of a randomized, double-blind, placebo-controlled trial. *Alcohol Alcohol.* 2011;46(3):312-317. doi:10.1093/alcalc/agr017.

219. Garbutt JC, Kampov-Polevoy AB, Gallop R, Kalka-Juhl L, Flannery B a. Efficacy and safety of baclofen for alcohol dependence: A randomized, double-blind, placebo-controlled trial. *Alcohol Clin Exp Res.* 2010;34(11):1849-1857. doi:10.1111/j.1530-0277.2010.01273.x.

220. The EMA and FDA Grant Orphan Drug Designation to Pharnext's PXT-3003 for the... -- PARIS, June 23, 2014 /PRNewswire/ --. http://www.prnewswire.com/news-releases/the-ema-and-fda-grant-orphan-drug-designation-to-pharnexts-pxt-3003-for-the-treatment-of-charcot-marie-tooth-disease-type-1a-264190171.html. Accessed June 26, 2015.

221. Padula A, McGuier N, Griffin W, Lopez M, Becker H, Mulholland P. Novel anticonvulsants for reducing alcohol consumption: A review of evidence from preclinical rodent drinking models. *OA alcohol.* 2013;1(1):1-11. doi:10.1016/j.biotechadv.2011.08.021.Secreted.

222. Aisen ML, Dietz M a, Rossi P, Cedarbaum JM, Kutt H. Clinical and pharmacokinetic aspects of high dose oral baclofen therapy. *J Am Paraplegia Soc.* 1992;15(4):211-216. http://www.ncbi.nlm.nih.gov/pubmed/1431867. Accessed April 3, 2015.

223. Smith CR, LaRocca NG, Giesser BS, Scheinberg LC. High-dose oral baclofen: experience in patients with multiple sclerosis. *Neurology.* 1991;41(11):1829-1831. doi:10.1212/WNL.41.11.1829.

224. Yamini D, Lee SH, Avanesyan A, Walter M, Runyon B. Utilization of Baclofen in Maintenance of Alcohol Abstinence in Patients with Alcohol Dependence and Alcoholic Hepatitis with or without Cirrhosis. *Alcohol Alcohol.* 2014;49(4):453-456. doi:10.1093/alcalc/agu028.

225. Brennan JL, Leung JG, Gagliardi JP, Rivelli SK, Muzyk AJ. Clinical effectiveness of baclofen for the treatment of alcohol dependence: A review. *Clin Pharmacol Adv Appl.* 2013;5:99-107. doi:10.2147/CPAA.S32434.

226. No Title. http://livertox.nlm.nih.gov/Baclofen.htm.

227. No Title. http://www.drugs.com/drug-interactions/baclofen.html.

228. Müller C a., Geisel O, Pelz P, et al. High-Dose Baclofen for the Treatment of Alcohol Dependence (BACLAD study): A Randomized, Placebo-Controlled Trial. *Eur Neuropsychopharmacol.* 2015. doi:10.1016/j.euroneuro.2015.04.002.

229. Plackett B. Baclomania: The Cult Of A Cure For Alcoholism. *Fix.* 2015. http://www.thefix.com/content/baclomania-cult-cure-alcoholism?page=all. Accessed April 30, 2015.

230. Szalavitz M. Treating Alcohol Addiction: Can a Pill Replace Abstinence? *Time Mag.* 2009. http://content.time.com/time/health/article/0,8599,1913016-2,00.html. Accessed May 13, 2015.

231. Arnst C. Can Alcoholism Be Treated? - Businessweek. *Bus Week.* 2005. http://www.bloomberg.com/bw/stories/2005-04-10/can-alcoholism-be-treated. Accessed May 18, 2015.

232. The B4a Baclofen Handbook: Phillip Thomas: 9781446640098: Amazon.com: Books. http://www.amazon.com/The-Baclofen-Handbook-Phillip-Thomas/dp/1446640094. Accessed December 17, 2015.

233. Masson N, Cunningham ML, Irnazarow MA, Chick PJ, Heydtmann M, Margaret Q. Baclofen at a Tailored Dose Reduces Alcohol Use , Craving and Adverse Consequences of Drinking in Alcoholics with Medical Disease due to Alcohol Dependence. *NHS Whitepaper.* 2011:243774.

234. de Beaurepaire R. The use of very high-doses of baclofen for the treatment of alcohol-dependence: a case series. *Front psychiatry.* 2014;5:143. doi:10.3389/fpsyt.2014.00143.

235. Leggio L, Zywiak WH, Edwards SM, Tidey JW, Swift RM, Kenna G a. A preliminary double-blind, placebo-controlled randomized study of baclofen effects in alcoholic smokers. *Psychopharmacology (Berl).* 2014;232(1):233-243. doi:10.1007/s00213-014-3652-9.

236. Lesouef N, Bellet F, Mounier G, Beyens M-N. Efficacy of

baclofen on abstinence and craving in alcohol-dependent patients: a meta-analysis of randomized controlled trials. *Therapie.* 2014;69(5):427-435. doi:10.2515/therapie/2014038.

237. Marsot A, Imbert B, Alvarez JC, et al. High Variability in the Exposure of Baclofen in Alcohol-Dependent Patients. *Alcohol Clin Exp Res.* 2014;38(2):316-321. doi:10.1111/acer.12235.

238. Muzyk AJ, Rivelli SK, Gagliardi JP. Defining the role of baclofen for the treatment of alcohol dependence: A systematic review of the evidence. *CNS Drugs.* 2012;26(1):69-78. doi:10.2165/11597320-000000000-00000.

239. Rigal L, Alexandre-Dubroeucq C, De Beaurepaire R, Le Jeunne C, Jaury P. Abstinence and "low-risk" consumption 1 year after the initiation of high-dose baclofen: A retrospective study among "high-risk" drinkers. *Alcohol Alcohol.* 2012;47(4):439-442. doi:10.1093/alcalc/ags028.

240. Evans SM, Bisaga A. Acute interaction of baclofen in combination with alcohol in heavy social drinkers. *Alcohol Clin Exp Res.* 2009;33(1):19-30. doi:10.1111/j.1530-0277.2008.00805.x.

241. Bucknam W. Suppression of symptoms of alcohol dependence and craving using high-dose baclofen. *Alcohol Alcohol.* 2006;42(2):158-160. doi:10.1093/alcalc/agl091.

242. Colombo G, Serra S, Vacca G, Carai M a M, Gessa GL. Effect of the combination of naltrexone and baclofen, on acquisition of alcohol drinking behavior in alcohol-preferring rats. *Drug Alcohol Depend.* 2005;77(1):87-91. doi:10.1016/j.drugalcdep.2004.07.003.

243. Flannery B a, Garbutt JC, Cody MW, et al. *Baclofen for Alcohol Dependence: A Preliminary Open-Label Study.*; 2004. doi:10.1097/01.ALC.0000141640.48924.14.

244. Stromberg MF. The effect of baclofen alone and in combination with naltrexone on ethanol consumption in the rat. *Pharmacol Biochem Behav.* 2004;78(4):743-750. doi:10.1016/j.pbb.2004.05.006.

245. Addolorato G, Caputo F, Capristo E, Colombo G, Gessa GL, Gasbarrini G. Ability of baclofen in reducing alcohol craving and intake: II--Preliminary clinical evidence. *Alcohol Clin Exp Res.* 2000;24(1):67-71. doi:10.1016/S1590-8658(00)80703-3.

246. Childress AR, Mozley PD, McElgin W, Fitzgerald J, Reivich M, O'Brien CP. Limbic activation during cue-induced cocaine craving. *Am J Psychiatry.* 1999;156(1):11-18. http://www.pubmedcentral.nih.gov/articlerender.fcgi?artid=2820826&tool=pmcentrez&rendertype=abstract. Accessed March 13, 2015.

247. Roberts DC, Andrews MM. Baclofen suppression of cocaine

self-administration: demonstration using a discrete trials procedure. *Psychopharmacology (Berl).* 1997;131(3):271-277. http://www.ncbi.nlm.nih.gov/pubmed/9203238. Accessed April 9, 2015.

248. Krupitsky EM, Burakov a M, Ivanov VB, et al. Baclofen administration for the treatment of affective disorders in alcoholic patients. *Drug Alcohol Depend.* 1993;33(2):157-163. doi:10.1016/0376-8716(93)90057-W.

249. Gerkin R, Curry SC, Vance M V, Sankowski PW, Meinhart RD. First-order elimination kinetics following baclofen overdose. *Ann Emerg Med.* 1986;15(7):843-846. http://www.ncbi.nlm.nih.gov/pubmed/3729110. Accessed May 18, 2015.

250. Cott J, Carlsson A, Engel J, Lindqvist M. Suppression of ethanol-induced locomotor stimulation by GABA-like drugs. *Naunyn Schmiedebergs Arch Pharmacol.* 1976;295(3):203-209. http://www.ncbi.nlm.nih.gov/pubmed/1012342. Accessed October 8, 2015.

251. Ahlenius S, Carlsson A, Engel J, Svensson T, Södersten P. Antagonism by alpha methyltyrosine of the ethanol-induced stimulation and euphoria in man. *Clin Pharmacol Ther.* 14(4):586-591. http://www.ncbi.nlm.nih.gov/pubmed/4723267. Accessed October 8, 2015.

252. Guglielmo R, Martinotti G, Quatrale M, et al. Topiramate in Alcohol Use Disorders: Review and Update. *CNS Drugs.* 2015;29(5):383-395. doi:10.1007/s40263-015-0244-0.

253. Blodgett JC, Del Re a. C, Maisel NC, Finney JW. A meta-analysis of topiramate's effects for individuals with alcohol use disorders. *Alcohol Clin Exp Res.* 2014;38(6):1481-1488. doi:10.1111/acer.12411.

254. Arbaizar B, Diersen-Sotos T, Gómez-Acebo I, Llorca J. Topiramate in the treatment of alcohol dependence: a meta-analysis. *Actas Esp Psiquiatr.* 2010;38(1):8-12.

255. Knapp CM, Ciraulo D a., Sarid-Segal O, et al. Zonisamide, Topiramate, and Levetiracetam. *J Clin Psychopharmacol.* 2015;35(1):34-42. doi:10.1097/JCP.0000000000000246.

256. Johnson B a., Ait-Daoud N, Akhtar FZ, Ma JZ. Oral topiramate reduces the consequences of drinking and improves the quality of life of alcohol-dependent individuals: a randomized controlled trial. *Arch Gen Psychiatry.* 2004;61(9):905-912. doi:10.1016/S0084-3970(08)70090-2.

257. Navarrete F, Rubio G, Manzanares J. Effects of naltrexone plus topiramate on ethanol self-administration and tyrosine hydroxylase gene expression changes. *Addict Biol.* 2013;19(5):862-

873. doi:10.1111/adb.12058.

258. Paparrigopoulos T, Tzavellas E, Karaiskos D, Kourlaba G, Liappas I. *Treatment of Alcohol Dependence with Low-Dose Topiramate: An Open-Label Controlled Study.*; 2011. doi:10.1186/1471-244X-11-41.

259. Rubio G, Ponce G, Jiménez-Arriero MA, Palomo T, Manzanares J, Ferre F. Effects of topiramate in the treatment of alcohol dependence. *Pharmacopsychiatry.* 2004;37(1):37-40. doi:10.1055/s-2004-815473.

260. Lingford-Hughes, Welch, Peters, Nutt. BAP updated guidelines: evidence-based guidelines for the pharmacological management of substance abuse, harmful use, addiction and comorbidity: recommendations from BAP. *J Psychopharmacol.* 2012;26(7):899-952. doi:10.1177/0269881112444324.

261. Jewell R. My Way Out - One Womans Remarkable Jouney. *Book.* 2005. http://amzn.to/1vD3eNc.

262. Kranzler HR, Covault J, Feinn R, et al. Topiramate treatment for heavy drinkers: moderation by a GRIK1 polymorphism. *Am J Psychiatry.* 2014;171(4):445-452. doi:10.1176/appi.ajp.2013.13081014.

263. Moore CF, Protzuk O a., Johnson B a., Lynch WJ. The efficacy of a low dose combination of topiramate and naltrexone on ethanol reinforcement and consumption in rat models. *Pharmacol Biochem Behav.* 2014;116:107-115. doi:10.1016/j.pbb.2013.11.013.

264. Edwards S, Kenna G a, Swift RM, Leggio L. Current and promising pharmacotherapies, and novel research target areas in the treatment of alcohol dependence: a review. *Curr Pharm Des.* 2011;17(14):1323-1332. doi:10.2174/138161211796150765.

265. Lynch WJ, Bond C, Breslin FJ, Johnson B a. Severity of drinking as a predictor of efficacy of the combination of ondansetron and topiramate in rat models of ethanol consumption and relapse. *Psychopharmacology (Berl).* 2011;217(1):3-12. doi:10.1007/s00213-011-2253-0.

266. Baltieri DA, Daró FR, Ribeiro PL, De Andrade AG. Comparing topiramate with naltrexone in the treatment of alcohol dependence. *Addiction.* 2008;103(12):2035-2044. doi:10.1111/j.1360-0443.2008.02355.x.

267. Flórez G, García-Portilla P, Álvarez S, Saiz P a., Nogueiras L, Bobes J. Using topiramate or naltrexone for the treatment of alcohol-dependent patients. *Alcohol Clin Exp Res.* 2008;32(7):1251-1259. doi:10.1111/j.1530-0277.2008.00680.x.

268. Johnson B a, Rosenthal N, Capece J a, et al. Topiramate for treating alcohol dependence: a randomized controlled trial. *JAMA.* 2007;298(14):1641-1651. doi:10.1001/jama.298.14.1641.

269. Johnson B a., Ait-Daoud N, Bowden CL, et al. Oral topiramate for treatment of alcohol dependence: A randomised controlled trial. *Lancet.* 2003;361(9370):1677-1685. doi:10.1016/S0140-6736(03)13370-3.

270. Anton RF, Voronin KK, Randall PK, Myrick H, Tiffany A. Naltrexone modification of drinking effects in a subacute treatment and bar-lab paradigm: influence of OPRM1 and dopamine transporter (SLC6A3) genes. *Alcohol Clin Exp Res.* 2012;36(11):2000-2007. doi:10.1111/j.1530-0277.2012.01807.x.

271. Oslin DW, Leong SH, Lynch KG, et al. Naltrexone vs Placebo for the Treatment of Alcohol Dependence: A Randomized Clinical Trial. *JAMA psychiatry.* 2015;72(5):10-11. doi:10.1001/jamapsychiatry.2014.3053.

272. Bilbao A, Robinson JE, Heilig M, et al. A Pharmacogenetic Determinant of Mu-Opioid Receptor Antagonist Effects on Alcohol Reward and Consumption: Evidence from Humanized Mice. *Biol Psychiatry.* 2015;77(10):850-858. doi:10.1016/j.biopsych.2014.08.021.

273. Garbutt JC. Efficacy and tolerability of naltrexone in the management of alcohol dependence. *Curr Pharm Des.* 2010;16(19):2091-2097. doi:10.2174/138161210791516459.

274. Attarian S, Vallat J-M, Magy L, et al. An exploratory randomised double-blind and placebo-controlled phase 2 study of a combination of baclofen, naltrexone and sorbitol (PXT3003) in patients with Charcot-Marie-Tooth disease type 1A. *Orphanet J Rare Dis.* 2014;9(1):1-15. doi:10.1186/s13023-014-0199-0.

275. Yoon G, Kim SW, Thuras P, Westermeyer J. Safety, tolerability, and feasibility of high-dose naltrexone in alcohol dependence: An open-label study. *Hum Psychopharmacol.* 2011;26(2):125-132. doi:10.1002/hup.1183.

276. Garbutt JC, Greenblatt AM, West SL, et al. Clinical and biological moderators of response to naltrexone in alcohol dependence: A systematic review of the evidence. *Addiction.* 2014;109(8):1274-1284. doi:10.1111/add.12557.

277. Various. The Cure for Alcoholism-The Medically .... *Amaz B Rev.* 2015.

278. Crowley P. Long-term drug treatment of patients with alcohol dependence. *Aust Prescr.* 2015;38(2):41-43.

279. O'Malley SS, Corbin WR, Leeman RF, et al. Reduction of Alcohol Drinking in Young Adults by Naltrexone. *J Clin Psychiatry.* 2015;(February):e207-e213. doi:10.4088/JCP.13m08934.

280. Verplaetse TL, Czachowski CL. Low-dose prazosin alone and in combination with propranolol or naltrexone: effects on ethanol

and sucrose seeking and self-administration in the P rat. *Psychopharmacology (Berl)*. 2015. doi:10.1007/s00213-015-3896-z.

281. Vuoristo-Myllys S, Lipsanen J, Lahti J, Kalska H, Alho H. Outcome predictors for problem drinkers treated with combined cognitive behavioral therapy and naltrexone. *Am J Drug Alcohol Abuse*. 2014;40(2):103-110. doi:10.3109/00952990.2013.853074.

282. Arias AJ, Gelernter J, Gueorguieva R, Ralevski E, Petrakis IL. Pharmacogenetics of naltrexone and disulfiram in alcohol dependent, dually diagnosed veterans. *Am J Addict*. 2013;23(3):288-293. doi:10.1111/j.1521-0391.2013.12102.x.

283. Laaksonen Esti V-MS. Predictors of Self-Reported Adherence to Naltrexone Medication in an Outpatient Treatment for Problem Drinking. *J Addict Res Ther*. 2013;04(04). doi:10.4172/2155-6105.1000159.

284. Miranda R, Ray L, Blanchard A, et al. Effects of naltrexone on adolescent alcohol cue reactivity and sensitivity: An initial randomized trial. *Addict Biol*. 2013;19(5):2014-2015. doi:10.1111/adb.12050.

285. Orrico a., Marti-Prats L, Cano-Cebrian MJ, Granero L, Polache A, Zornoza T. Improved effect of the combination naltrexone/D-penicillamine in the prevention of alcohol relapse-like drinking in rats. *J Psychopharmacol*. 2013;28(1):76-81. doi:10.1177/0269881113515063.

286. Rubio G, Jiménez-Arriero M a., Ponce G, Palomo T. Naltrexone versus acamprosate: One year follow-up of alcohol dependence treatment. *Alcohol Alcohol*. 2012;47(6):744. doi:10.1093/alcalc/ags114.

287. Anton RF, Myrick H, Wright TM, et al. Gabapentin combined with naltrexone for the treatment of alcohol dependence. *Am J Psychiatry*. 2011;168(7):709-717. doi:10.1176/appi.ajp.2011.10101436.

288. Bryson WC, McConnell J, Krothuis T, McCarty D. Extended-release naltrexone for alcohol dependence: persistence and healthcare costs and utilization. *Am J Manag Care*. 2011;17 Suppl 8:S222-S234.

289. Pettinati HM, Oslin DW, Kampman KM, et al. A double-blind, placebo-controlled trial combining sertraline and naltrexone for treating co-occurring depression and alcohol dependence. *Am J Psychiatry*. 2010;167(6):668-675. doi:10.1176/appi.ajp.2009.08060852.

290. Rösner S, Hackl-Herrwerth A, Leucht S, Vecchi S, Srisurapanont M, Soyka M. Opioid antagonists for alcohol dependence. *Cochrane Database Syst Rev*. 2010;(12):CD001867. doi:10.1002/14651858.CD001867.pub2.

291. Kranzler HR, Tennen H, Armeli S, et al. Targeted naltrexone for problem drinkers. *J Clin Psychopharmacol.* 2009;29(4):350-357. doi:10.1097/JCP.0b013e3181ac5213.

292. Kuzmin A, Stenback T, Liljequist S. Memantine enhances the inhibitory effects of naltrexone on ethanol consumption. *Eur J Pharmacol.* 2008;584(2-3):352-356. doi:10.1016/j.ejphar.2008.02.015.

293. Myrick H, Anton RF, Li X, Henderson S, Randall PK, Voronin K. Effect of naltrexone and ondansetron on alcohol cue-induced activation of the ventral striatum in alcohol-dependent people. *Arch Gen Psychiatry.* 2008;65(4):466-475. doi:10.1016/S0084-3970(08)79336-8.

294. Krishnan-Sarin S, Krystal JH, Shi J, Pittman B, O'Malley SS. Family History of Alcoholism Influences Naltrexone-Induced Reduction in Alcohol Drinking. *Biol Psychiatry.* 2007;62(6):694-697. doi:10.1016/j.biopsych.2006.11.018.

295. O'Malley SS, Garbutt JC, Gastfriend DR, Dong Q, Kranzler HR. Efficacy of extended-release naltrexone in alcohol-dependent patients who are abstinent before treatment. *J Clin Psychopharmacol.* 2007;27(5):507-512. doi:10.1097/jcp.0b013e31814ce50d.

296. Anton RF, O'Malley SS, Ciraulo D a, et al. Combined pharmacotherapies and behavioral interventions for alcohol dependence: the COMBINE study: a randomized controlled trial. *JAMA.* 2006;295(17):2003-2017. doi:10.1016/S0084-3970(08)70391-8.

297. Morley KC, Teesson M, Reid SC, et al. Naltrexone versus acamprosate in the treatment of alcohol dependence: A multi-centre, randomized, double-blind, placebo-controlled trial. *Addiction.* 2006;101(10):1451-1462. doi:10.1111/j.1360-0443.2006.01555.x.

298. Anton RF, Moak DH, Latham P, et al. *Naltrexone Combined with Either Cognitive Behavioral or Motivational Enhancement Therapy for Alcohol Dependence.*; 2005. doi:10.1097/01.jcp.0000172071.81258.04.

299. Garbutt JC, Kranzler HR, O'Malley SS, et al. *Efficacy and Tolerability of Long-Acting Injectable Naltrexone for Alcohol Dependence: A Randomized Controlled Trial.*; 2005. doi:10.1001/jama.293.13.1617.

300. Sinclair JD. Evidence about the use of naltrexone and for different ways of using it in the treatment of alcoholism. *Alcohol Alcohol.* 2001;36(1):2-10. doi:10.1093/alcalc/36.1.2.

301. Anton RF, Moak DH, Waid LR, Latham PK, Malcolm RJ, Dias JK. Naltrexone and cognitive behavioral therapy for the

treatment of outpatient alcoholics: Results of a placebo-controlled trial. *Am J Psychiatry*. 1999;156(11):1758-1764. http://www.ncbi.nlm.nih.gov/pubmed/10553740. Accessed May 8, 2015.

302. Oslin D, Liberto JG, O'Brien J, Krois S. *Tolerability of Naltrexone in Treating Older, Alcohol-Dependent Patients.*; 1997.

303. Sinclair JD. Drugs to decrease alcohol drinking. *Ann Med.* 1990;22(5):357-362. http://www.ncbi.nlm.nih.gov/pubmed/2291844. Accessed May 28, 2015.

304. Volpicelli JR, Davis MA, Olgin JE. Naltrexone blocks the post-shock increase of ethanol consumption. *Life Sci.* 1986;38(9):841-847. http://www.ncbi.nlm.nih.gov/pubmed/3951334. Accessed May 28, 2015.

305. Ross D, Hartmann RJ, Geller I. Ethanol preference in the hamster: effects of morphine sulfate and naltrexone, a long-acting morphine antagonist. *Proc West Pharmacol Soc.* 1976;19:326-330. http://europepmc.org/abstract/med/996000. Accessed May 28, 2015.

306. Points L, Commission E. Learning Points from Nalmefene / Selincro. 2015:1-5.

307. Spence D. Bad medicine: nalmefene in alcohol misuse. *BMJ.* 2014;348(feb14_1):g1531. doi:10.1136/bmj.g1531.

308. van den Brink W, Sørensen P, Torup L, Mann K, Gual A. Long-term efficacy, tolerability and safety of nalmefene as-needed in patients with alcohol dependence: A 1-year, randomised controlled study. *J Psychopharmacol.* 2014. doi:10.1177/0269881114527362.

309. Brink W Van Den, Strang J, Gual A, Sørensen P, Mann K. EPA - 0405 – Tolerability and safety of as - needed nalmefene in the treatment of alcohol dependence : results from the phase 3 programme. *Eur Psychiatry.* 2014.

310. van den Brink W, Strang J, Gual A, Sørensen P, Jensen TJ, Mann K. Safety and tolerability of as-needed nalmefene in the treatment of alcohol dependence: results from the Phase III clinical programme. *Expert Opin Drug Saf.* 2015;14(4):495-504. doi:10.1517/14740338.2015.1011619.

311. Gual A, He Y, Torup L, van den Brink W, Mann K. A randomised, double-blind, placebo-controlled, efficacy study of nalmefene, as-needed use, in patients with alcohol dependence. *Eur Neuropsychopharmacol.* 2013;23(11):1432-1442. doi:10.1016/j.euroneuro.2013.02.006.

312. Stevenson M, Pandor A, Stevens JW, et al. Nalmefene for Reducing Alcohol Consumption in People with Alcohol

Dependence: An Evidence Review Group Perspective of a NICE Single Technology Appraisal. *Pharmacoeconomics.* 2015;33(8):833-847. doi:10.1007/s40273-015-0272-0.

313. Sinclair J, Batel P, Kiefer F, Chick J, Sørensen P, Gual A. 1613 – As-needed use of nalmefene in the treatment of alcohol dependence. *Eur Psychiatry.* 2013;28:1. doi:10.1016/S0924-9338(13)76610-0.

314. van den Brink W, Sørensen P, Torup L, Mann K, Gual A. 1105 – Long-term efficacy of nalmefene as-needed in alcohol dependent patients with high drinking risk levels: results of a subgroup analysis. *Eur Psychiatry.* 2013;28:1. doi:10.1016/S0924-9338(13)76211-4.

315. van den Brink W, Aubin HJ, Bladström A, Torup L, Gual A, Mann K. Efficacy of As-Needed Nalmefene in Alcohol-Dependent Patients with at Least a High Drinking Risk Level: Results from a Subgroup Analysis of Two Randomized Controlled 6-Month Studies. *Alcohol Alcohol.* 2013;48(5):570-578. doi:10.1093/alcalc/agt061.

316. van den Brink W, Aubin H-J, Sørensen P, Torup L, Mann K, Gual A. 1108 – Esense 2 - randomised controlled 6-month study of as-needed nalmefene: subgroup analysis of alcohol dependent patients with high drinking risk level. *Eur Psychiatry.* 2013;28:1. doi:10.1016/S0924-9338(13)76213-8.

317. Mann K, Bladström A, Torup L, Gual A, van den Brink W. P-59 - Shifting the paradigm: reduction of alcohol consumption in alcohol dependent patients - a randomised, double-blind, placebo-controlled study of nalmefene, as-needed use. *Eur Psychiatry.* 2012;27:1. doi:10.1016/S0924-9338(12)74226-8.

318. Mann K, Bladström A, Torup L, Gual A, Van Den Brink W. Extending the treatment options in alcohol dependence: A randomized controlled study of As-needed nalmefene. *Biol Psychiatry.* 2013;73(8):706-713. doi:10.1016/j.biopsych.2012.10.020.

319. Arias AJ, Armeli S, Gelernter J, et al. Effects of opioid receptor gene variation on targeted nalmefene treatment in heavy drinkers. *Alcohol Clin Exp Res.* 2008;32(7):1159-1166. doi:10.1111/j.1530-0277.2008.00735.x.

320. Anton RF, Pettinati H, Zweben A, et al. A multi-site dose ranging study of nalmefene in the treatment of alcohol dependence. *J Clin Psychopharmacol.* 2004;24(4):421-428. http://www.ncbi.nlm.nih.gov/pubmed/15232334. Accessed June 2, 2015.

321. Drobes DJ, Anton RF, Thomas SE, Voronin K. Effects of naltrexone and nalmefene on subjective response to alcohol

among non-treatment-seeking alcoholics and social drinkers. *Alcohol Clin Exp Res.* 2004;28(9):1362-1370. http://www.ncbi.nlm.nih.gov/pubmed/15365307. Accessed June 2, 2015.

322. Mason BJ, Salvato FR, Williams LD, Ritvo EC, Cutler RB. A double-blind, placebo-controlled study of oral nalmefene for alcohol dependence. *Arch Gen Psychiatry.* 1999;56(8):719-724. doi:10.1001/archpsyc.56.8.719.Text.

323. Mason BJ, Ritvo EC, Morgan RO, et al. A double-blind, placebo-controlled pilot study to evaluate the efficacy and safety of oral nalmefene HCl for alcohol dependence. *Alcohol Clin Exp Res.* 1994;18(5):1162-1167. http://www.ncbi.nlm.nih.gov/pubmed/7847600. Accessed June 2, 2015.

324. Gal TJ, DiFazio CA, Dixon R. Prolonged blockade of opioid effect with oral nalmefene. *Clin Pharmacol Ther.* 1986;40(5):537-542. http://www.ncbi.nlm.nih.gov/pubmed/3533370. Accessed June 2, 2015.

325. Gabapentin (Neurontin) versus - eMedExpert.com. http://www.emedexpert.com/compare-meds/gabapentin.shtml#gaba_pregaba. Accessed June 29, 2015.

326. Bockbrader HN, Wesche D, Miller R, Chapel S, Janiczek N, Burger P. A comparison of the pharmacokinetics and pharmacodynamics of pregabalin and gabapentin. *Clin Pharmacokinet.* 2010;49(10):661-669. doi:10.2165/11536200-000000000-00000.

327. Häkkinen M. Abuse and Fatal Poisonings Involving Prescription Opiods - Revelations from postmortem toxicology. *Unpublished.* 2015.

328. FDA approves Horizant to treat restless legs syndrome. 2015:250188.

329. Sirven JI. New uses for older drugs: the tales of aspirin, thalidomide, and gabapentin. *Mayo Clin Proc.* 2010;85(6):508-511. doi:10.4065/mcp.2010.0267.

330. Gabapentin Effective Treatment for Alcohol Dependence | Psych Congress Network. http://www.psychcongress.com/article/gabapentin-effective-treatment-alcohol-dependence-14032. Accessed June 30, 2015.

331. Leung JG, Hall-Flavin D, Nelson S, Schmidt KA, Schak KM. The Role of Gabapentin in the Management of Alcohol Withdrawal and Dependence. *Ann Pharmacother.* 2015:1060028015585849. doi:10.1177/1060028015585849.

332. Martinotti G, Di Nicola M, Tedeschi D, et al. Pregabalin versus naltrexone in alcohol dependence: a randomised, double-blind,

comparison trial. *J Psychopharmacol.* 2010;24(9):1367-1374. doi:10.1177/0269881109102623.

333. Baird CRW, Fox P, Colvin LA. Gabapentinoid abuse in order to potentiate the effect of methadone: a survey among substance misusers. *Eur Addict Res.* 2014;20(3):115-118. doi:10.1159/000355268.

334. Edney A. Drugs for Alcoholism Don't Have to Lead to Sobriety. *Bloom Bus.* 2015. http://www.bloomberg.com/news/articles/2015-02-11/drugs-for-alcoholism-don-t-have-to-lead-to-sobriety-fda-says. Accessed April 3, 2015.

335. Guglielmo R, Martinotti G, Clerici M, Janiri L. Pregabalin for alcohol dependence: A critical review of the literature. *Adv Ther.* 2012;29(11):947-957. doi:10.1007/s12325-012-0061-5.

336. Brower KJ, Myra Kim H, Strobbe S, Karam-Hage M a., Consens F, Zucker R a. A randomized double-blind pilot trial of gabapentin versus placebo to treat alcohol dependence and comorbid insomnia. *Alcohol Clin Exp Res.* 2008;32(8):1429-1438. doi:10.1111/j.1530-0277.2008.00706.x.

337. Martinotti G, Nicola M, Tedeschi D, Mazza M, Janiri L, Bria P. Efficacy and safety of pregabalin in alcohol dependence. *Adv Ther.* 2008;25(6):608-618. doi:10.1007/s12325-008-0066-2.

338. Roberto M, Gilpin NW, O'Dell LE, et al. Cellular and behavioral interactions of gabapentin with alcohol dependence. *J Neurosci.* 2008;28(22):5762-5771. doi:10.1523/JNEUROSCI.0575-08.2008.

339. Furieri F a., Nakamura-Palacios EM. Gabapentin reduces alcohol consumption and craving: A randomized, double-blind, placebo-controlled trial. *J Clin Psychiatry.* 2007;68(11):1691-1700. doi:10.4088/JCP.v68n1108.

340. Bisaga A, Evans SM. The acute effects of gabapentin in combination with alcohol in heavy drinkers. *Drug Alcohol Depend.* 2006;83(1):25-32. doi:10.1016/j.drugalcdep.2005.10.008.

341. Karam-Hage M, Brower KJ. Open pilot study of gabapentin versus trazodone to treat insomnia in alcoholic outpatients. *Psychiatry Clin Neurosci.* 2003;57(5):542-544. doi:10.1046/j.1440-1819.2003.01161.x.

342. Gabapentin treatment for insomnia associated with alchohol dependence - ProQuest. http://search.proquest.com/openview/fa185dfc42ab42e98c4efc22eef95cf8/1?pq-origsite=gscholar. Accessed June 29, 2015.

343. Bankole A. Johnson. Patent - Serotonin transporter gene and treatment of alcoholism. *Google Patents.* 2014. https://www.google.com/patents/US20140206734. Accessed May 13, 2015.

344. Clark DB. Pharmacotherapy for adolescent alcohol use disorder. *CNS Drugs.* 2015;26(7):559-569. doi:10.2165/11634330-000000000-00000.

345. Moore CF, Lycas MD, Bond CW, Johnson B a, Lynch WJ. Acute and chronic administration of a low-dose combination of topiramate and ondansetron reduces ethanol's reinforcing effects in male alcohol preferring (P) rats. *Exp Clin Psychopharmacol.* 2014;22(1):35-42. doi:10.1037/a0035215.

346. Kenna G a., Zywiak WH, Swift RM, et al. Ondansetron Reduces Naturalistic Drinking in Nontreatment-Seeking Alcohol-Dependent Individuals with the LL 5'-HTTLPR Genotype: A Laboratory Study. *Alcohol Clin Exp Res.* 2014;38(6):1567-1574. doi:10.1111/acer.12410.

347. Kenna G a., Zywiak WH, Swift RM, et al. Ondansetron and sertraline may interact with 5-HTTLPR and DRD4 polymorphisms to reduce drinking in non-treatment seeking alcohol-dependent women: Exploratory findings. *Alcohol.* 2014;48(6):515-522. doi:10.1016/j.alcohol.2014.04.005.

348. Addolorato G, Mirijello A, Leggio L, Ferrulli A, Landolfi R. Management of alcohol dependence in patients with liver disease. *CNS Drugs.* 2013;27(4):287-299. doi:10.1007/s40263-013-0043-4.

349. Corrêa Filho JM, Baltieri DA. A pilot study of full-dose ondansetron to treat heavy-drinking men withdrawing from alcohol in Brazil. *Addict Behav.* 2013;38(4):2044-2051. doi:10.1016/j.addbeh.2012.12.018.

350. Johnson BA, Roache JD, Ait-Daoud N, Zanca NA, Velazquez M. Ondansetron reduces the craving of biologically predisposed alcoholics. *Psychopharmacology (Berl).* 2002;160(4):408-413. doi:10.1007/s00213-002-1002-9.

351. Overstreet DH, McArthur R. Alternatives to Naltrexone in Animal Models. *Alcohol Clin Exp Res.* 1996;20(s8):231a - 235a. doi:10.1111/j.1530-0277.1996.tb01782.x.

352. Johnson BA, Campling GM, Griffiths P, Cowen PJ. Attenuation of some alcohol-induced mood changes and the desire to drink by 5-HT3 receptor blockade: a preliminary study in healthy male volunteers. *Psychopharmacology (Berl).* 1993;112(1):142-144. http://www.ncbi.nlm.nih.gov/pubmed/7871004. Accessed June 8, 2015.

353. Erwin BL, Slaton RM. Varenicline in the Treatment of Alcohol Use Disorders. *Ann Pharmacother.* 2014;48(11):1445-1455. doi:10.1177/1060028014545806.

354. Litten RZ, Ryan ML, Fertig JB, et al. A double-blind, placebo-controlled trial assessing the efficacy of varenicline tartrate for alcohol dependence. *J Addict Med.* 2013;7(4):277-286.

doi:10.1097/ADM.0b013e31829623f4.

355. Ray L a, Courtney KE, Ghahremani DG, Miotto K, Brody A, London ED. Varenicline, naltrexone, and their combination for heavy-drinking smokers: preliminary neuroimaging findings. *Am J Drug Alcohol Abuse.* 2014;2990(00):1-10. doi:10.3109/00952990.2014.927881.

356. Ray LA, Courtney KE, Ghahremani DG, Miotto K, Brody A, London ED. Varenicline, low dose naltrexone, and their combination for heavy-drinking smokers: human laboratory findings. *Psychopharmacology (Berl).* 2014;231(19):3843-3853. doi:10.1007/s00213-014-3519-0.

357. Mitchell JM, Teague CH, Kayser AS, Bartlett SE, Fields HL. Varenicline decreases alcohol consumption in heavy-drinking smokers. *Psychopharmacology (Berl).* 2012;223(3):299-306. doi:10.1007/s00213-012-2717-x.

358. No Evidence Varenicline Raises Risk of Suicide, Accidents | Psych Congress Network. http://www.psychcongress.com/article/no-evidence-varenicline-raises-risk-suicide-accidents-22853. Accessed October 14, 2015.

359. Schacht JP, Anton RF, Randall PK, Li X, Henderson S, Myrick H. Varenicline effects on drinking, craving and neural reward processing among non-treatment-seeking alcohol-dependent individuals. *Psychopharmacology (Berl).* 2014;231(18):3799-3807. doi:10.1007/s00213-014-3518-1.

360. Vatsalya V, Gowin JL, Schwandt ML, et al. Effects of Varenicline on Neural Correlates of Alcohol Salience in Heavy Drinkers. *Int J Neuropsychopharmacol.* 2015:pyv068. doi:10.1093/ijnp/pyv068.

361. Fucito LM, Toll BA, Wu R, Romano DM, Tek E, O'Malley SS. A preliminary investigation of varenicline for heavy drinking smokers. *Psychopharmacology (Berl).* 2011;215(4):655-663. doi:10.1007/s00213-010-2160-9.

362. McKee SA, Harrison ELR, O'Malley SS, et al. Varenicline reduces alcohol self-administration in heavy-drinking smokers. *Biol Psychiatry.* 2009;66(2):185-190. doi:10.1016/j.biopsych.2009.01.029.

363. Steensland P, Simms JA, Holgate J, Richards JK, Bartlett SE. Varenicline, an alpha4beta2 nicotinic acetylcholine receptor partial agonist, selectively decreases ethanol consumption and seeking. *Proc Natl Acad Sci U S A.* 2007;104(30):12518-12523. doi:10.1073/pnas.0705368104.

364. Mayer M, Rogers J. Error in alcohol overuse article. *BC Med J.* 2012;54(1):1-2. http://www.bcmj.org/print/4423.

365. Functional Polymorphism of the Dopamine β-Hydroxylase Gene Is Associated With Increased Risk of Disulfiram-Induced

Adverse Effects in Alcohol-Dependent Patients. 2012. http://journals.lww.com/psychopharmacology/Citation/2012/0 8000/Functional_Polymorphism_of_the_Dopamine.26.aspx. Accessed July 6, 2015.

366. Fletcher K, Stone E, Mohamad MW, et al. A breath test to assess compliance with disulfiram. *Addiction.* 2006;101(12):1705-1710. doi:10.1111/j.1360-0443.2006.01602.x.

367. Nielsen CK, Simms JA, Pierson HB, et al. A Novel Delta Opioid Receptor Antagonist, SoRI-9409, Produces a Selective and Long-Lasting Decrease in Ethanol Consumption in Heavy-Drinking Rats. *Biol Psychiatry.* 2008;64(11):974-981. doi:10.1016/j.biopsych.2008.07.018.

368. Gilpin NW, Koob GF. Effects of adrenoceptor antagonists on alcohol drinking by alcohol-dependent rats. *Psychopharmacology (Berl).* 2010;212(3):431-439. doi:10.1007/s00213-010-1967-8.

369. Dd R, Le B, Cl K, Jc F. Combining the α1 adrenergic receptor antagonist, prazosin, with the β- adrenergic receptor antagonist, propranolol, reduces alcohol drinking more effectively than either drug alone. *Alcohol Clin Exp Res.* 2015;38(6):2014-2015. doi:10.1111/acer.12441.

370. Simpson TL, Malte C a, Dietel B, et al. A pilot trial of prazosin, an alpha-1 adrenergic antagonist, for comorbid alcohol dependence and posttraumatic stress disorder. *Alcohol Clin Exp Res.* 2015;39(5):808-817. doi:10.1111/acer.12703.

371. Meinhardt M, Sommer W. The postdependent state in rats as a model for medication development in alcoholism. *Addict Biol.* 2014;[accepted](1):1-21. doi:10.1111/adb.12187.

372. Froehlich JC, Hausauer BJ, Federoff DL, Fischer SM, Rasmussen DD. Prazosin reduces alcohol drinking throughout prolonged treatment and blocks the initiation of drinking in rats selectively bred for high alcohol intake. *Alcohol Clin Exp Res.* 2013;37(9):1552-1560. doi:10.1111/acer.12116.

373. Rasmussen DD, Alexander LL, Raskind M a., Froehlich JC. The α1-adrenergic receptor antagonist, prazosin, reduces alcohol drinking in alcohol-preferring (P) rats. *Alcohol Clin Exp Res.* 2009;33(2):264-272. doi:10.1111/j.1530-0277.2008.00829.x.

374. Knapp CM, Mercado M, Markley TL, Crosby S, Ciraulo DA, Kornetsky C. Zonisamide decreases ethanol intake in rats and mice. *Pharmacol Biochem Behav.* 2007;87(1):65-72. doi:10.1016/j.pbb.2007.04.001.

375. Knapp CM, Sarid-Segal O, Richardson M a, et al. *Open Label Trial of the Tolerability and Efficacy of Zonisamide in the Treatment of Alcohol Dependence.*; 2010. doi:10.3109/00952991003674812.

376. Arias AJ, Feinn R, Oncken C, Covault J, Kranzler HR. *Placebo-*

Controlled Trial of Zonisamide for the Treatment of Alcohol Dependence.; 2010. doi:10.1097/JCP.0b013e3181db38bb.

377. Rubio G, López-Muñoz F, Ferre F, et al. Effects of Zonisamide in the Treatment of Alcohol Dependence. *Clin Neuropharmacol.* 2010;33(5):250-253. doi:10.1097/WNF.0b013e3181f0ed9a.

378. Sarid-segal O, Knapp CM, Burch W, et al. The anticonvulsant Zonisamide Reduces Ethanol Self-Administration by Risky Drinkers. *Am J Drug Alcohol Abuse.* 2009;35(5):316-319. doi:10.1080/00952990903060150.The.

379. Alkermes plc - News Release. http://investor.alkermes.com/mobile.view?c=92211&v=203&d =1&id=2004543. Accessed October 23, 2015.

380. Littlewood R a, Claus ED, Arenella P, et al. Dose specific effects of olanzapine in the treatment of alcohol dependence. *Psychopharmacology (Berl).* 2014;232(7):1261-1268. doi:10.1007/s00213-014-3757-1.

381. Aubin HJ, Daeppen JB. Emerging pharmacotherapies for alcohol dependence: A systematic review focusing on reduction in consumption. *Drug Alcohol Depend.* 2013;133(1):15-29. doi:10.1016/j.drugalcdep.2013.04.025.

382. Gianoli MO, Jane JS, O'Brien E, Ralevski E. Treatment for comorbid borderline personality disorder and alcohol use disorders: a review of the evidence and future recommendations. *Exp Clin Psychopharmacol.* 2012;20(4):333-344. doi:10.1037/a0027999.

383. Hutchison KE, Ray L, Sandman E, et al. The effect of olanzapine on craving and alcohol consumption. *Neuropsychopharmacology.* 2006;31(6):1310-1317. doi:10.1038/sj.npp.1300917.

384. Hutchison KE, Wooden A, Swift RM, et al. Olanzapine reduces craving for alcohol: a DRD4 VNTR polymorphism by pharmacotherapy interaction. *Neuropsychopharmacology.* 2003;28(10):1882-1888. doi:10.1038/sj.npp.1300264.

385. Hutchison KE, Swift R, Rohsenow DJ, Monti PM, Davidson D, Almeida A. Olanzapine reduces urge to drink after drinking cues and a priming dose of alcohol. *Psychopharmacology (Berl).* 2001;155(1):27-34. http://www.ncbi.nlm.nih.gov/pubmed/11374333. Accessed November 16, 2015.

386. Conley RR, Kelly DL, Gale EA. Olanzapine response in treatment-refractory schizophrenic patients with a history of substance abuse. *Schizophr Res.* 1998;33(1-2):95-101. http://www.ncbi.nlm.nih.gov/pubmed/9783349. Accessed November 16, 2015.

387. Zoloft No Better Than Dummy Pill, Says Lawsuit - Medical

News Today. http://www.medicalnewstoday.com/articles/255782.php. Accessed November 19, 2015.

388. Hashimoto E, Riederer PF, Hesselbrock VM, et al. Consensus paper of the WFSBP task force on biological markers: biological markers for alcoholism. *World J Biol Psychiatry*. 2013;14(8):549-564. doi:10.3109/15622975.2013.838302.

389. Pettinati HM, Volpicelli JR, Luck G, Kranzler HR, Rukstalis MR, Cnaan A. Double-blind clinical trial of sertraline treatment for alcohol dependence. *J Clin Psychopharmacol*. 2001;21(2):143-153. http://www.ncbi.nlm.nih.gov/pubmed/11270910. Accessed June 5, 2015.

390. Keating GM. Sodium oxybate: A review of its use in alcohol withdrawal syndrome and in the maintenance of abstinence in alcohol dependence. *Clin Drug Investig*. 2014;34(1):63-80. doi:10.1007/s40261-013-0158-x.

391. D&A PHARMA Presents 3 Major Clinical Studies Which Confirm and Extend the Efficacy and Safety of ACOLVER® at the 14th Congress of ESBRA (European Society for Biomedical Research on Alcoholism), Warsaw | Business Wire. http://www.businesswire.com/news/home/20130906005437/e n/DA-PHARMA-Presents-3-Major-Clinical-Studies#.VbuGq_lViko. Accessed July 31, 2015.

392. Unknown. Sodium oxybate - Wikipedia. 2015:1-9.

393. GHB Legal Status. https://www.erowid.org/chemicals/ghb/ghb_law.shtml. Accessed July 31, 2015.

394. Unknown. Gamma -Hydroxybutyric Acid - Wikipedia. *Wikipedia*. https://en.wikipedia.org/wiki/Gamma-Hydroxybutyric_acid.

395. Griffiths CPG. Illicit gamma-hydroxybutyrate (GHB) and pharmaceutical sodium oxybate (Xyrem®): differences in characteristics and misuse. *Drug Alcohol Depend*. 2009;27(5):417-428. doi:10.1055/s-0029-1237430.Imprinting.

396. Pross N, Patat A, Vivet P, Bidaut M, Fauchoux N. Pharmacodynamic interactions of a solid formulation of sodium oxybate and ethanol in healthy volunteers. *Br J Clin Pharmacol*. 2015. doi:10.1111/bcp.12632.

397. LABORATORIO FARMACEUTICO CT Srl - R&D. http://www.labct.it/en/r-d-eng. Accessed October 23, 2015.

398. Mirijello A, Cibin M, Mosti A, et al. Novel strategies to treat alcohol dependence with sodium oxybate according to clinical practice. *Eur Rev Med Pharmacol Sci*. 2015:1315-1320.

399. Caputo F, Del Re A, Brambilla R, et al. Sodium oxybate in maintaining alcohol abstinence in alcoholic patients according to

Lesch typologies: a pilot study. *J Psychopharmacol.* 2014;28(1):23-30. doi:10.1177/0269881113504015.

400. Skala K, Caputo F, Mirijello A, et al. Sodium oxybate in the treatment of alcohol dependence: from the alcohol withdrawal syndrome to the alcohol relapse prevention. *Expert Opin Pharmacother.* 2014;15(2):245-257. doi:10.1517/14656566.2014.863278.

401. Leone MA, Vigna-Taglianti F, Avanzi G, Brambilla R, Faggiano F. Gamma-hydroxybutyrate (GHB) for treatment of alcohol withdrawal and prevention of relapses. *Cochrane database Syst Rev.* 2011;(2):CD006266. doi:10.1002/14651858.CD006266.pub2.

402. Alén F, Orio L, Gorriti MÁ, et al. Increased Alcohol Consumption in Rats After Subchronic Antidepressant Treatment . *Int J Neuropsychopharmacol* . 2013;16 (8):1809-1818. doi:10.1017/S1461145713000217.

403. Drake RE, Ph D, Mueser KT. Co-Occurring Alcohol Use Disorder and Schizophrenia. *Public Policy.* 2002;26(2):99-102.

404. Alén F, Serrano A, Gorriti MÁ, et al. The administration of atomoxetine during alcohol deprivation induces a time-limited increase in alcohol consumption after relapse. *Int J Neuropsychopharmacol.* 2014;17(11):1905-1910. doi:10.1017/S146114571400087X.

405. Kishi T, Sevy S, Chekuri R, Correll CU. Antipsychotics for primary alcohol dependence: A systematic review and meta-analysis of placebo-controlled trials. *J Clin Psychiatry.* 2013;74(7):642-654. doi:10.4088/JCP.12r08178.

406. Unknown A. ADial Pharmaceuticals LLC Announces Issuance of. *Globe Newswire.* 2015:2014-2015.

407. Warnock KT, Yang ARST, Yi HS, et al. Amitifadine, a triple monoamine uptake inhibitor, reduces binge drinking and negative affect in an animal model of co-occurring alcoholism and depression symptomatology. *Pharmacol Biochem Behav.* 2012;103(1):111-118. doi:10.1016/j.pbb.2012.07.014.

408. Which medication approaches could target the stress response in drug addiction? - ResearchGate. http://www.researchgate.net/post/Which_medication_approaches_could_target_the_stress_response_in_drug_addiction. Accessed October 23, 2015.

409. Should You Buy, Sell, Or Hold Reckitt Benckiser Group Plc's Spinoff, Indivior PLC? | The Motley Fool UK. https://www.fool.co.uk/investing/2014/12/29/should-you-buy-sell-or-hold-reckitt-benckiser-group-plcs-spinoff-indivior-plc/. Accessed October 16, 2015.

410. XenoPort Provides Highlights of HORIZANT Prescription

Trends and Update on Development for Alcohol Use Disorder | Business Wire. *BusinessWire.* 2015. http://www.businesswire.com/news/home/20150111005032/en/XenoPort-Highlights-HORIZANT-Prescription-Trends-Update-Development#.VXdbqflViko. Accessed June 9, 2015.

411. Brunetti M, Di Tizio L, Dezi S, Pozzi G, Grandinetti P, Martinotti G. Aripiprazole, alcohol and substance abuse: A review. *Eur Rev Med Pharmacol Sci.* 2012;16(10):1346-1354.

412. Li Y-L, Liu Q, Gong Q, et al. Brucine suppresses ethanol intake and preference in alcohol-preferring Fawn-Hooded rats. *Acta Pharmacol Sin.* 2014;35(7):853-861. doi:10.1038/aps.2014.28.

413. Manzardo AM, He J, Poje A, Penick EC, Campbell J, Butler MG. Double-blind, randomized placebo-controlled clinical trial of benfotiamine for severe alcohol dependence. *Drug Alcohol Depend.* 2013;133(2):562-570. doi:10.1016/j.drugalcdep.2013.07.035.

414. Manzardo AM, Pendleton T, Poje A, Penick EC, Butler MG. Change in psychiatric symptomatology after benfotiamine treatment in males is related to lifetime alcoholism severity. *Drug Alcohol Depend.* 2015;152:257-263. doi:10.1016/j.drugalcdep.2015.03.032.

415. Cui M, Qin G, Yu K, Bowers MS, Zhang M. Targeting the Small- and Intermediate-Conductance Ca2+-Activated Potassium Channels: The Drug-Binding Pocket at the Channel/Calmodulin Interface. *Neurosignals.* 2014;22(2):65-78. doi:10.1159/000367896.

416. Khokhar JY, Chau DT, Dawson R, Green AI. Clozapine Reconstructed: Haloperidol's Ability to Reduce Alcohol Intake in the Syrian Golden Hamster can be Enhanced Through Noradrenergic Modulation by Desipramine and Idazoxan. *Drug Alcohol Depend.* 2015. doi:10.1016/j.drugalcdep.2015.04.003.

417. Kalyoncu A, Mirsal H, Pektas O, Unsalan N, Tan D, Beyazyürek M. Use of lamotrigine to augment clozapine in patients with resistant schizophrenia and comorbid alcohol dependence: a potent anti-craving effect? *J Psychopharmacol.* 2005;19(3):301-305. doi:10.1177/0269881105051542.

418. Adamson SJ, Sellman JD, Foulds J a., et al. A Randomized Trial of Combined Citalopram and Naltrexone for Nonabstinent Outpatients With Co-Occurring Alcohol Dependence and Major Depression. *J Clin Psychopharmacol.* 2015;35(2):143-149. doi:10.1097/JCP.0000000000000287.

419. Seif T, Simms JA, Lei K, et al. D-Serine and D-Cycloserine Reduce Compulsive Alcohol Intake in Rats. *Neuropsychopharmacology.* 2015. doi:10.1038/npp.2015.84.

420. Kiefer F, Kirsch M, Bach P, et al. Effects of d-cycloserine on extinction of mesolimbic cue reactivity in alcoholism: a

randomized placebo-controlled trial. *Psychopharmacology (Berl)*. 2015;232(13):2353-2362. doi:10.1007/s00213-015-3882-5.

421. Shen Y, Lindemeyer AK, Gonzalez C, et al. Dihydromyricetin as a novel anti-alcohol intoxication medication. *J Neurosci*. 2012;32(1):390-401. doi:10.1523/JNEUROSCI.4639-11.2012.

422. Jin Z, Bhandage AK, Bazov I, et al. Selective increases of AMPA, NMDA, and kainate receptor subunit mRNAs in the hippocampus and orbitofrontal cortex but not in prefrontal cortex of human alcoholics. *Front Cell Neurosci*. 2014;8:11. doi:10.3389/fncel.2014.00011.

423. Author Unknown. Duloxetine Versus Pregabalin for Alcohol Dependence - Full Text View - ClinicalTrials.gov. *Clinicaltrials.gov*. 2014. https://clinicaltrials.gov/ct2/show/NCT00929344?term=The+Scripps+Research+Institute&rank=9. Accessed February 24, 2015.

424. Covault J, Pond T, Feinn R, Arias AJ, Oncken C, Kranzler HR. Dutasteride reduces alcohol's sedative effects in men in a human laboratory setting and reduces drinking in the natural environment. *Psychopharmacology (Berl)*. 2014;231(17):3609-3618. doi:10.1007/s00213-014-3487-4.

425. Karahanian E, Rivera-Meza M, Quintanilla ME, Munoz D, Fernandez K, Israel Y. PPAR Agonists Reduce Alcohol Drinking: Do They Act in the Brain or in the Liver? *Alcohol Alcohol*. 2015;(1988):1-2. doi:10.1093/alcalc/agv060.

426. Author Unknown. Piogliatazone for Alcohol Craving. *Clinicaltrials.gov*. 2015:1-5.

427. Simon O'Brien E, Legastelois R, Houchi H, et al. Fluoxetine, desipramine, and the dual antidepressant milnacipran reduce alcohol self-administration and/or relapse in dependent rats. *Neuropsychopharmacology*. 2011;36(7):1518-1530. doi:10.1038/npp.2011.37.

428. Kalinichev M, Palea S, Haddouk H, et al. ADX71441, a novel, potent and selective positive allosteric modulator of the GABAB receptor, shows efficacy in rodent models of overactive bladder. *Br J Pharmacol*. 2014;171(4):995-1006. doi:10.1111/bph.12517.

429. Unknown A. Addex Therapeutics: Addex and NIAAA Enter Collaboration to Evaluate ADX71441 in Alcohol Use Disorder. *Addextherapeutics.com*. 2015. http://www.addextherapeutics.com/investors/press-releases/news-details/article/addex-and-niaaa-enter-collaboration-to-evaluate-adx71441-in-alcohol-use-disorder/. Accessed April 3, 2015.

430. Li X, Kaczanowska K, Sturchler E, et al. KK-92A, a novel

GABAB receptor positive modulator, attenuates the rewarding effects of nicotine in rats (661.9). *FASEB J.* 2014;28(1_Supplement):661.9 http://www.fasebj.org/content/28/1_Supplement/661.9. Accessed October 16, 2015.

431. Vanderah T, Sandweiss A. The pharmacology of neurokinin receptors in addiction: prospects for therapy. *Subst Abuse Rehabil.* 2015;6:93. doi:10.2147/SAR.S70350.

432. Heillig M. Stress, Addiction, and Relapse Behaiours: The case of Alcoholism - Presentation. *Presentation.*

433. Ledford H. Drug eases cravings in stressed alcoholics. *Nature.* 2008. doi:10.1038/news.2008.575.

434. Rahman S, Engleman EA, Bell RL. Nicotinic receptor modulation to treat alcohol and drug dependence. *Front Neurosci.* 2014;8(January):426. doi:10.3389/fnins.2014.00426.

435. Tomasini MC, Borelli AC, Beggiato S, et al. GET73 Prevents Ethanol-Induced Neurotoxicity in Primary Cultures of Rat Hippocampal Neurons. *Alcohol Alcohol.* 2015:agv094 doi:10.1093/alcalc/agv094.

436. Loche A, Simonetti F, Lobina C, et al. Anti-Alcohol and Anxiolytic Properties of a New Chemical Entity, GET73. *Front psychiatry.* 2012;3:8. doi:10.3389/fpsyt.2012.00008.

437. Giuliano C, Goodlett CR, Economidou D, et al. The Novel μ-Opioid Receptor Antagonist GSK1521498 Decreases both Alcohol Seeking and Drinking: Evidence from a New Preclinical Model of Alcohol Seeking. *Neuropsychopharmacology.* 2015;(July). doi:10.1038/npp.2015.152.

438. Sofuoglu M, Rosenheck R, Petrakis I. Pharmacological treatment of comorbid PTSD and substance use disorder: Recent progress. *Addict Behav.* 2014;39(2):428-433. doi:10.1016/j.addbeh.2013.08.014.

439. Bell RL, Lopez MF, Cui C, et al. Ibudilast reduces alcohol drinking in multiple animal models of alcohol dependence. *Addict Biol.* 2015;20(1):38-42. doi:10.1111/adb.12106.

440. Development of Ivermectin for Alcohol Use Disorders - Full Text View - ClinicalTrials.gov. https://clinicaltrials.gov/ct2/show/study/NCT02046200?term=ivermectin&rank=1. Accessed October 19, 2015.

441. Baronio D, Gonchoroski T, Castro K, Zanatta G, Gottfried C, Riesgo R. Histaminergic system in brain disorders: lessons from the translational approach and future perspectives. *Ann Gen Psychiatry.* 2014;13(1):1-10. doi:10.1186/s12991-014-0034-y.

442. Penetar DM, Toto LH, Lee DY-W, Lukas SE. A single dose of kudzu extract reduces alcohol consumption in a binge drinking

paradigm. *Drug* *Alcohol* *Depend.* 2015. doi:10.1016/j.drugalcdep.2015.05.025.

443. Press Releases | News & Publications | Cerecor. http://cerecor.com/news-publications/news-publications-press-release-2015-02-20.php. Accessed October 27, 2015.

444. Kallupi M, Oleata CS, Luu G, Teshima K, Ciccocioppo R, Roberto M. MT-7716, a novel selective nonpeptidergic NOP receptor agonist, effectively blocks ethanol-induced increase in GABAergic transmission in the rat central amygdala. *Front Integr Neurosci.* 2014;8(February):1-11. doi:10.3389/fnint.2014.00018.

445. Kwako LE, Spagnolo PA, Schwandt ML, et al. The corticotropin releasing hormone-1 (CRH1) receptor antagonist pexacerfont in alcohol dependence: a randomized controlled experimental medicine study. *Neuropsychopharmacology.* 2015;40(5):1053-1063. doi:10.1038/npp.2014.306.

446. Ralevski E, Jane JS, O'Brien E, et al. Mecamylamine for Treatment of People With Dual Diagnoses of Depression and Alcohol Dependence. *J Dual Diagn.* 2013;9(4):301-310. doi:10.1080/15504263.2013.835163.

447. Guerrini I, Gentili C, Nelli G, Guazzelli M. A follow up study on the efficacy of metadoxine in the treatment of alcohol dependence. *Subst Abuse Treat Prev Policy.* 2006;1:35. doi:10.1186/1747-597X-1-35.

448. Leggio L, Kenna GA, Ferrulli A, et al. Preliminary findings on the use of metadoxine for the treatment of alcohol dependence and alcoholic liver disease. *Hum Psychopharmacol.* 2011;26(8):554-559. doi:10.1002/hup.1244.

449. Kwako LE, Schwandt ML, Sells JR, et al. Methods for inducing alcohol craving in individuals with co-morbid alcohol dependence and posttraumatic stress disorder: behavioral and physiological outcomes. *Addict Biol.* 2014. doi:10.1111/adb.12150.

450. Yoon SJ, Pae CU, Kim DJ, et al. Mirtazapine for patients with alcohol dependence and comorbid depressive disorders: A multicentre, open label study. *Prog Neuro-Psychopharmacology Biol Psychiatry.* 2006;30(7):1196-1201. doi:10.1016/j.pnpbp.2006.02.018.

451. de Bejczy A, Söderpalm B. The Effects of Mirtazapine Versus Placebo on Alcohol Consumption in Male High Consumers of Alcohol. *J Clin Psychopharmacol.* 2015;35(1):43-50. doi:10.1097/JCP.0000000000000259.

452. Joos L, Goudriaan AE, Schmaal L, et al. Effect of modafinil on impulsivity and relapse in alcohol dependent patients: A randomized, placebo-controlled trial. *Eur Neuropsychopharmacol.*

2013;23(8):948-955. doi:10.1016/j.euroneuro.2012.10.004.

453. Khemiri L, Steensland P, Guterstam J, et al. The Effects of the Monoamine Stabilizer (-)-OSU6162 on Craving in Alcohol Dependent Individuals: A Human Laboratory Study. *Eur Neuropsychopharmacol.* 2015. doi:10.1016/j.euroneuro.2015.09.018.

454. Wong CJ, Witcher J, Mallinckrodt C, et al. A Phase 2, Placebo-Controlled Study of the Opioid Receptor Antagonist LY2196044 for the Treatment of Alcohol Dependence. *Alcohol Clin Exp Res.* 2014;38(2):511-520. doi:10.1111/acer.12257.

455. Anderson RI, Becker HC, Adams BL, Jesudason CD, Rorick-Kehn LM. reduce ethanol self-administration in high-drinking rodent models. *Front Neurosci.* 2014;8:33. doi:10.3389/fnins.2014.00033.

456. Therapeutics. http://eolastherapeutics.com/therapeutics. Accessed October 22, 2015.

457. Mattson ME, Ph D, Collins JF, et al. A Double-Bind, Placebo-Controlled Trial to Asses the Efficacy of Quetiapine Fumarate in Very Heavy Drinking Alcohol- Dependent Patients. *Alcohol Clin Exp Res.* 2013;36(3):406-416. doi:10.1111/j.1530-0277.2011.01649.x.A.

458. Sherwood Brown E, Davila D, Nakamura A, et al. A randomized, double-blind, placebo-controlled trial of quetiapine in patients with bipolar disorder, mixed or depressed phase, and alcohol dependence. *Alcohol Clin Exp Res.* 2014;38(7):2113-2118. doi:10.1111/acer.12445.

459. Gulick D, Chau DT, Khokhar JY, Dawson R, Green AI. Desipramine enhances the ability of risperidone to decrease alcohol intake in the Syrian golden hamster. *Psychiatry Res.* 2014;218(3):329-334. doi:10.1016/j.psychres.2014.04.038.

460. Ray LA, Roche DJO, Heinzerling K, Shoptaw S. Opportunities for the development of neuroimmune therapies in addiction. *Int Rev Neurobiol.* 2014;118:381-401. doi:10.1016/B978-0-12-801284-0.00012-9.

461. Knapp CM, O'Malley M, Datta S, Ciraulo DA. The Kv7 potassium channel activator retigabine decreases alcohol consumption in rats. *Am J Drug Alcohol Abuse.* 2015. http://www.tandfonline.com/doi/abs/10.3109/00952990.2014.892951. Accessed June 9, 2015.

462. Sciascia JM, Mendoza J, Chaudhri N. Blocking dopamine d1-like receptors attenuates context-induced renewal of pavlovian-conditioned alcohol-seeking in rats. *Alcohol Clin Exp Res.* 2014;38(2):418-427. doi:10.1111/acer.12262.

463. Tekmira Expands Product Pipeline With RNAi Therapeutic for the Treatment of Alcohol Dependence (NASDAQ:ABUS).

http://investor.arbutusbio.com/releasedetail.cfm?releaseid=6530
67. Accessed October 16, 2015.

Printed in Great Britain
by Amazon

80546994R00366